AF781046

CONTENTS

FEBRUARY 13, 2007

WITNESSES

SUBMITTED MATERIAL

MARCH 22, 2007

WITNESSES

SUBMITTED MATERIAL

THE ADEQUACY OF FDA TO ASSURE THE SAFETY OF THE NATION'S DRUG SUPPLY

HEARINGS

BEFORE THE

SUBCOMMITTEE ON OVERSIGHT AND INVESTIGATIONS

OF THE

COMMITTEE ON ENERGY AND COMMERCE

HOUSE OF REPRESENTATIVES

ONE HUNDRED TENTH CONGRESS

FIRST SESSION

FEBRUARY 13, MARCH 22, 2007

Serial No. 110–5

Printed for the use of the Committee on Energy and Commerce

energycommerce.house.gov

U.S. GOVERNMENT PRINTING OFFICE

35–502 PDF WASHINGTON : 2007

For sale by the Superintendent of Documents, U.S. Government Printing Office
Internet: bookstore.gpo.gov Phone: toll free (866) 512–1800; DC area (202) 512–1800
Fax: (202) 512–2250 Mail: Stop SSOP, Washington, DC 20402–0001

COMMITTEE ON ENERGY AND COMMERCE

JOHN D. DINGELL, Michigan, *Chairman*

HENRY A. WAXMAN, California
EDWARD J. MARKEY, Massachusetts
RICK BOUCHER, Virginia
EDOLPHUS TOWNS, New York
FRANK PALLONE, Jr., New Jersey
BART GORDON, Tennessee
BOBBY L. RUSH, Illinois
ANNA G. ESHOO, California
BART STUPAK, Michigan
ELIOT L. ENGEL, New York
ALBERT R. WYNN, Maryland
GENE GREEN, Texas
DIANA DeGETTE, Colorado
Vice Chairman
LOIS CAPPS, California
MIKE DOYLE, Pennsylvania
JANE HARMAN, California
TOM ALLEN, Maine
JAN SCHAKOWSKY, Illinois
HILDA L. SOLIS, California
CHARLES A. GONZALEZ, Texas
JAY INSLEE, Washington
TAMMY BALDWIN, Wisconsin
MIKE ROSS, Arkansas
DARLENE HOOLEY, Oregon
ANTHONY D. WEINER, New York
JIM MATHESON, Utah
G.K. BUTTERFIELD, North Carolina
CHARLIE MELANCON, Louisiana
JOHN BARROW, Georgia
BARON P. HILL, Indiana

JOE BARTON, Texas
Ranking Minority Member
RALPH M. HALL, Texas
J. DENNIS HASTERT, Illinois
FRED UPTON, Michigan
CLIFF STEARNS, Florida
NATHAN DEAL, Georgia
ED WHITFIELD, Kentucky
BARBARA CUBIN, Wyoming
JOHN SHIMKUS, Illinois
HEATHER WILSON, New Mexico
JOHN SHADEGG, Arizona
CHARLES W. "CHIP" PICKERING, Mississippi
VITO FOSSELLA, New York
STEVE BUYER, Indiana
GEORGE RADANOVICH, California
JOSEPH R. PITTS, Pennsylvania
MARY BONO, California
GREG WALDEN, Oregon
LEE TERRY, Nebraska
MIKE FERGUSON, New Jersey
MIKE ROGERS, Michigan
SUE WILKENS MYRICK, North Carolina
JOHN SULLIVAN, Oklahoma
TIM MURPHY, Pennsylvania
MICHAEL C. BURGESS, Texas
MARSHA BLACKBURN, Tennessee

Professional Staff

Dennis B. Fitzgibbons, *Chief of Staff*
Gregg A. Rothschild, *Chief Counsel*
Sharon E. Davis, *Chief Clerk*
Bud Albright, *Minority Staff Director*

Subcommittee on Oversight and Investigations

BART STUPAK, Michigan, *Chairman*

DIANA DeGETTE, Colorado
CHARLIE MELANCON, Louisiana
HENRY A. WAXMAN, California
GENE GREEN, Texas
MIKE DOYLE, Pennsylvania
JAN SCHAKOWSKY, Illinois
JAY INSLEE, Washington

ED WHITFIELD, Kentucky
Ranking Minority Member
GREG WALDEN, Oregon
MIKE FERGUSON, New Jersey
TIM MURPHY, Pennsylvania
MICHAEL C. BURGESS, Texas
MARSHA BLACKBURN, Tennessee

THE ADEQUACY OF FDA TO ASSURE THE SAFETY OF THE NATION'S DRUG SUPPLY

TUESDAY, FEBRUARY 13, 2007

HOUSE OF REPRESENTATIVES,
SUBCOMMITTEE ON OVERSIGHT AND INVESTIGATIONS,
COMMITTEE ON ENERGY AND COMMERCE,
Washington, DC.

The subcommittee met, pursuant to call, at 9:15 a.m., in room 2123 of the Rayburn House Office Building, Hon. Bart Stupak (chairman of the subcommittee) presiding.

Members present: Representatives DeGette, Waxman, Green, Doyle, Schakowsky, Dingell [ex officio], Whitfield, Walden, Ferguson,Murphy, Burgess, and Barton [ex officio].

OPENING STATEMENT OF HON. BART STUPAK, A REPRESENTATIVE IN CONGRESS FROM THE STATE OF MICHIGAN

Mr. STUPAK. I call this hearing to order. Today we will have a hearing on the adequacy of the FDA to assure the safety of the Nation's drug supply. We will begin with opening statements. This is the first in a series of hearings this committee will be holding to evaluate the Food and Drug Administration's ability to safely approve new drugs and provide post-marketing surveillance of our Nation's drug supply.

This year Congress must reauthorize the Prescription Drug User Fee Act or PDUFA, as we call it, and the Pediatric Exclusivity law. PDUFA requires the FDA to quickly bring new drugs to the market. In its rush to approve new drugs, the FDA's ability to ensure a safe drug supply has been greatly compromised. Prior to PDUFA, seldom was the FDA forced to withdraw drugs from the market; within the first 3 years of PDUFA, seven drugs, resulting in more than a thousand deaths, had been removed. Those seven deadly drugs, rushed for approval under PDUFA, were not needed to save lives.

In the 108th Congress, serious questions were raised about the antidepressants SSRI's use in adolescents. SSRI's have not been proven effective in treating adolescent depression. To the contrary, their use may actually increase the suicide rate of young patients. In response to these reports of increased suicide rates with SSRI use, FDA officials suppressed their own post-marketing surveillance, prohibited FDA employees from discussing the report and launched an investigation to find the person who leaked the information to the press. Today, SSRI's remain on the market without a clear medical benefit to the patient.

In the 108th and 109th Congress, the COX2 pain relievers, Vioxx and Bextra, were the subject of hearings on the regulatory failure by the FDA. These pain relievers were supposed to be easier on the stomach and not cause ulcers for the chronic users. Post-marketing surveillance revealed serious cardiac side effects. Instead of focusing on these serious side effects, the FDA became entwined in a 14-month battle on how the cardiovascular risks should be labeled. FDA officials sided with the drug manufacturer and down played the warnings and the serious side effects of Vioxx. As a result, the FDA may have allowed thousands of patients to die prematurely because of its failure to believe its own scientist and his post-market surveillance findings.

Today we will hear from a panel of whistleblowers who will describe how Ketek was approved by the FDA, even though the FDA knew the large safety study it required was fraught with data irregularities. Ketek is prescribed for non-life threatening illnesses, but the rush to approve has resulted in serious and deadly consequences. There have been approximately 10 deaths related to Ketek's use.

With each of these drugs, it appears the FDA is not seriously questioning whether the risks outweigh the benefits of the new drug. One must ask if the FDA is not protecting its client, the American people, whose interest is being protected?

The problems with the FDA's drug approval and post-marketing surveillance cannot be totally blamed on PDUFA. While PDUFA may encourage a closer working relationship between regulators and drug companies, it is the FDA's leadership which has allowed the interaction to become incestuous. The FDA has blocked, misled and ignored congressional inquiries into its new drug and post-marketing surveillance programs.

Our first witness, Senator Charles Grassley, has been a champion in questioning, challenging and over-seeing the FDA's drug approval and post-marketing surveillance. As chairman of the Senate Finance Committee, Senator Grassley has fought, on behalf of the American people, to ensure our Nation's drug supply is safe. Instead of working with Senator Grassley, the FDA has obstructed, resisted and denied his congressional efforts to oversee and hold the FDA to its core mission of protecting Americans. The FDA has been so arrogant and emboldened that it ignores the Senate Finance Committee's subpoenas. If the FDA willfully ignores a U.S. Senate subpoena issued by the committee of jurisdiction, whose interest and mission is the FDA protecting?

Our second panel is made up of whistleblowers who will testify how their efforts to disclose serious medical risks with Ketek were ignored, covered up or dismissed by FDA officials. In order for these brave individuals to appear before this committee, each individual was subpoenaed.

Our final panel, Dr. Steven Nissen and Dr. David Graham, who was also subpoenaed, will state that FDA officials ignored their well-documented evidence, especially on Vioxx, and compromised patient safety in the new drug approval and post-marketing surveillance programs.

The FDA has lost sight of its mission. When the U.S. Congress or FDA scientists or experts in the medical field try to inject safety into the FDA drug approval process and post-marketing surveillance, these individuals are ignored, ridiculed or silenced.

As I stated earlier, this is the first of several hearings this committee will be conducting on the FDA drug approval process. Congress must confront the FDA and return it to its core mission of protecting the American consumer, not the pharmaceutical industry.

Members of this committee should keep in mind these questions: Has the culture at the FDA lost sight of its core mission? Has PDUFA made the FDA more beholden to the pharmaceutical industry? Are the drug approval time limits found in PDUFA contributing to drugs being rushed to market without understanding the extent of the medical risks and benefits? Does the FDA adequately provide post-marketing surveillance?

While Ketek and its FDA approval is the focus of this hearing, the American people and this Congress, must remain vigilant in shaping public policy and re-writing PDUFA to restore the FDA's core mission of ensuring America's drug supply is safe for all Americans.

With that, I next turn to the ranking member of this subcommittee, the gentleman from Kentucky, Mr. Whitfield, for an opening statement, please.

OPENING STATEMENT OF HON. ED WHITFIELD, A REPRESENTATIVE IN CONGRESS FROM THE COMMONWEALTH OF KENTUCKY

Mr. WHITFIELD. Thank you, Chairman Stupak, for convening this important hearing on drug safety and the FDA's role in assuring the safety of the drug supply. As Chairman Stupak said, this will be the first in a series of hearings on this important issue. The safety of our Nation's drug supply and how it affects the health and well-being of our fellow citizens. Questions have been raised for many years about the FDA's management of safety issues with respect to the approval and post-market surveillance of drugs, including questions raised by this sub-committee with respect to the use of anti-depressant drugs among children and studies showing that their use was linked to increased risk of suicide.

While FDA's management of drug safety has received increased scrutiny, this is certainly, as I have said, not a new issue. In fact, in a 2006 report requested by then-chairman, Joe Barton, and Senator Chuck Grassley, the Government Accountability Office stated that problems have been raised about the FDA's management of drug approval and post-market surveillance for the last 30 years.

These are certainly complex issues and often involve complicated scientific debate and judgment. Issues raised by the FDA's approval of the drug Ketek, which we will learn more about from today's witnesses, certainly demonstrate this. The debate within FDA about the Ketek drug application was not simply a matter of approving or disapproving the drug. Instead, the Ketek application raised larger public health questions that were debated by doctors and scientists within the FDA with respect to the approval of antibiotics and about what types of studies should be performed to demonstrate a drug safety inefficacy.

At what point should data collected during drug trials be included or disqualified from the study? How should data regarding resistance to antibiotics be interpreted? And how should this affect the availability of antibiotics? These are questions about which scientists, physicians and experts continue to debate. While it is critical that we examine drug safety and whether FDA's decision making processes are suited to ensure the safety of our drug supply, it is also critical that we do so in a careful and deliberate way.

Today we will hear from two witnesses, Dr. David Ross and Dr. John Powers, who were employed by the FDA when Ketek's application was pending and who were involved, actually, in reviewing the application. We will also hear from a third witness, Ann Marie Cisneros, who was employed by a contractor for a Ketek sponsor, Sanofi-Aventis. It is my understanding that these witnesses disagree with the actions of the FDA, Sanofi-Aventis or both with respect to how that application was handled.

Today's witnesses have expertise and first-hand knowledge of the events that took place, but it is also important to note whom we are not hearing from today. Ketek's sponsor, Sanofi-Aventis, is not present today to offer its side of the story, nor are other FDA officials who took part in approving Ketek, but who do not share the views of today's witnesses about the approval decision or agency processes here to defend their decisions. But they will be asked to testify at a later hearing.

So we are at the beginning of our inquiry. We just sent a document request to FDA and after obtaining additional records by a hearing from all sides, we will be able to determine whether mistakes were made during the FDA's examination of Ketek and if so, what those mistakes were and whether those mistakes were simply an aberration or a sign of a systemic problem in the way FDA manages drug safety.

The GAO report, the Institute of Medicine report, FDA's response to these reports and recent actions, today's testimony, evidence collected by the subcommittee during previous investigations and Senator Chuck Grassley and his committee's investigation of Ketek all confirm that there is certainly room for improvement in FDA's management of drug safety.

So the subcommittee will be keeping an open mind looking at the evidence, and I look forward to the hearing and certainly I would be remiss if I did not thank Senator Grassley for joining us this morning. He and his staff on the Senate Committee on Finance have spent considerable time investigating the FDA's oversight of drug safety and we look forward to his testimony.

Mr. STUPAK. I thank the gentleman. He is right; we will have the FDA and the manufacturer of this drug at a later hearing. Exactly when that will be will probably depend upon the cooperation we get from the FDA to open their files, so that could be some time, but we expect them to testify. I next recognize the gentleman from Pittsburgh, Mr. Doyle, for an opening statement.

Mr. DOYLE. Thank you, Mr. Chairman. I want to thank you for convening this important hearing and I am going to waive my opening statement.

Mr. STUPAK. OK. The gentlewoman from Colorado.

OPENING STATEMENT OF HON. DIANA DEGETTE, A REPRESENTATIVE IN CONGRESS FROM THE STATE OF COLORADO

Ms. DEGETTE. Thank you very much, Mr. Chairman. I want to thank you for calling this hearing and thank you also for committing to making this the first of many hearings that we will have about drug safety and the FDA's handling of new drug applications and also post-market review of adverse side effects.

As the public's watchdog on prescription drugs, the FDA plays a critical role in protecting us from drugs whose risks outweigh their benefits. I also want to thank you for asking Dr. Steven Nissen to testify today. I met Dr. Nissen last fall when I was in Cleveland and his work, in 2004, on the FDA advisory panel about the safety of Vioxx led us to a much better understanding about the dangers of the drug.

Mr. Chairman, I remember hearings this committee convened in 2004 to examine antidepressant use of pediatric populations and at that time we talked about the need for the FDA to fulfill its mission, to conduct objective studies with rigorous scientific inquiries. When risks are identified, it is essential that they be communicated to the public. And at that hearing we talked about why there had been delays in presentation of data on the link between suicides and antidepressants. The system clearly had broken down.

I also remember when Vioxx was found to dramatically increase the risk of heart attacks for those taking this medication. We discovered that the FDA process was lacking as the valid concerns of FDA scientists were overruled by high-ranking officials. Again, the system had broken down. I hope, Mr. Chairman, as we address concerns about FDA's apparent mishandling of yet another drug review, that we can begin to move towards systemic change and not more lip service.

I am confident that our witnesses today will provide us with a comprehensive description of the inherent problems with the FDA system, but beyond that, I think, Mr. Chairman, we need to move far beyond talking about the problem and begin to develop a real solution. Once all of us here have been on this committee for a long time and these issues keep coming up again and again, the FDA issue, the Los Alamos issues that we had hearings on just a week or two ago. I think it is really time for Congress to identify these issues but then move beyond that and start to work in collaboration, of course, with the FDA and others to begin the solve the problems and I look forward to doing that and yield back my time.

Mr. STUPAK. I thank the gentlewoman. Gentleman from New Jersey, Mr. Ferguson, for an opening statement.

OPENING STATEMENT OF HON. MIKE FERGUSON, A REPRESENTATIVE IN CONGRESS FROM THE STATE OF NEW JERSEY

Mr. FERGUSON. Thank you, Mr. Chairman. I appreciate you convening this hearing today. I thank Mr. Whitfield and our panelists and our guest for being here this morning. I strongly believe that one of the most vital functions played by any of our Government agencies is that of the Food and Drug Administration's responsibility to ensure the safety and efficacy of pharmaceuticals for our citizens.

I would venture to say that at some point in almost every American's life, when they are sick, they will turn to an FDA-approved drug to make them better. Therefore, almost every American will put their trust in the testing and the scientific review done by the FDA. They must also trust that the drug was approved with their best interests in mind, weighing the relative risks and the benefits that that drug might bring.

I have long been interested in the issue of responsibility for drug safety carried out by the FDA. This issue has been brought my attention both by constituents in my district, but also it has been my own very interests to ensure that our Nation's drug supply is not only on the cutting edge of medicine, but also is the safest in the world. I believe information is vital for patients to make informed decisions and I have urged, through letters and conversations with FDA officials that they make available to patients necessary items like medication guides when they are necessary.

Over the past few years news reports, some generated by some of the panelists that we have here today, have chipped away at the public's confidence in the ability of the FDA to protect them. We need the FDA to be the worldwide gold standard. Coupled with our leadership role in research and development, the FDA must have the full and complete confidence of the public to protect them. Cutting edge medicines can only live up to their full potential when accompanied by public confidence in the FDA. Therefore, I believe this conversation that we are having today is a necessary one and I am very pleased that we are looking into these issues.

But as I look at the list of panelists today, I note a stark absence of other stakeholders that I view to be very necessary to this conversation. For instance, we don't have anybody today here who is speaking officially on behalf of the FDA. We don't have anybody here who is speaking on behalf of the patient community or the patient advocacy community. We don't have anybody here today talking, representing the Institute of Medicine, who have made some important examinations and recommendations.

I doubt that the opportunity we will have today, that we will have the necessary give and take to constructively talk about what is wrong and what is going right and what we need to do to fix the problems that we see. And I am hopeful that in the future, Mr. Chairman, as you mentioned, that we will have those opportunities.

Our conversation is particularly timely because we are quickly approaching the end of the authorization of the Prescription Drug User Fee Act or PDUFA, and looking through the testimony offered today, some assail PDUFA, but let us not forget why PDUFA was created in the first place. Before PDUFA existed, there was the commonly held belief that life-saving therapies were taking way too long to be approved by the FDA. Advocates for patients with cancer, HIV-AIDS and many other diseases cried out for a way to get drugs to market faster, while safely weighing the relative risks and benefits that those drugs might bring.

Let us not go back to the days when access to drugs was the most important problem that we faced. Last year the Institute of

Medicine, at the behest of the FDA, completed a thorough review of the state of drug safety at the agency. They issued a number of recommendations and there are many ideas that we ought to consider when we go through the reauthorization of PDUFA this year. But again, the absence of a proper give and take today will really preclude us from having the conversation today, anyway, to help us to do the job that we need to do properly.

Mr. Chairman, once again, this is a good conversation to be having, although today it is incomplete, and I look forward to, hopefully, in the future, that we will have an opportunity to have a more complete, a more thorough and more comprehensive examination of these issues so we will be able to move forward and do the right thing for our constituents and for the American people because at the end of the day, their confidence and the safety of our drug supply is perhaps one of the most important things we can be doing.

I appreciate, Mr. Chairman. I yield back.

Mr. STUPAK. I thank the gentleman for his comments. Next we turn to the chairman of the full committee, Mr. Dingell of Michigan. It should also be noted, before Mr. Dingell begins, Members will be moving back and forth as we have a climate change hearing also going on under Mr. Dingell's leadership where we have five hearings this week, so we are a busy committee this week. With that, Mr. Dingell.

OPENING STATEMENT OF HON. JOHN D. DINGELL, A REPRESENTATIVE IN CONGRESS FROM THE STATE OF MICHIGAN

The CHAIRMAN. Mr. Chairman, thank you, and thank you for holding this oversight investigation and for holding the first hearing of this Congress on drug safety and the Food and Drug Administration. I commend you. This subcommittee has a long history of FDA oversight and oversight of other agencies, too, and by and large, FDA is a fine organization where many people do good work for the American people.

Unfortunately, from time to time this committee has had to address problems before that agency. It seems every so often FDA loses its way, sometimes because of the work of scoundrels and sometimes because of poor management or other unfortunate events. But sometimes it is because of a more serious breakdown in the policies and procedures that are critical to assure the safety of food, drugs, blood and medical devices that are so essential to the health of the American people.

Today's hearing will deal with just such a fundamental breakdown in the policies and procedures for evaluating the safety of drugs. It is clear from the work that Chairman Stupak has already performed, which will be the subject of today's hearings, that FDA is badly broken. I expect that before this investigation is finished, and it is now just getting underway, that we will discover whether the problems we have found are due to the work of scoundrels, irrational penny-pinching or because the doors to the FDA hen house have been thrown open to foxes. It is possible that it will be a combination of all three.

What we do know, from our dear friend, Senator Grassley, who is going to be here this morning to testify and for whom we have the greatest respect and extend a very warm welcome, is that this administration appears to be engaged in hiding wrongdoing at FDA. We see this in other Federal agencies, as well. Today we will hear a warning from Senator Grassley that during his investigation, that his committee was confronted by obfuscation and delay and that this committee will face a similar problem with an agency that seems to try to hide its poor decision making behind the specious veil of Executive Privilege, a matter with which this committee has some familiarity over the years.

Those with the ear of the Secretary and the Commissioner of the FDA may erroneously believe that the committees of competent jurisdiction can be denied documents and interviews to obtain information that Congress must have to fulfill its constitutional obligations. They will find that that is an error. There are those who may be counseling the Secretary and the Commissioner that Congress may not interview or call to testify Department of Health and Human Services and FDA employees under any circumstances. There may even be those who are tempted to think that it is possible to deliberately mislead us. I warn them, these are dangerous thoughts.

I promise those in charge of HHS and any other department that chooses to deny this committee the information and access to proper personnel that is needed for oversight, as is our responsibility, that they will not succeed. I promise them, however, fair treatment if they will cooperate. I hope enthusiastically, but at least they will cooperate. There is an easy way to be investigated and there is a hard way, and I can assure, all in authority, that the hard way is not the better way.

Mr. Chairman, I thank you for your recognition.

Mr. STUPAK. I thank the gentleman for his statement. We next move to the ranking member of the full committee, the gentleman from Texas, Mr. Barton, for an opening statement.

OPENING STATEMENT OF HON. JOE BARTON, A REPRESENTATIVE IN CONGRESS FROM THE STATE OF TEXAS

Mr. BARTON. Thank you, Mr. Chairman. We on the minority side of this subcommittee support this particular investigation. We must have an objective and balanced FDA. The agency serves the American people and makes life and death decisions every day that affect our public health. Any credible concern that FDA's objectivity is in question must be examined.

We are at the very beginning of this particular investigation; document requests have been made and are about to be made; witnesses are being interviewed. We should have additional hearings, including witnesses from the FDA and the affected industry. Today we are at a very preliminary stage. The subcommittee is going to be hearing serious allegations and concerns about an antibiotic called Ketek, which is produced by Sanofi-Aventis. Individuals, including some other former FDA officials, who took part in this particular review, have charged that the safety data presented by the company in support of Ketek's approval was compromised or unreliable. They contend that the company knew it, that the FDA knew it and that although concerns were raised about the drug's safety, the FDA went ahead and approved the drug anyway.

These allegations go to the heart of FDA's professionalism, integrity, and the agency's mission. In fairness, I must note that some representatives from the FDA and the company who briefed the committee staff dispute some of the points that are going to be made today. We have been assured by the majority that additional witnesses from the FDA and the company will be heard.

Given the life and death consequences that flow from the FDA's decisions on drugs like this and from public information about prescription drugs, this subcommittee needs to pursue these issues very carefully, not attack the delicate and complicated matters with a sledgehammer.

Having said that, it is important that we keep an open mind today as we wait for the investigation to unfold. Until we assemble the most complete and thorough record possible, we should not draw premature conclusions about peoples' judgments, motivations and integrity. Complicating our work is the fact that debates over drug safety and the FDA decision making process involve complex and sometimes abstract issues for science and scientific judgment.

The FDA's decision with respect to Ketek's new drug application took place against the backdrop of an ongoing debate about antibiotic resistance, whether it is possible for certain types of studies, such as non-inferiority trials, to demonstrate a drug's effectiveness. Before we can determine whether Ketek should serve as a case study of how the FDA's management of drug safety is ineffective or worse, broken, we must review the evidence in context and with perspective.

This is a very good investigation to be instigating. I want to commend Mr. Dingell and Mr. Stupak and Mr. Whitfield for their leadership on this. I look forward to working with him and the other members of the subcommittee as we pursue this important piece of work before our Oversight subcommittee.

With that, Mr. Chairman, I yield back.

Mr. STUPAK. Thank you, Mr. Barton. Next, 5 minutes for opening statements, Ms. Schakowsky of Illinois.

OPENING STATEMENT OF HON. JAN SCHAKOWSKY, A REPRESENTATIVE IN CONGRESS FROM THE STATE OF ILLINOIS

Ms. SCHAKOWSKY. Thank you, Mr. Stupak, for holding this hearing and for your efforts to improve drug safety. The Oversight and Investigations Subcommittee has been a leader in investigating problems and pushing for solutions at the FDA and within the pharmaceutical industry. Ensuring the safety and efficacy of prescription drugs remains a top priority and I am glad that we are continuing our investigation on a bipartisan basis.

I also want to thank Senator Grassley and his staff for their efforts on the issue. It is clear we share a desire to return to evidence-based decision making and to ensure that FDA advisory groups, Congress and the public receive accurate and science-based information about prescription drugs. It is also clear that we have all faced enormous difficulty in getting the information that we need from the Bush administration.

I hope that we will be able to work together to solve all of these problems and protect the lives of our constituents. The evidence that we are going to hear today about the Ketek approval process and the failure to report potentially fatal effects is extremely serious. What is more troubling is that, as several witnesses will testify, Ketek is not an anomaly. These same problems, the culture of secrecy and hiding of significant health threats are mirrored in other drug application experiences and they appear to be ongoing, despite past investigations.

The testimony we will hear from Dr. Ross indicates that last summer FDA scientists were still being told to be "team players" and not report safety problems to those outside of the FDA. This occurred after our subcommittee's hearings on childhood antidepressants raised serious problems about the lack of disclosure by drug companies and the FDA.

Last year the Union of Concerned Scientists and Public Employees for Environmental Responsibility surveyed FDA scientists. According to their survey, nearly one in five scientists have been asked for nonscientific reasons to inappropriately exclude or alter technical information in an FDA scientific document. Sixty percent knew of cases where FDA political appointees and commercial interests had inappropriately influenced FDA actions. Only 49 percent agreed that the FDA leadership was as committed to product safety as to bringing products to the market. And only 47 percent believed FDA routinely provides complete and accurate information to the public.

What frightens me is that a survey taken today could show the same results. One of my constituents whose mother committed suicide after participating in an adult antidepressant trial wrote me that "there is a gaping hole between the data the FDA is collecting and the information reaching the general public." Today's hearing shows that the public is not alone. FDA's own advisory committees have been kept in the dark. Data has been falsified and manipulated and serious safety concerns have been kept hidden from Congress, as well as physicians and patients.

Mr. Chairman, it is time for full accountability and for serious change. I look forward to hearing the recommendations of our witnesses. I yield back.

Mr. STUPAK. I thank the gentle lady. The gentleman from Pennsylvania, Mr. Murphy.

OPENING STATEMENT OF HON. TIM MURPHY, A REPRESENTATIVE IN CONGRESS FROM THE COMMONWEALTH OF PENNSYLVANIA

Mr. MURPHY. Thank you, Mr. Chairman. Thank you for holding this important hearing. We all want new drugs and new therapies to cure diseases and save lives and we are thankful that so many have come out of the research in this Nation. However, we need to do so in a way that is scientifically reliable and valid, and when errors are made in that reliability and validity and errors are made in reporting problems with research, so much comes into question of the organizations that perform those studies and those that manufacture the medications.

Today's hearing is an essential part of the ongoing congressional role of oversight of the FDA. Well, there is a continuing demand from the public, however, and our doctors, for new drugs and we understand the prescription drugs, by their nature, all have some risk associated with them. We must ensure that the risks do not outweigh the benefits, thus accurate research for new drugs is absolutely vital to continue our efforts to discover the next generation of life saving treatments or treatments for mental illness or treatments for cancer or diabetes.

On the one hand, however, there is a constant pressure on the FDA by many patients and families eager to realize the hope these drugs may provide to review these medications quickly and it is important that we do not succumb to that pressure just for the sake of bringing out a medication if we do not yet have the scientific data to tell us what those risks and benefits are. This must be balanced. And this hearing is important to review that balance because we must have accurate and reliable research on medications so we can determine those risks and benefits to restore confidence in the drug programs of the Food and Drug Administration.

To do so, however, Congress must also approach these hearings demanding the same scientific integrity and comprehensive review of ourselves that we demand of the FDA. Now, there are some concerns that perhaps this committee is not receiving information yet from the administration. To my knowledge, I don't think we have yet requested information from the administration and the FDA and when we do so, my assumption is we will get accurate and cooperative information. If we do not, then we should act accordingly.

However, in the meantime, I believe that what the American people expect of us is to keep the pressure on for scientific integrity here; that all of us must review the studies, ourselves; to bring out the truth, whatever that may tell us about these medications, because at the very least, physicians and patients and families want to know that that prescription filled by their pharmacist and taken by themselves or a family member, maintains a gold standard of quality that we can trust and our Food and Drug Administration and all involved in that process.

We are not here to stop research, we are not here to rush drugs to market that are not ready, we are not here to stop medication that is needed. We are here, however, to make sure that integrity is what returns to the FDA and that all the patients and physicians in America demand that and I look forward to the results of this hearing to make sure we do look at this information accurately. Thank you, Mr. Chairman.

Mr. STUPAK. Next, for an opening statement, Mr. Green from Texas.

OPENING STATEMENT OF HON. GENE GREEN, A REPRESENTATIVE IN CONGRESS FROM THE STATE OF TEXAS

Mr. GREEN. Thank you, Mr. Chairman, for holding the hearing today on the Food and Drug Administration drug safety procedure. It is a pleasure to return to the Oversight and Investigation Committee. I look forward to working with you and our chairman, Chairman Dingell, on an aggressive oversight investigation agenda to increase accountability among all Federal agencies within our jurisdiction.

The first, though, in our subcommittee hearings of the 110th Congress, the continuation of good work this subcommittee is performing on drug safety in the 108th and 109th Congresses on a bipartisan basis. The investigation of the antibiotic, Ketek, is particularly timely. In fact, it appears that the FDA has been paying close attention to our hearing schedule, since it made a significant announcement yesterday about label and indication changes for Ketek.

Specifically, the FDA removed two of the three previously approved indications from the drug's label leaving acquired pneumonia as the only remaining indication for which Ketek is appropriate. I think most of my colleagues on the committee agree that it is too little too late. Three years after a flawed advisory committee process paved the way for approval for Ketek, the FDA has finally taken a step that represents its commitment to serve the public's interest regarding Ketek.

The FDA's action yesterday is not the final word on the matter and certainly does not rule out our need to analyze the problems associated with the approval of Ketek. If anything, we need to look at this case even closer to determine where the problems lie in the approval process for new drugs and what actions need to be taken to restore the public's confidence. Certainly, a question arises whether non-inferiority studies are appropriate, to begin with, as opposed to traditional clinical trials where a drug is tested against a placebo, the non-inferiority study simply tests whether a new drug is as effective as a drug already approved for its specific indication.

I look forward to a robust discussion on this issue, on the use of these studies, in particular, and which cases are appropriate and necessary. Despite that question of methodology, I have significant concerns of the specific manner in which this non-inferiority study was implemented. It doesn't take a room full of scientists to know that it was completely inappropriate for the full data to Study 3014 to be presented to the FDA advisory committee, especially in the criminal investigations being initiated on one physician investigator and serious questions have been raised about data from other sites with significant enrollment levels.

The Ketek investigation gives us tremendous insight in the cultural failings of the FDA regarding drug safety. Although this investigation may elicit more questions than answers, I hope we can learn from Ketek case studies as we seek to address the FDA's larger drug safety issues and implement policies to ensure that the agency has the necessary tools to appropriately weigh the risks and benefits of particular drugs for the American people.

Mr. Chairman, I would like to thank the witnesses for appearing today and offering us insight, and it is difficult in a highly technical case, and I also look forward, as a member of the Health Subcommittee, looking at FDA reform, Mr. Chairman, so I know these studies for the last, this third Congress, will hopefully significantly affect the FDA reform. I yield back my time.

Mr. STUPAK. I thank the gentleman from Texas. The other member from Texas, Mr. Burgess, is recognized for 5 minutes.

OPENING STATEMENT OF HON. MICHAEL C. BURGESS, A REPRESENTATIVE IN CONGRESS FROM THE STATE OF TEXAS

Mr. BURGESS. Thank you, Mr. Chairman, and I thank the chairman and the ranking member for opening this hearing. This committee has a vital role in providing meaningful oversight and investigations over important public health issues. As a physician, I take this role extremely seriously and I thank the leadership of this committee for their vigilant pursuit of truth in regard to our Nation's healthcare issues.

Today we are here to discuss the FDA's process for the approval of new and important life saving drugs. While I appreciate the whistleblowers being here to discuss their observations of the approval process of Ketek, I do find it curious that the FDA isn't able to present their side of the story today. The whistleblowers are making serious allegations, allegations that need to be heard and deserve to be heard, but I am disappointed that neither the FDA nor the manufacturers of Ketek, Sanofi-Aventis, were invited to answer these serous allegations and tell their side of the story.

Now, I do understand that there is another hearing scheduled for later in March, but unfortunately, we all know, with the shortened press cycle in this town, that the damage will be done long before the weekend comes. We have heard some discussion of fairness this morning. We really can't talk about fairness. It is not reasonable to talk about an administration stonewalling a document request that, frankly, has not yet been made.

The question always comes down, in these hearings, what did they know and when did they know it. That is important information and this committee should dedicate itself toward answering that question, but an independent review of internal documents is going to be necessary before those questions could be answered. I would also like to remind members of this committee that we must be cautious not to come to conclusions today.

It is merely the opening side of a preliminary investigation. Today we will only hear one side of the story, an important side, to be sure, but it is still only one side. We must be cognizant of the fact that the power of oversight is, in effect, the power to destroy, therefore it is crucial this issue be fully vetted and that all sides are heard before conclusions are drawn.

Mr. Chairman, as a physician, I have long had a love/hate relationship with the FDA. I was concerned that they wouldn't bring medications quickly enough to benefit my patients. It seemed that other countries in the world could get newer medications on a much faster timeline and yet, at the same time, we look to the FDA to protect and ensure the certainty of safety of drugs in this country. Most of us don't question when a prescription is written, torn off the pad and put in our hands. We don't question the validity or the safety of that medication and that is a good thing, and we want that certainty that surrounds the FDA to be assured.

The FDA has no small task. This is a Physician's Desk Reference. I don't even know how many medications are listed in this reference; the print is very small, the pages are very thin and there is a lot of information in here. We charge the FDA with staying up to date on all of those medicines and assuring their safety. It is a big task. Do we fund it properly? That is surely a question that is going to have to be answered before these hearings are drawn to a conclusion.

Well, Mr. Chairman, as long as we are mindful of these issues and truly diligent in the work to obtain real answers and real conclusions, I am supportive of this investigation. And I will yield back the balance of my time.

Mr. STUPAK. I thank the gentleman. The gentleman from Washington, State of Washington, Mr. Inslee, for an opening statement.

Mr. INSLEE. I will waive, Mr. Chair.

Mr. STUPAK. OK, that concludes our opening statements. We

We now turn to our first witness, the Honorable Charles Grassley, United States Senator from the State of Iowa. Senator, it is a great pleasure to welcome you today, here today as our lead witness in the first of what I predict will be many hearings that this subcommittee will hold this Congress, that will look into improving the way the FDA protects the American people.

Before starting your prepared testimony, I would like to note that it has been a long tradition of the Oversight and Investigation Subcommittee to swear all witnesses, whether they be private citizens, Cabinet members or Senators. I believe, if my memory serves me correct, the last Senator to appear before us was your colleague, Senator Hatch, in 1991, who was sworn in and testified under oath before us on drug safety issues. So accordingly, Senator, please rise and raise your right hand to take the oath.

[Witness sworn.]

Mr. STUPAK. Thank you, Senator. I believe that you have a prepared statement for the record, as well as a shorter statement to present this morning. Before starting, let me advise my colleagues the Senator has a limited time and we will take questions, 10 minutes on each side for questioning of the Senator this morning. And Senator, again, thank you for being here and thank you for your work on drug safety issues throughout your career.

TESTIMONY OF HON. CHARLES GRASSLEY, A SENATOR FROM THE STATE OF IOWA

Senator GRASSLEY. Well, it is very much a privilege for me to be invited here and I appreciate that invitation and I had a chance to hear many members of this committee give opening statements and I particularly want to thank Chairman Dingell, Chairman Stupak, ranking members Barton and Whitfield for their statements and most importantly, to all of you who are involved in oversight because it is such an important constitutional responsibility, one that I don't think we talk enough about or do enough about, but it is important that you do the work you are doing on this hearing and particularly, a hearing on drug safety and particularly, the role of the Food and Drug Administration.

During the last 3 years, I conducted extensive oversight of the Food and Drug Administration while I was chairman of the Senate Finance Committee and as you probably know, we have jurisdiction over both Medicare and Medicaid. I view my role as working to ensure the safety and well-being of the more than 80 million Americans who are beneficiaries of these programs. The Medicare and Medicaid programs spend a lot of money on prescription drugs and medical devices, and that money should be spent on drugs and devices that are safe and effective.

In the course of my oversight of the Federal bureaucracy, I have developed many good relationships with whistleblowers. And it was FDA whistleblowers and concerned FDA scientists who first drew my attention to the problems of the Food and Drug Administration.

It started in early 2004 with an FDA psychiatrist named Dr. Andrew Mosholder, who realized, through his work, that there was a serious suicide risk for teenagers taking certain antidepressants. He wanted to make a presentation about his findings to an FDA advisory committee. But for some reason, FDA supervisors didn't want this information out. They canceled Dr. Mosholder's presentation and instructed him to write a script, approved by his supervisors, that he would use if anybody asked him why he was no longer presenting.

This fall, I held a hearing, or that fall, which was 2004, I held a hearing on drug safety in the aftermath of Vioxx, the blockbuster pain medication, being pulled off the market by its manufacturer, rather than by the Food and Drug Administration. The testimony at my hearing turned a bright spotlight on problems with the FDA's post-marketing surveillance effort. The Food and Drug Administration works tirelessly, as it should, to approve new life saving and life enhancing drugs, but it could do a lot better job of keeping track of developments with these drugs after they get out onto the market. Reviewing what happened inside the FDA with Vioxx and also working with a number of whistleblowers who bravely stuck their necks out and came to me after that landmark hearing, I have identified problems at the FDA that consistently fit into a few themes.

First, scientific dissent is discouraged, quashed and sometimes muzzled inside the FDA. Second, the FDA's relationship with drug makers is too cozy. The FDA worries about smoothing things over with the industry much more than it should with its regulatory responsibilities. Third, inside the FDA there is widespread fear of retaliation for speaking up about problems. And fourth, the public safety would be better served if the agency was more transparent and more forthcoming with drug safety and drug risks. These problems involve, then, the culture at the Food and Drug Administration. Those problems are not isolated, but are systemic and they can be partly attributed to the organizational structure at the FDA.

My concerns are not isolated, either. During the last year, they have been validated by highly regarded Institute of Medicine, as well as the independent Government Accountability Office and more importantly, or as importantly, respected medical journals. What is at stake is public safety and public confidence in our Nation's world-renown Food and Drug Administration.

My investigations of FDA issues have also revealed a deeply troubling disregard for Congress' responsibility to conduct oversight of the executive branch of Government, getting right to the heart of whether or not the checks and balances of the 225-year history of our Government are functioning properly, to see that the laws we passed are faithfully executed and to see that the money that we appropriate is spent in accordance with Congress intent. The FDA and the Department of Health and Human Services have put up so much resistance to my efforts to find out what happened inside the Food and Drug Administration with a relatively new antibiotic called Ketek, that I can only wonder what there is to cover up. Every excuse under the sun has been used to create roadblocks, even in the face of congressional subpoenas requesting information and access to FDA employees.

In denying access to documents responsive to the subpoenas, the Department and the Food and Drug Administration have claimed the official words "Prosecutorial deliberative process," another one "confidential communication," another one, "agency prerogative to determine who will be interviewed or testify before jurisdictional committees." That strikes right at the heart of the work you are doing here, Mr. Chairman, today. Yet, during my years in the Senate, my investigators have obtained access to every single one of these categories of so-called confidential information, even from HHS, as well as other executive branch agencies. So why now?

Further, I asked the Congressional Research Service to look into the Department's policies regarding this matter and CRS told me that there is, in their words, "no legal basis" for the Department's executive branch assertions.

Nevertheless, the Department and FDA not only withheld documents that do not appear to be privileged, but they also won't say what has been withheld and why. The subpoenas compel a privilege log, but the Department and the FDA will not provide one.

The Department and the FDA say that they have been responsive to the Finance Committee's Ketek investigation because they made available millions of pages of documents. But what they provided is quantity, not quality.

They delivered hundreds of pages simply marked, for example, "57 pages removed" or "43 pages removed," and that is in attachments 1 through 5 that you will have. Other documents have whole pages, paragraphs and sentences redacted with no explanation for what has been held or redacted or why. In fact, listen to this, the FDA redacted some of the same documents differently and they even redacted one of my own letters to them on a different matter, and that is attachment 6.

When I point out the absurdities in the Department's response to my request for documents and interviews related to Ketek, the Department argues it could not provide access to information and individuals related to criminal investigations, just like that was what I was trying to do. But I didn't ask for access to open criminal investigations. I don't want to jeopardize a criminal matter; you folks don't, either. The Department and the FDA know that, yet they keep using that excuse anyway.

Even so, what I have learned about what happened with Ketek troubles me. I have learned that FDA gave its advisory committee questionable data on Ketek and did not tell them about problems with that data. I sent a letter to the FDA in December regarding my findings on this matter and I am still awaiting a response. The FDA approved Ketek without much safety data from the U.S. The agency relied almost exclusively on foreign post-marketing safety data. And lastly, Ketek's sponsor, in all likelihood, was aware of the fact that it submitted some questionable data to the FDA regarding its large safety study. The sponsor was informed of problems with one of the study sites prior to the date of submission to the FDA. However, according to the FDA reviewers, the sponsor never raised these problems with the FDA. FDA learned about them after his own investigators inspected the site.

During the last 3 years, I have also tried to work in a productive way with the Commissioners and Acting Commissioners of the FDA. It will take bold leadership to get on top of the FDA's problems and to turn the agency around. So far, lip service has been fine; the reality has been a lot less.

Last month, Senator Chris Dodd and I introduced two reform bills that we proposed in 2005 to get the safety, to fix the safety shortcomings at FDA. Our first bill would elevate and empower the office with the FDA that is responsible for monitoring FDA-approved drugs after they are on the market. It would make the post-market safety function within the FDA independent, but within the FDA, instead of under the thumb of the office and the center that puts the drugs on the market in the first place and that is the way it is today.

I want to point your attention to the Wall Street Journal in regard to Chairman Dingell. It is reported that he is intrigued by the idea of drug safety center within the FDA. I appreciate that view. It doesn't make any sense that the FDA officials who are supposed to monitor the safety of a drug on the market serve only as consultants to the FDA officials who approve the drug in the first place. The officials who approve the drug would obviously be conflicted in making a judgment that approval is no longer appropriate or was a mistake in the first place. Kind of like having egg on your face. A separate center for drug safety within the FDA is a vital lynchpin when it comes to meaningful reform and improvement of the agency's post-marketing surveillance.

The second bill that Senator Dodd and I have introduced would expand an existing public data base by mandating the registry of all clinical trials and the results of those trials. This reform is key to establishing greater transparency regarding clinical trials, the good ones and the bad ones, and to hold drug makers and drug regulators accountable and to give doctors all the information they can to their patients. Both of these legislative initiatives would make drug information used by doctors and patients more complete and more accessible.

American consumers should not have to second guess the safety of pills in their cabinet. I appreciate the attention that all of you are giving to this important national issue with this hearing. You will hear from some of the heroic whistleblowers who have helped my work, without whom my work would not have been possible. Two of the whistleblowers have left FDA, outstanding scientists, outstanding investigators, people that want to get to the bottom of something, something that an agency like FDA can't afford to lose people like that. It is a tremendous loss for our country when an agency like the FDA gets so dysfunctional that specialists like these whistleblowers are forced to leave the agency to avoid retaliation.

Whistleblowers are like a skunk at a picnic. They ought to be considered, though, by us, as patriotic Americans just wanting to do what the law requires them to do and spend money according to the way Congress wants it spent. I want to work closely with you, Mr. Chairman, to make sure that FDA whistleblowers can communicate with Congress without fear. We got laws that protect them, but it doesn't protect them enough.

In addition, the existing agreement between the Inspector General of HHS and FDA gives too much power to the FDA when it comes to how allegations of criminal misconduct by FDA employers are being investigated. And we have an attachment F on that. That agreement should be revisited. I look forward to reform opportunities in the year ahead. There is no doubt that the FDA needs additional tools and resources in its work. The FDA also needs an overhaul to make the agency more transparent, more forthcoming and more independent minded.

I look forward to working with this committee and particularly, with the leaders of the committee, both Republican and Democrat, subcommittee as well as the full committee. And I thank you and as you indicated, I will be glad to stay and answer questions.

Mr. STUPAK. Well, thank you, Senator. We appreciate your time effort in appearing here today. We are going to take 10 minutes on each side. I will begin the questioning. I am going to ask two questions. I will turn it over to Mr. Dingell and we will move on.

Senator Grassley, you mentioned once again, in your testimony about the agreement between the Office of Inspector General for the Department of Health and Human Services and the Food and Drug Administration. In that agreement, certain responsibilities were given to the FDA when it comes to how allegations of criminal misconduct by FDA employees are investigated and you mentioned in your testimony, whistleblowers, the retaliation. We still have some brave scientists within the FDA who come forward and assist us in our work and they are still there and I am concerned about the retaliation. Could you explain that a little bit more what you think should be done in this area on this agreement, how it should be restructured?

Senator GRASSLEY. Well, obviously it gets back to what is very basic about Inspectors General; great deal of independence over anything within the agency; only very remotely connected with the administration of the agency; to do, basically, what you and I do as individual Congressmen or as chairmen of committees, to make sure that laws are faithfully executed and an agency is doing what it is supposed to do; to basically get down to being independent, to ferret out things that are wrong.

And so it seems to me that what we have here is the Office of Internal Affairs in the FDA engaging what is abused of power and an example of that, I referred to Dr. Mosholder. Two or 3 years ago he was threatened with being prosecuted, like Martha Stewart, as an example. We saw the office used as a tool by drug companies to investigate a safety review by the FDA's Center for Veterinary Medicine and when the Office of Inspector General was trying to do its work, it was reported to me that they are concerned about the weaknesses that they uncovered in that agency within FDA. So I can only say that, bottom line, just get back to Inspectors General being able to do what they are supposed to do and not see the FDA as an institution unto itself.

Mr. STUPAK. Thank you. On your testimony, you catalog your personal experience with FDA's suppression of independent researchers' opinions, harassment of whistleblowers, persistent refusal to produce documents in response to your request in your capacity as chairman of the Senate Finance Committee. So with respect to Ketek, you say that you learned that the FDA gave its advisory committee questionable data on Ketek and did not tell them about the problems with the data. FDA approved Ketek without much safety data from the U.S., that Ketek's sponsor, in all likelihood was aware of the fact that it had submitted some questionable data to the FDA regarding its large safety study.

Senator, your experience with the FDA simply refusing to respond to subpoenas, refusing to produce documents and other information to aid your investigation is astonishing. I gather this was not an isolated incident, but occurred on numerous occasions and that the FDA is still refusing to give you information that you requested on the Ketek investigation?

Senator GRASSLEY. Without a doubt. And what is really miraculous about that approach on their part, we asked for the log that I have already referred to in my statement, so in a sense, we don't even really know what is being held, withheld from us, why it is being withheld, and we happen to be aware, through information we get from inside, of some documents that could be responsive and don't appear to be privileged, but still being withheld from us. But see, there is no reason why we can't at least have that log so we can separate where maybe there is a legitimacy to their point of view or something. Maybe it deals with proprietary information, as an example. Although, if that doesn't get out to the public, that shouldn't even be withheld.

Mr. STUPAK. Senator, do you have any thoughts on the fact that the FDA reported that it is changing the label on Ketek and that changes include the removal of two of the three previously approved indications, bacterial sinuses and acute bacterial chronic bronchitis, from the drugs label? According to news reports, the FDA determined that the balance of benefits and risk no longer support approval of the drug for these indications, being the sinus and the bronchitis. So now Ketek will remain on the market for the treatment of community acquired pneumonia of mild to moderate severity. In addition, the FDA said it would work with the company to update the product labeling with a boxed warning, FDA's strongest form of warning. Any comments on that?

Senator GRASSLEY. Well, I think it is quite evident, since it just come out yesterday, you are having this hearing today, that finally the heat in the kitchen got a little bit too hot and they decided to move out of the kitchen. But also, it is perfect evidence that eventually when you push the envelope enough, they do show some respect for the scientific process, but in all of this, whether it is Ketek or Vioxx or a lot of others, it is a lack of respect for the scientific process that I think is basic to what is wrong with some of these drugs getting on the market and not getting there and when there is dissidence, a dissident point of view, or let us say an alternative point of view, not a dissident point of view, alternative point of view among scientists.

All you got to do is let science operate. If Scientist Grassley has a view and it has got to be reviewed by Scientist Stupak and you don't quite agree with me, then it is out there for peers to take action. Everything in science might not be perfect, but it sure is a heck of a lot perfecter than the subjective judgment of a few administrators stepping in, for some reason or other, to short circuit the scientific process. So if we get the FDA back to proper respect for the scientific process, I don't know whether you and I would have to be here today.

Mr. STUPAK. Last month the FDA proposed an increase in annual user fees paid to the agency by pharmaceutical companies to improve drug safety oversight, the post-marketing surveillance we speak of, to speed approval time for the new drugs and monitor direct to consumer advertising. Do you think user fees give companies too much influence over the FDA?

Senator GRASSLEY. Well, from that standpoint, it is kind of, since money is fungible, I suppose it shouldn't, but when you have got an agency getting their money directly from the industry that they are regulating, it is hard for the public and maybe for us, and it causes us to be a little more suspicious here in the Congress, but for the public that is unsophisticated about how Government works, it is sure going to appear to them of undue influence. But more importantly than just the user fees, I can make reference to a lot of e-mails that we have had access to from within the FDA that would say things along this line, and I don't have a specific reference. I could have my staff get you a specific reference, but things that said well, if there is any question about this or that, some specific drug they would mention, talk to us first or let us have an opportunity to explain, et cetera. It is almost like the pharmaceutical companies feel like they have a seat at the table and maybe this fee business makes them feel that way. I don't know for sure. But the point is, there should only be one person across the table from the FDA and that is John Q. Public, not members of the pharmaceutical industry.

Mr. STUPAK. Senator, you went all the way to the Department of Health and Human Services to talk to an agent regarding Ketek. Has HHS finally given you access to that agent?

Senator GRASSLEY. Absolutely not and there is not reason to, but their excuse is that there is a criminal investigation or there is an investigation generally, see, an investigation generally. And I will tell you how absurd this gets. Now, they referred to the fact that the Department of Justice is advising them accordingly, see? So I am sitting in Judiciary Committee in the United States Senate on an entirely different issue and Senator Kennedy, with more seniority, goes ahead of me and he says something to somebody from the Department of Justice, I want to ask these line agents some questions. Well, you can have access to these line agents.

Well, a light bulb goes off that Chuck Grassley can't have access to a line agent because somebody in the Justice Department told HHS that I couldn't talk to Agent West. So I talked to the Justice Department about the situation right after Senator Kennedy gets done and they said I could have access the same way Kennedy had access, to other agents in some other department. I still don't have access to Agent West. So if the Justice Department is advising

HHS that you can't have access to Agent West but the Justice Department, in a similar case of a line agent says Senator Kennedy has, well, what is the policy of this administration on having access to line agents? Is it one policy for Kennedy, a Democrat, and another policy for Grassley, a Republican?

Mr. STUPAK. I understand. I want to respect your time. I am done with my 10 minutes. Any comments, Mr. Green? Ms. DeGette? Thank you. Thank you. Mr. Whitfield, please, for 10 minutes.

Mr. WHITFIELD. Thank you, Mr. Stupak, and I have one question and then we will let the other Members on our side expend the 10 minutes.

Senator, we appreciate you being here. In your testimony, you brought attention to one of the basic tenets of our Government and that is the responsibility of oversight by the legislative branch and I would just ask you a question because I think you have touched on a significant issue, just the difficulty that you had in obtaining information from a branch of the Government on the executive side. Did you consider using a subpoena at any time to, not only a subpoena, but holding them in contempt?

Senator GRASSLEY. In the Senate, you get to this place. We considered that, yes. But you have to have a majority vote of the committee. You have to have a majority vote of the Senate for that to happen and so we did not decide to go that route because we thought there were other routes we could go. Obviously, the other routes have not been successful, either.

Mr. WHITFIELD. Well, we appreciate very much your bringing attention to this issue and we look forward to working with you as we try to address it and——

Senator GRASSLEY. Well, let me suggest to you, Chairman, or Ranking Member Whitfield, that you can be very helpful. This double standard in this administration, that a Democratic Senator, supposedly not as friendly with the administration as I am, maybe they don't consider me friendly anymore, but the point is if Senator Kennedy can get access to line agents why can't Senator Grassley get access to a line agent, when I have already had access to line agents over the years? So some sort of new policy?

Mr. WHITFIELD. Yes, I understand. I get frustrated. I find the appropriators sometimes have access to things I don't have access to and it is very frustrating. Since I guess I am controlling the time on our side, at this time I recognize Mr. Ferguson, Mr. Burgess and then Mr. Walden.

Mr. FERGUSON. Thank you, Mr. Whitfield. Senator, thank you very much for being here today. I can fully identify with your frustration in not always getting information that you are looking for. I know you were commenting before on whether the administration considers you a friend or not, we all certainly here consider you a friend and we very much appreciate your being here.

Senator GRASSLEY. Well, sometimes I wonder why I spent 2 days in the car with President Bush riding around the cold of Iowa to help him get nominated in the year 2000, as an example.

Mr. FERGUSON. I wish I could shed more light on that for you but maybe I ought to stick to my topic. Senator, you mentioned before the Mosholder investigation on SSRI's with children. That was a very, very important topic for this subcommittee, something that I was very involved with personally and really highlights the importance of this topic, this issue of post-market analysis and I know, in your bill, your approach in the bill that you have introduced would move this issue of post-market review out of CDER, out of the Center for Drug Education or Evaluation and Research.

Would you just comment on the differences between your approach and the approach that was suggested by the recommendations of the Institute of Medicine? I don't want to bring up Senator Kennedy's name, because that seems to raise your ire, but I know in the bill that Senator Kennedy has introduced, his approach seems to be, anyway, more consistent with the recommendation that the Institute of Medicine had suggested. Would you just comment on those differences, please?

Senator GRASSLEY. In a very general way, I think that the main difference is that I want, within FDA—because some people think we are setting up something outside FDA, so I want to emphasize, we are doing it within FDA—report directly to the Director so that there is no doubt that even though, on a chart of organization, the Office of New Drugs is separate from the post-marketing, the Office of Drug Safety, but as I indicated, it is not really so. So I want to get this box over here, wherever this box is located, I want it not to be under the thumb of this agency, even though the chart doesn't show it that way, reporting directly to it. And I think that Senator Kennedy's approach, and it is probably a bipartisan bill, so it is not a political, partisan issue, is that we are going to still have a cloudy relationship, not the black and white separation that I call for under the bill that came out of committee last year. Now, I don't know whether Senator Kennedy, in his new bill, is going the same direction this year or not, but last year, that is the way it was and we just want guaranteed independence in reporting directly so that we don't have these people in the Office of New Drugs that says this drug is safe, trying to quash out here when somebody says it isn't safe. And I don't want what happened to some of your witnesses who are patriotic Americans, wanted to make sure the scientific process works, being blackballed and ruined professionally because of that. It doesn't need to be. It compromises too much and there is too much found out in post-marketing surveillance that needs to have an independent judgment of it. And I don't think that in the bill that Senator Kennedy has that it goes far enough.

Mr. WHITFIELD. We have less than 4 minutes left. Dr. Burgess, did you have a question?

Mr. BURGESS. Yes, Mr. Whitfield. Senator, thank you for being here. On perhaps just a side note. Yesterday in the Wall Street Journal there was an op-ed article about clinical trials and patients who have reached the end of their therapeutic ropes, if you will, who are denied access to drugs that are in phase 2 trials. It raises a separate issue with the FDA, but physicians and clinical staffs who apply for exceptions to get their patients into these clinical trials find the statistical issues raised by the FDA staff aimed at the applying physician can sometimes rival receipt from the IRS.

Clearly, that is an interference in getting new cutting edge medications to patients, again, who have exhausted all therapeutic activity, so I hope, Mr. Chairman, we can perhaps spend some time looking at that, as well. I guess I am most interested, Senator, and I do agree with you, the proper respect for the scientific process needs to be paramount in our minds. Line Agent West, whom you referenced, were you ever able to establish contact with this individual and if not, Mr. Chairman, are we planning on asking for similar access to Line Agent West? Senator?

Senator GRASSLEY. Well, I have not personally had access to him in the way that makes any difference. I think maybe I better not speak beyond that because I don't want to get anybody in trouble, but we have some information, but we need to get the information in an open, transparent way. And I don't want to imply we got information, that we just want to be more transparent. We don't have all the information we can get if we can talk to him.

Mr. BURGESS. But I judged from your tone and demeanor you felt that this individual had some pretty important information?

Senator GRASSLEY. Oh, absolutely. Without a doubt.

Mr. BURGESS. Thank you, Mr. Chairman. I will yield.

Mr. WHITFIELD. Mr. Walden.

Senator GRASSLEY. Can I? On the first thing you brought up, I don't think you meant to imply this, but just in case; I don't want any misunderstanding. I hope, in all of my testimony, that I don't want to interfere with the things that you were bringing up that were in the Wall Street Journal in the sense of special opportunities for people who are willing to be guinea pigs because it is the end of the life, it might save their life, it might not save their life. Where an individual is totally aware of every gamble he is taking and he is educated in that and he is will to take it and everything is transparent, I don't want to stand in the way of that.

Mr. WHITFIELD. Mr. Walden.

Mr. WALDEN. Thank you. Thank you, Mr. Chairman. Senator, welcome. We appreciate your work on this issue. I want to touch on one topic and that is that Memorandum of Understanding that I understand exists between the IG's office and HHS and the FDA.

Senator GRASSLEY. Yes.

Mr. WALDEN. To allow the FDA to investigate itself, basically, on employee misconduct issues. And I am just curious. I know that is an issue you have been concerned about, Senator, and I wondered if you or your staff has learned anything new regarding the status of that MOA?

Senator GRASSLEY. Well, I think I better look at my staff, but I don't think we have anything more than we are just recommending that it should be reviewed and rewritten. I don't know that we're in the process of thinking it is being reviewed and rewritten. Yes. We have asked the IG to examine it. He has come up with some recommendations. But your question to me is, is it being rewritten and the answer is no. OK?

Mr. WALDEN. All right. It is just a concern I think we share.

Senator GRASSLEY. Well, yes, and it would be nice if—this is an extremely powerful committee you have here and the extent to which you can push that, it would be much appreciated by me, but more importantly, the people's safety is at stake here and independence from industry being regulated would be enhanced by it, as well, I think.

Mr. WALDEN. I think we concur with that.

Senator GRASSLEY. And maybe less pressure brought against whistleblowers, too.

Mr. STUPAK. Well, Senator, there is concern on that memorandum that the FDA is using it under a criminal pretext to suppress scientific opinion on drugs that are being approved. It appears, from the SSRI, Vioxx and others, when a scientist within the FDA or a whistleblower is going to speak out, they suddenly find themselves under some kind of criminal investigation from the FDA underneath this Memorandum of Understanding. It seems like it is a form of retaliation and harassment on scientists willing to speak up and speak out.

Senator GRASSLEY. Yes. And let me tell you, you have stated it better than I could and as a matter of emphasis, and more importantly, because you are chairman of this subcommittee, I hope people listen, from that point of view, and you pursue that because you are absolutely right.

Mr. STUPAK. Thank you. Mr. Dingell, anything for Senator Grassley?

The CHAIRMAN. Mr. Chairman, only this. I want to thank our old friend for coming over here. Thank you, Senator, very much for being here. I would ask that perhaps if I send you a little letter requesting some information on your statement today and your comments on some questions before us related to this matter. Perhaps maybe you would respond and I would ask unanimous consent that that response be put in the record.

Senator GRASSLEY. Yes, we will do that, Chairman Dingell, and thank you for your leadership and I look forward to a return to the days of your aggressive oversight work where almost every agency knew that you were going to get to the bottom of things and that they ought to cooperate.

The CHAIRMAN. Thank you. Well, you have set a good example and I will certainly try to follow it, but we have an outstanding chairman in this subcommittee, Senator, in the person of Mr. Stupak and he will do a superb job of helping folks understand that we all work for the taxpayers and the people, as do you, sir. Thank you very much for being here.

Senator GRASSLEY. That last statement he made, if I could comment on it. We all work for the taxpayers and we have got institutions, not just FDA. Maybe the example I always use is the FBI more than the FDA in this manner, but we have got too many agencies around here that talk about it as our agency or our institution. In the case of the FBI, it was our institution.

I got tired of the director saying that all the time at a meeting we were in, our institution, and I said that is what is wrong with the FBI and maybe that is what is wrong with the FDA, although I haven't heard that from them, but the point is that I said we all work for the American people. It is not your agency, it is not my agency, it is the people's agency and we are all working for the American people and the sooner we understand we are working for the American people and not for our institution, the better we are going to do our job.

Mr. STUPAK. Well said. Any other comments? Senator, thank you once again. Thank you for your time and thank you for your work and we look forward to working with you.

Senator GRASSLEY. Thank you.

Mr. STUPAK. We will call our second panel up to testify.

Mr. BURGESS. Mr. Chairman, while the second panel is seating, can I ask for a unanimous consent request? I ask unanimous consent that yesterday's op-ed from the Wall Street Journal be submitted as part of the record?

Mr. STUPAK. Hearing no objection, it will be made part of the record.

Mr. STUPAK. The second panel will consist of Dr. David Ross, National Clinical Health Programs, U.S. Department of Veterans Affairs; Ann Marie Cisneros, Independent Clinical Research Associate; and Dr. John Powers, Scientific Applications International Corporation. If they would come forward, please. It is the policy of this subcommittee to take all testimony under oath. Please be advised that witnesses have the right, under the rules of the House, to be advised by counsel during testimony. Do any of the witnesses before us, this panel, have counsel at this time? Do you want to introduce your counsel, Dr. Ross?

Dr. ROSS. My counsel is Mr. Mark Cohen of the Government Accountability Project.

Mr. STUPAK. OK. Ms. Cisneros?

Ms. CISNEROS. My counsel is the same.

Mr. STUPAK. Same. Dr. Powers?

Dr. POWERS. Same.

Mr. STUPAK. OK. Please rise and raise your right hand to take the oath.

[Witnesses sworn.]

Mr. STUPAK. OK, record shall reflect the witnesses have been sworn and Dr. Ross, we will begin with your opening statement, please.

TESTIMONY OF DAVID ROSS, M.D., NATIONAL CLINICAL HEALTH PROGRAMS, U.S. DEPARTMENT OF VETERANS AFFAIRS

Dr. ROSS Good morning, Mr. Chairman, Mr. Ranking Member and members of the committee. Thank you for the opportunity to speak before this committee. I am here today to speak about the drug Ketek.

My name is David Ross. For purposes of identification only, I am National Director of Clinical Public Health Programs for the U.S. Department of Veterans Affairs. I am here today as a private citizen. I was trained as a medical doctor at New York University and Yale and am Board certified in internal medicine and infectious diseases. I take care of patients at my local VA hospital and teach medical students and residents.

I served for 10 years at the FDA in positions ranging from primary reviewer of new drug applications to a member of the senior leadership team of FDA's Office of New Drugs. I served as both the primary safety reviewer and the safety team leader for Ketek. FDA approved Ketek despite knowing that it could kill people from liver damage and that tens of millions of people would be exposed to it, despite FDA knowing that the drug's maker submitted fabricated data, and despite knowing that Ketek is no better than any other antibiotics and may not even work.

Why does Ketek matter? Because FDA broke its own rules and allowed Ketek on the market. Because dozens of patients have died or suffered needlessly. Because FDA allowed Ketek's maker to experiment with it on children over reviewers' protests. Because FDA ignored warnings about fraud. And because FDA used data it knew were false to reassure the public about Ketek's safety. In March 2000, when Ketek was submitted to FDA, reviewers were alarmed over a patient treated with Ketek who had developed severe liver damage, an even that could mean hundreds or thousands of deaths every year.

In April 2001, a Federal advisory committee was so concerned about Ketek's potential to kill patients, that it required a large safety study before the drug could be approved. In October 2002, FDA reviewers, examining the safety study found serious and pervasive misconduct point at fraud. In December 2002, Ketek's manufacturer admitted that it had known about issues at its largest enroller but hadn't told the FDA. The company claimed that there were no other issues with the study, even though every study site inspected by FDA turned out to have major problems, an unprecedented situation in my experience.

In January 2003, over reviewer's protests, FDA managers hid the evidence of fraud and misconduct from the advisory committee, which was fooled into voting for approval. Starting the same month, FDA managers also pushed to use uncontrolled, unreliable side effect reports from overseas supplied by the drug's manufacturer. FDA's own division of scientific investigations concluded that none of the safety study data were reliable. One week later, FDA managers approved Ketek. They repeatedly cited it was evidence of Ketek's safety.

In February 2005, 7 months after Ketek's launch, FDA managers received the first reports of fatal Ketek-related liver failure. They did nothing. In February 2006, I and other reviewers warned senior FDA managers, in writing, about the problems with Ketek, including reviewers being pressured to change their opinions. The managers did nothing. In March 2006, FDA managers received new warnings from criminal investigators. They did nothing. In May 2006, FDA managers received warnings from safety reviewers that Ketek was much more dangerous than comparable antibiotics. They did nothing.

Only after congressional subpoenas, which FDA resisted, and stories in the news media about Ketek and fraud, did FDA managers finally do anything. They reworded the label. In late June 2006, FDA reviewers, including myself, were summoned to a meeting with Commissioner von Eschenbach in which he compared the FDA to a football team and told reviewers that if they told anyone outside the FDA about the problems with Ketek, they would be traded from the team. Rather than be silenced, I chose to move on to my current position.

How did this happen? The FDA reviewers did their job. This is not their fault. Ketek can be laid directly at the door of senior FDA managers who knew better because they were told repeatedly by reviewers and criminal investigators, but chose to look the other way. Their behavior was worse than being in a state of denial. FDA managers were so bent on approving Ketek, that they suppressed evidence of fraud and pressured reviewers, including myself, to change their reviews.

What is the bottom line? An unsafe drug got past the system despite warning after warning about fraud, liver damage and death because FDA managers at the highest levels refused to listen. Will this happen again? Yes. Without significant changes in our drug safety system and in FDA, we are certain to see more Keteks. Thank you. The views presented here are my own. I will be happy to answer any questions from the committee.

[The prepared testimony of Mr. Ross appears at the conclusion of the record.]

Mr. STUPAK. Thank you, Dr. Ross. Ms. Cisneros, for a 5 minute opening statement.

TESTIMONY OF ANN MARIE CISNEROS, INDEPENDENT CLINICAL RESEARCH ASSOCIATE

Ms. CISNEROS. Sure. Good morning, Mr. Chairman and members of the committee. I am honored that you are giving me the opportunity to tell my story.

My name is Ann Marie Cisneros. I am currently an independent clinical research associate. I was trained in the United States Air Force as a medical technologist, have a Bachelors of Science Degree in Occupational Education from Wayland Baptist University and a Masters of Business Administration Degree from Pfieffer University.

I have worked as a clinical research associate for approximately 8 years. My first 3 years in this industry I spent at PPDI, a contract research organization, where I monitored a number of protocols that included Study 3014. At the time of Study 3014 I was a senior clinical research associate and was asked to assist with the monitoring of Dr. Anne Kirkman-Campbell's site.

Dr. Kirkman-Campbell is currently serving a 57-month prison sentence for fraud associated with Study 3014. In addition, she was ordered by the court to pay restitution to the drug sponsor, Aventis, which had paid her $400 per patient enrolled.

Mr. Chairman, based upon what I observed and learned in monitoring the Kirkman-Campbell site, Dr. Kirkman-Campbell indeed had engaged in fraud. But what the court that sentenced her did not know is that Aventis was not a victim of this fraud. On the contrary. Let me explain.

Even before conducting the Kirkman-Campbell site visit, a number of red flags were apparent. I knew that Dr. Campbell had enrolled over 400 patients, or 1 percent of the adult population of Gadsden, Alabama. By comparison, another site in Gadsden had enrolled just 12 patients. In a recent quality assurance audit by Aventis, several Informed Consent issues were noted, as well as significant under-reporting of adverse events and no reports of serious adverse events. No patients had withdrawn from the study and no patients were lost to follow up, an unusual occurrence given the number of subjects. She enrolled patients within minutes of each other and upwards of 30 patients per day. She enrolled patients at times and on days when the office was closed.

Once we started reviewing patient charts, we discovered that every informed consent had a discrepancy. Most of the consents looked like they had been initialed by someone other than the patient. A lot of the consents were dated by someone other than the subjects. One consent was a blatant forgery. There date discrepancies as to when patients were enrolled in the study, had their blood drawn or signed their consent. Most patients diagnosed with bronchitis either had no history of the ailment or not have a chronic condition. She enrolled her entire staff in the study.

Frankly, all Kirkman-Campbell seemed really interested in was getting more business from Aventis as an investigator. At one point during my site visit, she told Aventis project manager Nadine Guenthe that I could only stay if Nadine got her other studies at Aventis and Nadine agreed. It is my understanding that when the FDA audited Kirkman-Campbell's site, she was participating in another Aventis clinical trial.

While at the site, I was so concerned about patient safety, I called Copernicus Independent Review Board to express my concerns and seek guidance. An IRB, which is under contract to the drug sponsor, has as its primary purpose as patient advocacy. It is allowed to contact patients directly and is duty-bound to report to the FDA any unanticipated problems involving risks to subjects and serious noncompliance with regulations. I spoke with the president of the company and was told that while she shared my concerns, she preferred to wait and see what actions Aventis took. I never heard from the IRB again and to my knowledge, Copernicus never did audit, blacklist the site or report any irregularities to the FDA.

I e-mailed a summary of my site findings to Robert McCormick, head of quality assurance at PPD and copied Aventis personnel. I also participated in a teleconference between PPD and Aventis at which I discussed issues identified in my visit. At some point after that, I understand that Aventis took site management responsibilities away from PPD because Kirkman-Campbell would not cooperate with anyone but the sponsor.

I subsequently left PPD but learned that the Kirkman-Campbell site was being audited by the FDA. In preparation for the audit, Aventis' Nadine Guenthe coached Dr. Campbell with leading questions on how to explain away improper conduct. Nadine would say, for example, is the reason you enrolled so many patients in 1 day because that is when your supply of drug came in? I was told about this by a trusted and distressed former colleague of PPD who witnessed the prepping.

In my 8 years in clinical research work, this is the only instance I have come across such bad behavior by a drug sponsor. I feel I can speak for those who agonized over this situation when I say we are pleased that Dr. Campbell is serving prison time for her actions. But what brings me here today is my disbelief at Aventis' statements that it did not suspect that fraud was being committed. Mr. Chairman, I knew it, PPD knew it and Aventis knew it. Thank you.

[The prepared testimony of Ms. Cisneros appears at the conclusion of the hearing.]

Mr. STUPAK. Thank you. Ms. Cisneros. Dr. Powers, opening statement, please.

TESTIMONY OF JOHN POWERS, M.D., SCIENTIFIC APPLICATIONS INTERNATIONAL CORPORATION

Dr. POWERS. Thank you, Mr. Chairman, and members of the committee. Good morning. My name is John Powers. I am a physician-scientist who worked at the Food and Drug Administration for 8 years, the last 5 of which I was the Lead Medical Officer for Antimicrobial Drug Development and Resistance Initiatives. I really do not consider myself as having "blown a whistle," but having done my job, since I appropriately raised the issues that I will discuss with you today to my supervisors at FDA. I chose to leave the agency to pursue other research opportunities after over half a decade of attempting to advance the science of clinical trials and infectious diseases, feeling I could better serve the public outside the agency. There are numerous individuals in both the FDA and the drug industry who work hard appropriately evaluating and I learned a tremendous amount while I was at FDA. I would still be there today if I felt I could perform my job in the way it should be done.

Many of the recent discussions regarding evaluation of new drugs have focused on their safety, but there are also important issues with the evaluation of drug effectiveness, especially with antibiotics. In 1962, Congress amended the Food, Drug and Cosmetic Act to state that there must be substantial evidence of effectiveness from adequate and well-controlled trials in order to justify the adverse events that are inherent with all drugs. In the absence of substantial evidence of effectiveness, any adverse effect, no matter how rare, is not justifiable.

The approval of Ketek is a symptom of a larger problem. Over the last 25 years FDA has approved approximately 68 new drug applications for ear, sinus and bronchial infections, which are mostly self-resolving. All of these drugs were approved based on so-called non-inferiority trials. The word itself, non-inferior, means not worse, but the purpose of these trials is to rule out an amount by which the new drug's effectiveness may, in fact, be worse compared to an older drug. Showing a new drug is potentially worse than an old drug whose effectiveness, itself, is unclear in the setting of a given trial. It is like the Billy Preston song, "nothing from nothing leaves nothing."

Previous placebo control trials show 12 of 17 studies in sinus infections and 9 of 14 studies in bronchial infections lack evidence of a benefit for antibiotics and the situation is similar for ear infections, therefore showing that Ketek may be less effective than older drugs is not evidence that Ketek is effective at all in sinus and bronchial infections and this was clear at the time the drug was approved in 2004.

While non-inferiority trials are justifiable in serious infections where the benefits of antibiotics are clear, even here the trial must be done properly in order to provide meaningful results. The major problem is that many of the safeguards and trials that protect against false conclusions are less useful in the setting of non-inferiority trials. For instance, trials in pneumonia may enroll patients who don't have pneumonia, but instead have the common cold. This says nothing about the new drug's effectiveness in pneumonia, but the new drug may appear to be similar in effectiveness to the old drug. This is like testing a new parachute against an older proven parachute when all the people are jumping out of a plane that is standing still and only two inches off the ground. Everyone will do well, but it says nothing about how the new parachute will work in a real life situation.

Lack of effectiveness is a more important problem in antibiotics than it is for other types of drugs. If a non-antibiotic doesn't work, it only affects the person who takes it. If an antibiotic doesn't work, it affects the person who takes it and other people, by spreading resistance to that drug and to other related drugs, as well. Antibiotic resistance is a safety issue and lack of effectiveness of antibiotics can promote the problem of resistance we are actually trying to combat. Why would FDA continue to allow approval of antibiotics without substantial evidence of effectiveness?

Drug sponsors have exited the field of antibiotic development over the last few decades and this was an attempt to provide an economic incentive for sponsors to develop drugs where we really need them, in serious and life threatening diseases. We do need new antibiotics, but approval of ineffective and therefore inherently unsafe drugs is not a proper or effective incentive for drug development. Exposing children who might not even have a bacterial infection to Ketek in the setting of a non-inferiority trial is not the way to develop new drugs, as children will be exposed to harm without the ability to determine the drug's effectiveness. Despite the approval over the last two decades of scores of antibiotics whose effectiveness remains unclear, there has been no boom in antibiotic development and developing economic incentives to promote development is needed, but it is the province of Congress, not the FDA.

In summary, FDA needs to require sponsors to perform placebo control trials and self-resolving diseases. For serious diseases, FDA needs to require appropriately designed, conducted and analyzed trials to give clinicians the information they need to make appropriate decisions for patients. FDA needs to address the drugs that still carry approvals for self-resolving diseases without substantial evidence of effectiveness. FDA needs to promptly publish new guidances based on appropriate scientific and regulatory principles and remove the old guidances from its Web site now, since they continue to mislead drug sponsors.

Mr. Chairman, the bottom line is we must preserve the effectiveness of antibiotics, which are among the marvels of modern medicine, and that means they must be studied in trials that tell us whether they truly help people, not just have activity in test tubes. Thank you.

[The prepared testimony of Dr. Powers appears at the conclusion of the hearing.]

Mr. STUPAK. Thank you. Before we begin questions, in order to proceed in a more orderly and efficient manner, I would propose that instead of minutes for each Member for questioning, that each Member will have 10 minutes to use for questioning during this hearing. If there is no objection, I propose we do this this morning. Mr. Whitfield, do you have any comments or thoughts on that, going to 10 minutes?

Mr. WHITFIELD. I don't have any objections.

Mr. STUPAK. No objections? So ordered.

Dr. Ross, if I may start with you, please. In your testimony, as powerful and as forceful as it was, you indicated, in January 2003, over viewers protest, FDA managers hid the evidence. You went on and talked about FDA managers pushed to use uncontrolled, unreliable side effect reports from overseas. You indicated throughout your testimony that they did nothing, that FDA managers didn't review things; FDA managers were aware of things but did not act. Who are these FDA managers?

Dr. ROSS. There are specifically six individuals I would——

Mr. STUPAK. And we are just talking about Ketek right now?

Dr. ROSS. We are just talking about Ketek, yes, sir. There are six individuals I would point to: Dr. John Jenkins, the director of the Office of New Drugs; his deputy, Dr. Sandra Kweder; the director of the Office of Antimicrobial Products, Dr. Mark Goldberger; his deputy, Dr. Edward Cox; his associate director, Mr. David Roeder; and the division director for the Division of Anti-infective and Ophthalmologic Drug Products, Dr. Janice Soreth.

Mr. STUPAK. OK. What rules did the FDA break in it approval of Ketek? Now, you were there for 10 years, you were a senior analyst on these drugs.

Dr. ROSS. I was the safety team leader for Ketek and——

Mr. STUPAK. Would that be like the medical review officer assigned to Ketek?

Dr. ROSS. It would be. I served at different points, two roles.

Mr. STUPAK. OK.

Dr. ROSS. One was as the primary safety reviewer or the person actually looking at the data, and during the second review cycle, I directed a team of safety reviewers.

Mr. STUPAK. OK.

Dr. ROSS. And then later on in my career at FDA, I was a member of what is called the senior leadership team for the Office of New Drugs. So in terms of rules that FDA broke with respect to Ketek, it approved Ketek based on a study that its own investigators said was worthless, which breaks the rule about needing adequate and well-controlled trials. When I say a rule, that is a statutory requirement under the Food, Drug and Cosmetic Act. It used uncontrolled foreign safety reports to answer a critical safety question that should have been answered by an adequate and well-controlled trial. It failed to assess the overall integrity of the Ketek application, despite warnings about potential systemic fraud.

Mr. STUPAK. Warnings from whom?

Dr. ROSS. Warnings from reviewers and warnings from criminal investigators.

Mr. STUPAK. Warnings from yourself?

Dr. ROSS. Yes. And warnings, as well, from members of the Office of Criminal Investigations.

Mr. STUPAK. OK.

Dr. ROSS. It failed to verify the integrity of foreign data submitted to it before approving Ketek. It allowed managers to violate

Federal law by coercing reviewers into removing disagreements from the administrative record. Title 21, part 10.70 of the Code of Federal Regulations provides that disagreements on the provability of an application shall be entered in the administrative record. Finally, the FDA failed to carry out its responsibilities to enforce parts 50 and 56 of title 21 of the Code of Federal Regulations by failing to hold the Institutional Review Board for Dr. Kirkman-Campbell is responsible for its actions. To this date, as far as I am aware, there has been no action by FDA taken against that IRB.

Mr. STUPAK. What evidence is there that the FDA used the safety data from Study 3014 in its approval of Ketek? From what I can gather, the FDA denies that it relied upon that study in its approval process of Ketek. Can you shed any light on that?

Dr. ROSS. Yes. Let me just refer first off to yesterday's action by the FDA in changing the labeling for Ketek and at the press conference for that, Dr. John Jenkins, the director of the Office of New Drugs, stated unequivocally that they did not rely on Study 3014 for the approval. Let me quote from an e-mail that his own deputy sent on March 21, 2006 to myself and another reviewer.

> In speaking with the division about this, they did not completely ignore the data from the 3014 study, but assessed those AEs,

that is adverse events,

> that were identified to qualitatively assess patterns of toxicity.

Let me say the relevant clause again.

> They did not completely ignore the data from the 3014 study.

Second, FDA cited the safety study when it first issued a public health advisory about Ketek's potential to cause liver damage. It is still citing it on that same public health advisory as a large safety study. If they didn't use it for approval, why are they citing it on their own Web site?

Finally, I have been told that in making the decision about how and whether to prosecute Dr. Kirkman-Campbell, OCI asked CEDR if it had used the study in making the approval decision and the answer was yes.

Mr. STUPAK. Dr. Ross, were you present at all three advisory meetings for the approval of Ketek?

Dr. ROSS. Yes.

Mr. STUPAK. Why, at any one of these meetings, any one of these three advisory meetings, did you not speak up about your concerns about this study and how the approval process was moving forward on Ketek?

Dr. ROSS. Well, at the first advisory committee meeting, I gave a presentation on the overall safety of Ketek and at that point I did make my concerns very clear to the committee.

Mr. STUPAK. And is that when the committee voted, then, to do a larger study?

Dr. ROSS. That is correct.

Mr. STUPAK. OK.

Dr. ROSS. At the second advisory committee, we had been told by supervisors that the committee was not going to hear about the fraud issues. If I had spoken about that, I would have been fired immediately.

Mr. STUPAK. So before the second one you were told by FDA you were not allowed to bring up the fraud issue about, and this would be Study 3014?

Dr. ROSS. That is correct. We were told we are not going to discuss it with the committee.

Mr. STUPAK. OK. And you felt that if you would have brought up that issue, the fraud in the study—obviously the FDA knew about it then—you would have been fired?

Dr. ROSS. There is no doubt in my mind and I think I likely would have been subject to investigation by OCI that would have been initiated.

Mr. STUPAK. OK, then that is the approval of Ketek. Then there was a third advisory meeting?

Dr. ROSS. Yes. At that third committee meeting I appeared as a private citizen and spoke at the open public hearing.

Mr. STUPAK. Were you still an FDA——

Dr. ROSS. No. At that point I was not. I took leave from my current position for that day, so I was only appearing for myself and I made facts known to the committee that they had not been told by FDA.

Mr. STUPAK. Thank you. Ms. Cisneros, in your testimony you state that Aventis performed a quality assurance audit of the Kirkman-Campbell site. Who, at Aventis, would have seen the results of this audit?

Ms. CISNEROS. Nadine Guenthe, who was the project manager for Aventis and Ron Gincosly, who was the auditor.

Mr. STUPAK. You also indicated, in your testimony, that even before the visit to the Kirkman-Campbell site, a number of red flags were apparent, you said. Would Aventis have known of the these red flags?

Ms. CISNEROS. Absolutely. I spoke with the in-house CRA that managed Dr. Campbell's site and she had told me that she was communicating with her superiors on almost a daily basis about the oddities that were occurring at her site and it is my understanding that the project manager at PPD would be having discussions with Nadine Guenthe at Aventis about those issues.

Mr. STUPAK. OK. There is a large binder right there. There is exhibit No. 15, if you would look at that for me. In that document, exhibit No. 15, it is sent to Nadine Guenthe of Aventis attached to an e-mail dated February 27, 2002 by Jessica Lasley of PPDI. A number of issues were raised with regard to the Kirkman-Campbell site. For example, one item says all subjects were 100 percent compliant with study medication. Have you ever seen a study in which a hundred percent of the subjects, in this case, some 400 people, were compliant with the study medication?

Ms. CISNEROS. No, I have not. And in this note that I gave to Aventis, this referred to the 30 patients that I had monitored at this site.

Mr. STUPAK. OK. And you said you gave this to Aventis, so this would have been February 27, 2002 or thereabout, so that is some 2 years before Ketek was ever approved for the general population?

Ms. CISNEROS. Correct.

Mr. STUPAK. In your last statement, I would like to shed a little light on it, if you may. In your testimony you indicate that you knew there were problems with the Ketek study with this site; the FDA new and Aventis knew, and the PPD.

Ms. CISNEROS. PPD knew.

Mr. STUPAK. Right.

Ms. CISNEROS. Right.

Mr. STUPAK. How are you saying that Aventis knew of the problems? You make a very emphatic statement at the end.

Ms. CISNEROS. They could not have not known. The data, the evidence was clear. They just had to prove a suspicion of fraud. They didn't have to necessarily prove the fraud. They just have to report a suspicion of fraud. And the evidence that I brought back from my site visit, the evidence that was discovered at the quality assurance audit, was pretty extraordinary.

Mr. STUPAK. So if I understand this correctly, if Aventis knew there was suspicion of fraud in any of——

Ms. CISNEROS. Right.

Mr. STUPAK. Even a suspicion, you have to report that to the FDA?

Ms. CISNEROS. Correct.

Mr. STUPAK. And that is required underneath your contract to do this service?

Ms. CISNEROS. I believe it is in the Code of Federal Regulations, yes.

Mr. STUPAK. Thank you. Mr. Whitfield for 10 minutes.

Mr. WHITFIELD. Thank you. Thank you, Mr. Stupak, and I thank the three witnesses for being with us this morning, as well. Dr. Ross, in your testimony, you went through a number of pages here talking about how FDA managers had information, and did nothing. They were warned by criminal investigators about possible fraud, and did nothing. They received records from the company that raised further concerns, and did not review them. The FDA's own division of scientific investigation concluded that none of the safety study data was reliable and then they went on one week later and approved Ketek. Through a number of very strong statements and as a citizen, a Member of Congress, has oversight.

When these people are appointed in leadership positions, at certainly FDA, they all are professionals; they are physicians, they are scientists, they have great responsibility that has an impact on all of our society in their decision. This seems to be, from your testimony and the other testimony, so blatant. Why would FDA managers do something like this? What would be your best guess?

Dr. ROSS. That is an outstanding question and it is something I have been wracking my brains about. My best guess is that there is two things. Overall, there is a culture of approval that if you can get a product on the market, and this was particularly egregious in this particular office, then you find some way of doing it. The second thing that I have concluded, and this is speculation on my part, but I do want to bring it to the committee's attention, it is inconceivable to me that after receiving a warning in July 2003 from an experienced criminal investigator, that a decision to not have an investigation was made at this level. I am also have been told that Dr. Kweder was also briefed by OCI about the need for a multi-jurisdictional task force. It is my belief that the decision not to have an investigation was made at a higher level and that would most likely be the Office of Chief Counsel.

Mr. WHITFIELD. And how long were you at FDA? Ten years?

Dr. ROSS. Yes, sir.

Mr. WHITFIELD. And you left simply because, as a physician, you felt like you could not work at an agency with that kind of culture, would that be safe to say?

Dr. ROSS. One thing I have to say is FDA has wonderful physicians and scientists who are public health heroes. They really are dedicated to doing the best job possible. In the office I was in, before I left, the Office of Oncology Drug Products was one where I felt the managers were very committed to doing the right thing, to getting life saving products out quickly to the American public, but overall, seeing how the senior managers, the individuals who I mentioned, were dealing with what was clearly a horrible situation and not dealing with it, I felt I couldn't, in good conscience, continue to work at the agency and I gave them a chance to do this before I left. A year ago, I met with Dr. Jenkins and Dr. Kweder in the presence of a witness and followed this up with e-mails and told them about what was going on and I said we have got a huge problem here, but we can turn it around. We can solve this problem.

I gave them steps to follow, a corrective action plan about Ketek and about the problems with scientific culture and I said please do this. If we don't, we are going to get crucified. They really didn't do anything. I told them survey the reviewers, find out what the problem is. They didn't do that. I said get everybody together in a room so we are not sullying information about Ketek and let us see what the fraud situation is. They said well, we will look into this. I found out later that Dr. Kweder concealed my briefing that I had given to her from the Office of Compliance within CEDR. So at that point I felt I can't be in an agency that has a culture like this even if I like the people and the work that I am doing.

Mr. WHITFIELD. Now, you named one, two, three, four, five, six people that were so-called senior management, that is Dr. Jenkins and Dr. Kweder?

Dr. ROSS. Yes, sir.

Mr. WHITFIELD. And then Mark Goldberger.

Dr. ROSS. Dr. Goldberger.

Mr. WHITFIELD. And Dr. Cox.

Dr. ROSS. Dr. Cox. Mr. Roeder and Dr. Soreth.

Mr. WHITFIELD. OK. And Dr. Powers, now, tell me again how long were you at the agency?

Dr. POWERS. I was there for 8 years.

Mr. WHITFIELD. Eight years. And you certainly heard the testimony of Dr. Ross and the same question I asked him I would ask you: why would they approve a drug like Ketek, assuming that the facts that you have stated and that Dr. Ross has stated are true, what would be your best guess? Now, he said that there is a culture of approval.

Dr. POWERS. Let me answer specifically about this drug, first. I think, first of all, that there were economic issues regarding antibiotic development that were pressuring FDA from the outside.

Mr. WHITFIELD. Now, what do you mean by that?

Dr. POWERS. So over the last 20 years several large pharmaceutical companies had decided that they were no longer going to participate in either discovering or developing new antibiotics. And this was occurring at a time when we really do need new antibiotics because of rising resistance and when I say need, what I mean is in serious and life threatening diseases where people could die if they don't get appropriate therapy. In 2001 a member of the pharmaceutical industry and a prominent academician wrote a letter in the journal Clinical Infectious Diseases and that letter was titled "The U.S. Food and Drug Administration and the End of Antibiotics". And in it they outlined that if FDA made any moves to increase the rigor of scientific studies in the area of antibiotics, that we would be perceived as a scientific disincentive.

And I remember having a meeting about this and this is clearly something we need to take account of and we do need to make studies more efficient. In fact, placebo control trials can be done with fewer numbers of patients. But that really seemed to cause a lot of uproar within the agency, as well. I think there is a second reason, though, and I think that there is a bias about antibiotics, in general, and that is we tend to focus on microorganisms instead of people. It is very clear that antibiotics can kill microorganisms and they are very effective in preventing death in serious diseases like pneumonia. The question is what do they do for a disease like a sinus infection where your own immune system gets you better, even though they have a huge effect on bacteria, what do they do for people? And I think a lot of scientists in this area have this bias that if it affects the bug, that is all we need to know.

And then there is the third issue and that is there were a number of antibiotics approved in this method and it is just human nature to sort of not want to go back and say whoa, wait a minute. Maybe perhaps we need to readdress all of this. That is a huge undertaking, actually. So I think that there is just a human aspect to it, as well.

Mr. WHITFIELD. Now, in the article that was written about the FDA being responsible for the ending of antibiotics, research and development, what year was that article written?

Dr. POWERS. It was published in early 2002, I believe.

Mr. WHITFIELD. And you say drug companies were letting it be known that they were going to stop developing antibiotics?

Dr. POWERS. Some already had and this is an issue that has gone back to the 1980's, actually, where some companies had decided to stop antibiotic discovery.

Mr. WHITFIELD. And the reason for that was just the rigors of the approval process?

Dr. POWERS. No. Actually, antibiotics have the highest approval rate of any therapeutic class of drugs and in some ways the studies are shorter and easier to do. You don't have to study people for like arthritis for a year.

Mr. WHITFIELD. Yes.

Dr. POWERS. The issue is that antibiotics are usually given for a short period of time and therefore, the returns on actually investing in an antibiotic are not as great as they would be for a drug that you would take for your lifetime. And there is also a lot of generic competition, as well.

Mr. WHITFIELD. Now, Ketek, of course is still on the market and was originally approved for three conditions and now it is being used or approved for only one and that is pneumonia, is that correct?

Dr. POWERS. Yes.

Mr. WHITFIELD. Now, somewhere I read or someone told me that in some of the studies on Ketek that it said only 23 out of 10 million would be expected to suffer any kind of liver damage. Am I just imagining this figure or is there any basis for that at all?

Dr. POWERS. Let me go into that number. In May 2006, what was then the Office of Drug Safety, presented an analysis of a number of cases of acute liver failure that had been reported and put that in the context of the number of prescriptions that had been written. And let me just say in terms of the number of prescriptions that have been written—I did a quick, back of the envelope calculation last night. I would say at this point, a Ketek prescription is written in this country every 22 seconds and this is after all of the publicity. Last year it was every 4 or 5 seconds. There were, at the time, 12 cases of acute liver failure that had been reported and without boring members of the committee, acute liver failure is an extremely serious condition that can lead to death or the need for liver transplantation. Thirty percent of the patients dies.

So 12 cases probably doesn't sound like a lot, but the problem is most serious liver events are never reported. If you look at a study that was done in France, and this is the only study of its type I am aware of, where researchers said how many serious liver events actually get reported compared to how many actually occur, they found that physicians only reported one out of every 24,000 liver injuries and out of serious liver injuries, things where people were dying from liver failure, it was still one out of every 16. So for each one of those 12 cases, there are many patients who we don't know about.

So 23 out of 10 million, you could say well, that may not sound like very much. If you compare that to other antibiotics, for example a comparable antibiotic for the same indications, the rate was only two per 10 million. Twenty-three per 10 million is a lot when you are talking about an antibiotic that does not save lives.

Mr. STUPAK. The gentlewoman from Colorado, Ms. DeGette.

Ms. DEGETTE. I thank you very much, Mr. Chairman. Actually, Mr. Whitfield's question about how did this happen and why does it happen was the first question I was going to ask, so I am just going to follow up on that very excellent line of questioning.

Dr. Powers, you gave three reasons why you thought maybe this type of thing could happen and it is that there have been disincentives to antibiotic development, that there is not a focus on people and that people didn't want to have to go back and revisit the whole thing. That might be a good explanation, except for the fact that over the years in this committee, we have seen similar problems at the FDA with respect to other types of drugs that are not antibiotics. And so we begin to wonder is the problem not just a drug specific problem, but really a culture at the FDA that we have to figure out how to fix for patient safety. Wouldn't you agree with that?

Dr. POWERS. I think so and I have to say my experience with this was actually quite confusing to me in terms of when this became an issue, we had several public meetings before Ketek was ever approved, in 2002 and 2003 where we addressed these issues related to these kinds of studies. And the general agreement was that really they didn't provide substantial evidence of effectiveness and yet, we still got to the point where, in 2004, we were approving drugs like Ketek.

When I went to people, my supervisors and then their supervisors, I have to be honest and say there were people that were very rightfully concerned. Why that never translated into a change was really a mystery to me.

Ms. DEGETTE. And Dr. Ross, in your written testimony, you said that Ketek was approved despite the FDA knowing that the drug's maker submitted fabricated data, is that correct?

Dr. ROSS. Yes.

Ms. DEGETTE. Now, how do you know that they knew that there was fabricated data?

Dr. ROSS. First off, the results of the initial inspections from Study 3014 were available in the fall of 2002 and it was clear at that point, it was clear as day that there were serious, serious problems.

Ms. DEGETTE. And why do you think that they went forward with this anyway?

Dr. ROSS. I have never gotten a good explanation.

Ms. DEGETTE. Well, what is your opinion? What do you think? Why would they do this knowing that data was fabricated and knowing that the risks of the liver failure could be quite high?

Dr. ROSS. As I said, there is a culture of approval and let me explain what I mean by that. Under the Prescription Drug User Fee Act there are obviously goals, which everybody knows. And FDA is fond of saying that that doesn't mean that we are going to approve it, but the bottom line is the fastest way to deal with a drug application, meet that deadline, is not to raise too many questions and approve it. That is No. 1.

Number 2, FDA has limited resources and Dr. Jenkins is very, been very vocal about how we have to stop having multiple cycle reviews and I think the feeling was let us just get this thing out of the way.

Ms. DEGETTE. Well, as Dr. Powers says, maybe you don't need to have as large or many reviews, but you certainly have to have thorough reviews that aren't fraudulent, right? You could restructure the way you do the reviews.

Dr. ROSS. I agree. One of the things that is missing right now from the review process is any measure of quality. Once a manager who has got sign off authority for a product writes a review, nobody else looks at it and says what were you thinking? So there is no measure of the quality of decision making that goes on.

Ms. DEGETTE. Well, later this year we are going to be reauthorizing PDUFA and I am wondering is, Dr. Powers, I would also like to ask you this question, is do you think that tying the user fees to the drug review is causing a bias in the system and if so, what can we think about doing when we reauthorize the Act to eliminate that bias?

Dr. ROSS. Let me first say I do not believe we can go back to the days in which we had 3 to 4 year reviews. We all know that.

Ms. DEGETTE. Everybody knows that, that is right.

Dr. ROSS. But I just want to put that on the record. But I am mindful of a sign I saw in a repair shop once, "fast, good, cheap. Pick any two." And I think right now what we have got, I hate to say it, is we are trying to do things on the cheap at FDA. We need more resources and more reviewers and higher standards there. And I think we are never going to get things perfect, but we can have fast and good. It won't be cheap, though.

Ms. DEGETTE. Dr. Powers.

Dr. POWERS. I often think about when my medical license comes up for renewal, I have to pay a fee to get that license renewed. It seems clear to me that when a drug sponsor asks an agency to review all of this information, it makes logical sense to pay a fee. But I don't tell the medical licensing board what they can do with my money. And I think the issue is this negotiating of what the money gets used for, I think, is an issue, in terms of PDUFA.

The second thing, I think, is that I don't know a single reviewer at FDA who says gee, my paycheck is coming from a drug company, I have to do what they say. That is not the way it works and reviewers are really doing an excellent job, for the most part. The question is his work done and some accountability for when that work is not done properly. And if that was built into the PDUFA system, it would be very helpful.

Ms. DEGETTE. Ms. Cisneros, I was struck in your testimony about what you saw about the real fraud in the patients that Dr. Kirkman-Campbell were seeing and I wanted to ask you a couple of questions about that. Do you think that the fraud was that she was enrolling all of these people and she wasn't enrolling them? Or was she actually giving the drug to all of these people who may be more sick? What was the problem?

Ms. CISNEROS. Well, it came out in the FDA audit that they never did find out what she did with the drug. She never disclosed that and refused to do so. Now, I think they called all 400 patients and she had actually enrolled maybe 50.

Ms. DEGETTE. OK.

Ms. CISNEROS. And all of the other patients were fabricated.

Ms. DEGETTE. So I guess the good news is she wasn't really killing all of those people.

Ms. CISNEROS. Yes.

Ms. DEGETTE. The bad news is she wasn't doing the job.

Ms. CISNEROS. The concern that I had when I was at the site is I didn't know what she was doing with the drug and she was giving a potentially harmful investigative medication to patients and not following them.

Ms. DEGETTE. Something else that piqued my interest, because I have been working for a long time on the issue of patient protection and patient notification, was when you called the Copernicus IRB to talk to them and my question is—and actually this is something both of the doctors could answer too, is if we beefed up the IRB process in these drug reviews, would that help maybe ensure the efficacy of some of these independent studies?

Ms. CISNEROS. Well, I am not quite sure who dropped the ball here with the IRB issue. They did nothing. They did not audit the site, they did not black list the site, even though they should have received information about her data. That is not usual for an IRB. I don't know what went wrong there.

Ms. DEGETTE. Was this a private IRB?

Ms. CISNEROS. No, they are a central IRB.

Ms. DEGETTE. OK.

Ms. CISNEROS. Yes.

Ms. DEGETTE. What about Dr. Ross? Do you think it would help if we beefed up the IRB system in these cases?

Dr. ROSS. Yes, I think there is two fundamental problems here. One is the IRB system nationally is broken. IRBs don't know what their responsibilities are. They don't know what they are supposed to do when there is a problem. It is No. 1, so we need to fix that. Number 2 is the enforcement side of things, that FDA basically has cut its enforcement to the bone and beyond. Just one example for the committee. We had a situation in Texas, when I was a deputy office director, where an investigator, a physician injected women with breast cancer with a radioactive substance without getting proper informed consent. When this came to our attention we jumped on it, but it took FDA over a year to take any kind of action on this. So you have an IRB system that is broken and then the enforcement office at FDA with good people who basically are being not supported by leadership.

Ms. DEGETTE. Dr. Powers, do you——

Dr. POWERS. Yes, I am going to concentrate on the scientific end of the IRB process. How does an IRB approve a non-inferiority trial for Ketek in little children with ear infections? So when you think about that, it says, well, what are the people at the IRB thinking about? And when I was at FDA, we actually got a letter back from an IRB, from a drug sponsor who actually tried to do the right thing and tried to do a placebo-controlled trial, saying we don't think you should be doing these kinds of trials, and says there is a lack of scientific understand at the IRB level, too.

Ms. DEGETTE. Mr. Chairman, I just asked those questions as a commercial announcement for my legislation, the Patient Protection Act, which I introduced the last two Congresses with Mr. Greenwood when he was here, and we are working on this bill and I have been talking to Mr. Dingell. I would hope that if you folks had some ideas about ways we could work on this legislation to make it effective. We do intend to move forward with it. Thank you, Mr. Chairman.

Mr. STUPAK. The gentleman from Texas, Mr. Burgess.

Mr. BURGESS. Thank you, Mr. Chairman, and I too want to thank the witnesses for being here this morning and particularly thank you for the efforts you have done ensure that we have safe and reliable medications in this country. Dr. Powers, let me just pick up on something that you were discussing with Ms. DeGette. In the PDUFA system, you mentioned that the barriers, or what the requirement was, that we have full transparency and accountability. What in your opinion are the barriers to transparency and accountability in the PDUFA system?

Dr. POWERS. I think it is interesting for me now, as no longer working for the FDA, what do I want to see as a physician out there in the community? What I would like to see is that when a drug gets approve, that all of the documents which went into that approval, all of the data, including the decision-making process, the meeting minutes, et cetera, go up on the FDA's Web site within, say, 7 working days of when the drug gets approved. Then everybody could look at this information and be able to make those kinds of decisions. Right now that kind of information gets up there and it is spotty at best and when you see an advisory committee, you see enormous amounts of information. That level of detail should be available for every kind of drug as well. And then, if there is scientific discussion within the review team and some people have differences of opinion, those could also go into there. Doctors could read those and be able to make their own decisions about those things.

Mr. BURGESS. Well, certainly if you made that a searchable database, it would improve the information that is out there, but I will also say, having been in a busy practice, you don't always have time to avail yourself of those things and unfortunately, like many people do, you rely on the other information that is available to you, which may come through post-marketing advertising. Dr. Ross, you talked about Dr. Kweder, who concealed the briefing that you all had. Do you know why this would've happened?

Dr. ROSS. I assume she didn't want them to know about it.

Mr. BURGESS. And what ultimately would have been the benefit to either the FDA or Dr. Kweder about concealing that briefing?

Dr. ROSS. I think, in any bureaucracy, the one thing you don't want are problems and the best way of making problems go away is by controlling information and concealing them and that is what I think was going on here.

Mr. BURGESS. Well, I will just say, from my own experience, I haven't been up here that long, but from my own experience, it seems the function of bureaucracy is to consume dollars and erode value, but that is from our hearings on Katrina, Chairman. I just have to say, Dr. Ross, I am astounded by your figures on the liver failure. Twenty-three cases of liver failure attributable to Ketek in this country, is that correct?

Dr. ROSS. No, I am sorry, sir. Right now what the most current figures we have are 13 reported cases.

Mr. BURGESS. Thirteen reported.

Dr. ROSS. And that is what we know about. Of course, as I said, most cases are never reported.

Mr. BURGESS. Yes. And how does that happen? How do you not report a case of acute liver failure requiring a transplant or facing death? It is hard to miss the clinical symptoms.

Dr. ROSS. When I say report, I mean report it to the MedWatch Program at FDA and that is a structural hole, it is a gaping hole that everyone, including FDA, says we have with our current post-marketing system and what we need is much better data. The reason that we have trouble making the right decisions is that we don't have the right data systems in place. And FDA just announced, after years of urging, that it is going to have partnerships with the Veterans Health Administration as well as other agencies that have large databases that can be used for prospective collection of safety data. But it is the sad fact that, except for devices where there is mandatory reporting of problems, most drug events, even very serious ones, never get reported.

Mr. BURGESS. With how many cases of acute liver failure requiring transplantation or resulting in patient death occur with acetaminophen?

Dr. ROSS. Acetaminophen is certainly the most common cause of drug-induced liver injury. However, it is important to remember that those events generally occur in the setting of intentional overdose or in the setting of co-consumption of alcohol, and if you correct that for the amount of acetaminophen that is prescribed in this country or taken over the counter, the rate is going to be lower, I believe, than with Ketek and I believe that Dr. Graham may be able to address this later. But I think this is not the only toxin on the market. But if I could use a medical example, there is an antibiotic that we as physicians are all familiar with, chlorenphenocol, it is a lifesaving drug in the right circumstances.

Mr. BURGESS. Absolutely.

Dr. ROSS. But it is rarely used right now because of the risk of aplastic anemia, and I have only used it twice in my career. That has a lower rate of aplastic anemia than Ketek does of acute liver failure.

Mr. BURGESS. I am embarrassed to tell you that I am old enough to have taken chlorenphenocol as a child.

Dr. ROSS. I am glad you are still with us, Dr. Burgess.

Mr. BURGESS. Does the FDA hold periodic meetings, regulatory briefings, that serve as an opportunity for different views or questions to be heard on drug safety? Do you guys all get together in a room and talk about this stuff?

Dr. ROSS. They do but the problem is that it reminds me of a cartoon I saw, where a bureaucrat is telling somebody on the phone, I can assure you that your problem is being ignored at the very highest level. The most recent example that I am aware of occurred in April 2006, where a product called daptomycin was discussed at a regulatory briefing and everybody unanimously, with the exception of the division director, said this product should not be approved for this indication. Everyone had their say and then the division director, who happened to have been Dr. Soreth, politely listened and ignored them. Again, there is no accountability. You can simply ignore good science and you won't be held to account for it.

Mr. BURGESS. Let me ask you a question because you have brought up the issue of post-marketing data and that is not all bad, because also being old enough to have taken chlorenphenocol, I am old enough to remember when Falitimide was held up in this country because of, not post-marketing data, but post-marketing data from other countries. Obviously the experience in Europe tempered the judgment of the FDA at that time, as to whether or not to release that medicine in this country. So it is not all bad that the post-marketing data comes from other countries.

Dr. ROSS. No, I would never say that, but it is a question of the quality of the data and on what do we want to be making our decision. If I can go to a building analogy, which I am fond of, in——

Mr. BURGESS. Well, let me interrupt you before you make the analogy. The inclusion of exacerbations of myosenic gravis and the labeling of Ketek, did that not occur from an assessment of post-marketing foreign experience with that medication?

Dr. ROSS. I think the problem is that, while you can pick up a signal, when you say, well, there is no signal here, there is nothing going on, that is where we get into trouble.

Mr. BURGESS. On the issue of foreign post-marketing surveillance of adverse events, you referenced the study of the adverse liver events and was that not a French study?

Dr. ROSS. That is correct, but that used a prospective database to determine what was going on.

Mr. BURGESS. Thank you. Dr. Powers, let me just ask you about the non-inferiority issue with the antibiotics. Like you I am concerned about the emergence of multiply-resistant strains of what previously were relatively easily disposed of bacteria. Does Ketek play any of challenging these more aggressive organisms?

Dr. POWERS. I think the answer to that is we don't know. We would like to know. We know that Ketek can kill some organisms in a test tube that are not killed by other kinds of antibiotics. The question is, has Ketek actually been shown to be superior in people, in folks who are infected?

Mr. BURGESS. Well, let me interrupt you on that point. Now, say you did a side-by-side comparison of Ketek and Augmentin and found that the Ketek was identical to Augmentin, would there then be no reason to approve the Ketek because Augmentin is going to do a good job?

Dr. POWERS. If you were going to approve Ketek for Augmentin-resistant organisms, that wouldn't make a whole lot of sense.

Mr. BURGESS. What about for people who are allergic to penicillin?

Dr. POWERS. Well, that is the issue, is you want to actually then—but then you are saying that Ketek has a safety benefit, not an effectiveness benefit. That is changing the question.

Mr. BURGESS. On the question of the institutional review boards—I was involved with clinical studies back when I was a resident, but it was a long time ago and they were generally a pain in the neck because you had so much paperwork to fill out. And the institutional review board was basically—for me it was Parkland Hospital. Is it not the institution that is sponsoring the study that is responsible for that institutional review board, or is that just a misconception on my part?

Dr. POWERS. No, I think that the name comes from an era in which most research was conducted at academic institutions.

Mr. BURGESS. So your example of the breast cancer injections, was that just done in someone's clinic and not part of an institution?

Dr. POWERS. No, that was done at an institution.

Mr. BURGESS. In Texas?

Dr. POWERS. Yes, sir.

Mr. BURGESS. All right. Well, off line you can tell me which one and it will be funded. Thank you, Mr. Chairman. Ms. Cisneros, just before we leave, in March 2002, when did you become aware that the fraud that was being perpetrated by the physician who was doing the investigation for Aventis?

Ms. CISNEROS. Well, we always had suspicion and I think that it was actually confirmed at the quality assurance audit by Aventis.

Mr. BURGESS. And was that the reason that you left the company that you were working with at the time, PPD?

Ms. CISNEROS. No, I left for a different reason.

Mr. BURGESS. OK. Thank you, Mr. Chairman.

Mr. STUPAK. Thank you. We have three or four Members who would still like to question this panel, but we have four votes on the floor pending right now. In fact, we have less than 10 minutes to vote on this first one, so let us recess this hearing until 12:30 and let everyone stretch their legs, grab something. Our witnesses, if you would come back at 12:30 and we will finish up with the Members who have not yet asked questions and then we will move to our last panel.

[Recess]

Mr. STUPAK. We will resume our questioning with the panel of Dr. Ross, Ms. Cisneros and Dr. Powers. Please come forward. I would remind the witnesses that they remain under oath. I appreciate your patience. They took care of one other matter on the floor and it made us a few minutes late. But with that, I would like to recognize the gentleman from Texas, Mr. Green for 10 minutes for questions.

Mr. GREEN. Thank you, Mr. Chairman, and I have a number of questions, Mr. Chairman, and I don't know if we can get them all in. Can we submit questions to the panel for later response? Is that possible?

Mr. STUPAK. Yes, there will be written questions and there will be an appropriate time to do them later.

Mr. GREEN. OK. Thank you. Dr. Ross, how unusual is it to see fraud in a clinical trial?

Dr. ROSS. Well, it happens but it is unprecedented, in my experience, to see it at this scope and scale.

Mr. GREEN. Why was the study considered unreliable?

Dr. ROSS. Well, first off, out of 10 sites that were inspected, all had serious problems that made their data completely unreliable. FDA's investigators concluded that if these sites which were high unrolling sites, which supposedly the company had been keeping close tabs on the doctors, were unreliable. The rest of the sites couldn't be relied on either.

Mr. GREEN. What do you mean that every site inspected by FDA had problems?

Dr. ROSS. Of the 10 sites inspected, every single one was found to have significant violations of what are called good clinical practices, the rule book for conducting clinical trials. Four the 10, 40 percent, were referred for criminal investigation. It is an outstanding percentage.

Mr. GREEN. Let me back up just a little bit, then. The advisory committee, in 2001, was first concerned about liver damage from Ketek, was that only concern, was the liver damage?

Dr. ROSS. No, there were also concerns over effects of Ketek on the heart and on vision, as well as Ketek's potential for interaction with many other drugs.

Mr. GREEN. What exactly was the misconduct found in the safety study?

Dr. ROSS. Well, the largest enroller, as we have heard, was convicted of fraud and this was not sophisticated or subtle fraud. It was absolutely blatant. The second and third largest enrollers had significant violations of procedure that called into question the reliability of data from those sites. And I think it is interesting to note that the third largest enroller was arrested shortly after the study on cocaine and weapons possession charges and this is not the type of investigator—the study physician, rather, that FDA likes to see in clinical trials.

Mr. GREEN. I can imagine. Coming from Texas, we don't mind the weapons possession, but the cocaine bothers me. Ms. Cisneros, what came out of your teleconference with Aventis and regarding irregularities in the Kirkman-Campbell site. Did they seem concerned about it?

Ms. CISNEROS. No, they really just glossed over all the issues. Nadine had an excuse for every irregularity that we found. I walked away from it being astounded at the laisse-faire attitude that they had about the issues that we found at the site.

Mr. GREEN. To your knowledge, did anyone from RBPPD or Aventis call the FDA to report the site?

Ms. CISNEROS. To my knowledge, when I spoke with the FDA auditor, she said that the reason for audit was because Dr. Campbell was such a high enroller. There was not a for cause audit.

Mr. GREEN. What made Dr. Campbell fraud so apparent to you and not Aventis, as they are claiming?

Ms. CISNEROS. Because the fraud wasn't sophisticated. And Dr. Campbell was not a practicing research physician, so a lot the mistakes she made were very obvious.

Mr. GREEN. In your experience, what would have been done once fraud was suspected?

Ms. CISNEROS. Normally, the site is closed immediately to further enrollment of patients and the FDA and the IRB are notified.

Mr. GREEN. Dr. Powers, some people argue that the placebo-controlled trials in these self-resolving diseases would be unethical. Is this really a problem?

Dr. POWERS. Well, it is really not unethical to give people a placebo in a situation where you are not really sure about the effectiveness of the old drug in the first place. I think the second issue is that these are diseases that people commonly don't take antibiotics for. I had a sinus infection myself last week. I didn't take anything for it and got better, anyway. And third, people will sign a proper informed consent in these studies. They know that they might be getting a placebo. And fourth, there is actually some benefits to being on the placebo group. You might get better anyway and yet not be exposed to adverse effects. So the last thing is the real issue of doing a placebo-controlled trial is, is there a question to be answered, a thing called equipoise, and that question still remains unanswered as to in whom and when are antibiotics effect for these self-resolving diseases.

Mr. GREEN. Would there be any specific benefits evaluating antibiotics in placebo-controlled trials?

Dr. POWERS. I think, again, part of this is people would not be exposed to adverse events. The other issue, we would finally be able to figure out how beneficial these drugs actually are. And in a placebo-controlled trial, you could also weigh the adverse effects of those drugs as well. So say that we do find out that antibiotics do decrease symptoms of ear infections in kids by 2 percent compared to placebo. If they cause diarrhea in 10 percent of kids, then we would be able to actually make that assessment and make an overall risk benefit.

Mr. GREEN. Don't clinicians and patients want to know how new drugs stack up against the old drugs in terms of safety and effectiveness?

Dr. POWERS. I think that is an important question and the issue is, do we really just want to know that a drug is better than a placebo? And that is why people do these kinds of trials where they compare one drug to another. But the problem with these trials is we miss the overall question of is it effective at all? So if FDA had the authority to require three group trials, that is, compare a new drug to old drug to placebo, we could actually answer both of those questions, make sure that both drugs are better than a placebo, and how one drug stacks up against another one.

Mr. GREEN. The FDA doesn't have the authority to do that right now?

Dr. POWERS. Right now the only thing FDA has the authority to say is, is the drug is effective compared to nothing. And they are very fond of reminding us that there is no relative efficacy standard. So all you have to do is be better than nothing and that is actually the complaint some people have about placebo-controlled trials, is some people say, well, this just tells me it is better than nothing and that is not what I really want to know.

Mr. GREEN. Thank you. Again, I would hope, out of this oversight hearing, we will see FDA reform legislation and it would be addressed in that through our committee process. Ms. Cisneros, during the investigation of the three highest enrollment sites, the Division of Scientific Investigation determined that Dr. Salerno, the third highest enroller, had been placed on probation by the State Medical Board and later during the study had his medical license suspended. While I understand your experience with this case was limited to Dr. Kirkman-Campbell, can you speak to the typical measures taken to ensure that the physicians participating in the usual care settings are reputable? And do contract research organizations check out the credentials of their enrolling physicians?

Ms. CISNEROS. It is my understanding that the IRB is supposed to do that and in my review of Copernicus, they are actually given $600 per PI to investigate that physician. And in my working with PPD, I believe we did review physician licenses as well. It is a very simple process. It is on the Internet. There is nothing to it.

Mr. GREEN. Dr. Ross, can you speak on this question from the FDA's perspective?

Dr. ROSS. Yes. There is a requirement that a drug that is approved will be approved via adequate and well-controlled investigations by investigators who are qualified by training and experience.

A physician who is on probation, medical probation, which is a matter of public record, is not what I would call a physician who is qualified by training or experience.

Mr. GREEN. Dr. Ross, according to the FDA e-mail cited in Senator Grassley's letter to FDA Commissioner von Eschenbach, regarding irregularities associated with Ketek, and FDA employee status states a total of 72 sites enrolled more than 50-patient maximum.

Dr. ROSS. Yes, that is correct.

Mr. GREEN. The FDA goes on to ask in this e-mail, is it common for companies to allow centers to enroll beyond the allowable limit? Is this viewed as acceptable?

Dr. ROSS. It is not. It is something that should immediately trigger concerns and it is something that, internally, I send e-mails to people in management about, pointing out the high enrollers who are enrolling at rates that were far greater than what would be expected in a normal trial.

Mr. GREEN. Does the FDA have any enforcement mechanism to promote the compliance by these drug sponsors?

Dr. ROSS. Yes, if they choose to use them.

Mr. GREEN. And in your experience, has there been recent history of that, using them on the drug sponsors?

Dr. ROSS. No. For example, Dr. Kirkman-Campbell the FDA did not even more to disqualify her from conducting clinical studies until after Ketek hit the news. As of this point, although she is in prison, in a Federal correctional facility, this physician is still eligible to conduct clinical trials.

Mr. GREEN. Ms. Cisneros, do you have any additional light in the last 30 seconds I have?

Ms. CISNEROS. There is definitely a fault in the system and there was a breakdown on the Sierra level, on the IRB level and there are people that were interested in coming here today but felt, due to repercussions, they didn't feel comfortable doing so.

Mr. GREEN. Mr. Chairman, I know your experience in upper Michigan and our experience with depending on the FDA and drug approval, compared to other countries, that it is really shocking and I think it is shocking to our constituents to see what is happening, because we depend Ms. Cisneros on FDA when we deal with imported pharmaceuticals, but it is just not there. So I guess the committee—again, being back on the subcommittee after about three terms, I am just shocked and I hope we can deal with it during the authorizing legislation.

Mr. STUPAK. I thank the gentleman. Mr. Walden from Oregon for 10 minutes.

Mr. WALDEN. Thank you very much, Mr. Chairman, and I want to thank our witnesses, all of them, today for sharing your stories with us. It is most helpful as we do our oversight work. Dr. Ross, you indicated in your testimony that you were pressured to change your view and I am just curious. Was that pressure from the supervisor, uniformly in the direction of not being as stringent on safety as the lower-level official?

Dr. ROSS. That is correct. It might be helpful for the committee if I outlined the sequence of events.

Mr. WALDEN. Yes, that would be good. Thanks.

Dr. ROSS. In January 2003, the FDA issued an approval letter to Aventis outlining requirements for Ketek to be approved. I had been the safety team leader for that review cycle. I finished my safety team leader memo, in September of 2003. which was about 8 months later and that was because I had another priority review to work on. I gave that to my division director. She called me into her office, I think, a couple weeks later and said, could you soften this to give Mark, that is Mark Golderberger, and Ed, that is Ed Cox, more wiggle room? I knew from previous experience that if I refused, she would get very angry. A number of colleagues advised me to comply lest she retaliate.

I decided that I would comply, but I also sent an e-mail to the office above hers, outlining what had happened. I put this in writing. This was sent to Mr. David Roeder, who was Mark Goldberger's associate director. I did not get any response in writing, or otherwise, from Dr. Goldberger. When I didn't get any response, I took my original review, without the changes that Dr. Soreth had requested, put it in an electronic archive and added a note about what would happen in case there was any question down the line about the situation. I did that and signed off on it on March 16, 2004. That was almost 3 years before this committee hearing and it was almost 2 years before Ketek hit the news.

Mr. WALDEN. Mr. Chairman, do we have any of the e-mail traffic or any of that for the record?

Mr. STUPAK. There is some e-mail traffic right in the big binder there. You should have one right there.

Mr. WALDEN. OK. So we have a copy of the e-mail Dr. Ross has referenced?

Mr. STUPAK. The one that Dr. Ross has, yes, we do have that e-mail.

Mr. WALDEN. OK. Because I was just provided with a story out of the Wall Street Journal, I guess, where Dr. Soreth denies ordering the change and says, "If he felt strongly, he was free to keep it," she says, adding that the review didn't reflect Aventis' final submission to the agency. In both versions, Dr. Ross' examination says Ketek could be approved for a third condition, pneumonia. And I am just curious. Obviously, it is a he said/she said from our vantage point. Why would she say that?

Dr. ROSS. Because she would get in trouble if she admitted to it. That would be a serious infraction to pressure a reviewer to change their reviews. I do not want to get distracted on this, because while personally it was angering to me, I think the real question is, why did FDA use this fraudulent data? I will just say, however, that I documented, at the time, what was happening. That was the only thing I knew what to do.

Mr. WALDEN. No.

Dr. ROSS. I went to upper management as well and said here is what is going on.

Mr. WALDEN. And that seems like the responsible thing to do and it is most helpful as we look at it. I am just trying to figure out how all this works inside this particular box within the agency.

Dr. ROSS. Understood.

Mr. WALDEN. You state in your testimony that the FDA reviewers, including yourself, were pressured to change reviews by FDA managers. Were you pressured to change any reviews for Ketek, and if so, which ones?

Dr. ROSS. It was my team leader memorandum for the second review cycle. The key change was that initially I had said that it was doubtful that Ketek could be approved for the lesser indications of acute bacterial sinusitis and acute exacerbation of chronic bronchitis, the two indications that FDA just removed, even if there was more safety data, given the fact that these are self-resolving infections, with many other antibiotics available, I changed that——

Mr. WALDEN. Was that for pneumonia?

Dr. ROSS. I am sorry. Pneumonia. I said I thought, with additional safety data, it could be approved, although I said I did not think it could be approved for a particular type of resistant bug, mainly because of the lack of data.

Mr. WALDEN. All right, all right. Good. And you have indicated that you objected when you were asked to change your data even though you changed it, you did notify her supervisor.

Dr. ROSS. Yes.

Mr. WALDEN. All right. Why do you believe, as you put in your testimony, that the FDA managers were so bent, I think was the word you used, to approve Ketek? What was driving this?

Dr. ROSS. I think there is a fear of being seen as holding up new products.

Mr. WALDEN. Right.

Dr. ROSS. And frequently there is a perception that just because something is new, it must work, otherwise why would the company be submitting it? And the sad fact is, for example, in cancer therapies, 95 percent of therapies that start trials never make it because they don't work. But I think, in this instance and others, FDA managers were afraid of being perceived as holding up an important drug and so they felt really pressured to find some way to approve it.

Mr. WALDEN. And as you talk to other reviewers, I assume you all run in circles where you are talking, I don't know that for a fact——

Dr. ROSS. No, it is——

Mr. WALDEN [continuing.] But I assume that. Is this an isolated piece of FDA, the way this whole thing unfolded? Is this what is happening in every division? Is it happening that way in oncology?

Dr. ROSS. No.

Mr. WALDEN. Is this an isolated incident?

Dr. ROSS. Let me answer that. First off, it does not happen in every division and I would certainly say, in oncology, when I told my managers there about what had happened, they were appalled. I cannot imagine this sort of thing happening in the Office of Oncology. Having said that, however, there is a number of instances that I saw in the Office of Antimicrobial Products, in which reviewers were pressured, either directly or more subtly, to kind of get with the program and find some way of approving a product, even if they had reservations. Now, I have to say that if a reviewer says don't approve this and a manager disagrees, the manager is fully free to write their own review and overrule that reviewer and put it on the record, and everybody accepts that.

Mr. WALDEN. And that can go both ways, right?

Dr. ROSS. That can go both ways.

Mr. WALDEN. Have you seen instances where it has gone the other way?

Dr. ROSS. I have not.

Mr. WALDEN. OK.

Dr. ROSS. I will say, for example, for Gemzar, which was approved for treatment of metastatical ovarian cancer and oncology. The primary reviewer said, I don't think should be approved, and the division director wrote a very carefully reasoned memorandum saying I disagree. I am going to approve it. And it was on the record for everyone to look at.

Mr. WALDEN. So your issue is that approach versus one where the supervisor tells you to rewrite your report?

Dr. ROSS. It is a way for the supervisor to avoid taking responsibility.

Mr. WALDEN. Now, I note that you cite senior FDA medical advisor Dr. Robert Temple in footnote 6 of your written testimony. Do you consider Dr. Temple a reputable and credible witness on clinical trial matters? And perhaps I think both Dr. Powers and Dr. Ross, are any of you familiar with Dr. Temple?

Dr. ROSS. Absolutely. I have enormous respect for Dr. Temple. I have to say that he privately has condemned the use of noninferiority trials, but publicly will not condemn the agency's approach. That is No. 1. Number 2, I can tell you that he has disparaged the idea that reviewers are pressured. He has openly said—and this is in meetings of senior management—do we ever know that this really happens? And I would go up to him as a member of the senior leadership team and said, Bob, it happened to me.

Mr. WALDEN. What would he say?

Dr. ROSS. Just nothing. I think there is an air of disbelief.

Mr. WALDEN. Do you think he would be a good witness for this subcommittee to call?

Dr. ROSS. I think it would be helpful to the committee to get his perspective and raise these issues with him.

Mr. WALDEN. Dr. Powers, do you want to comment on Dr. Temple?

Dr. POWERS. I wanted to link the question about Dr. Temple to a previous one you asked, about how systemic is this?

Mr. WALDEN. Right.

Dr. POWERS. I consider that the agency wouldn't even be in as good a position as they are now, in terms of the evaluation of drug products, if it wasn't for people like Dr. Temple. And in fact, Dr. Temple was one of the first people to write about the issues with noninferiority trials back in the early 1980's. I actually approached Dr. Temple several years ago about some of these very issues with noninferiority trials and he was in agreement. I think, then, the question becomes what is the systematic issue when someone of his stature, who is a director of the Office of Medical Products, is still unable to alter or change the way things that were done in an office below him, in the Office of Antimicrobial Products? And I think that is where you get to the systemic issue and I know for a fact that if he was capable of changing this, he would have.

Mr. WALDEN. So I guess the question is, he would probably be a good person for us to ask under oath what is going on below him, above him, around him?

Dr. POWERS. Yes.

Mr. WALDEN. All right. Thank you, Mr. Chairman, and I want to again thank our witnesses today. It is most helpful.

Mr. STUPAK. We are joined now by Mr. Markey, a member of the full committee who has asked to sit in on this hearing and I know he has been bouncing around between the global climate change hearing and this one. So I would like to enter his opening statement for the record. Without objection, that will be entered.

[The prepared statement of Mr. Markey follows:]

PREPARED STATEMENT OF HON. EDWARD J. MARKEY, A REPRESENTATIVE IN CONGRESS FROM THE COMMONWEALTH OF MASSACHUSETTS

Chairman Stupak, thank you for allowing me to participate in today's hearing.

The FDA is clearly in desperate need of oversight and reform. Like Senator Grassley, I have been working on FDA reform with whistleblowers for several years and asking the FDA questions about Ketek since May, 2006. The FDA refused to answer my requests for information.

It appears that the FDA has finally responded to congressional oversight. It is not a coincidence that FDA finally took action to protect the public from Ketek by making changes to the label the day before this hearing.

But the FDA's long overdue actions on Ketek do not eliminate the threat to the American people.

Although the FDA has acted to warn the public about Ketek, we have no idea exactly how many dangerous products like Ketek the FDA has allowed on the market and put our families at risk every day. The FDA's problems are systemic and it is in dire need of reform.

Today we will hear about the truly frightening problems at the FDA including:

- a culture of suppression and intimidation;
- a lack of transparency into the review process;
- the inaction of FDA management in response to serious drug risks; and
- a lack of scientific freedom and the inability of FDA Reviewers to have their concerns heard by senior management, FDA advisory committees and the public.

It is clear from the testimony that the FDA is a deeply troubled agency that has failed to act in the best interest of the public. We need the FDA to be a watchdog for public health, not a lapdog for the industry.

We need to bring transparency, accountability and scientific integrity back to the FDA through a combination of increased oversight and legislative reform.

Today we begin the oversight and later this week I will reintroduce my bill, the Swift Approval, Full Evaluation (SAFE) Drug Act to address many of these problems.

We need to act now—not only to protect the public health but also to restore the public's confidence in the FDA. A Harris Poll conducted last year found that 80 percent of adults say they are concerned about the FDA's ability to make independent decisions that will ensure that patients have access to safe and effective medicines.

We need to turn this agency around now and I look forward to working with my colleagues on this committee to make the changes necessary to ensure that the FDA can protect the public health.

Mr. STUPAK. The gentleman is recognized for 10 minutes.

Mr. MARKEY. Thank you, Mr. Chairman, and thank you for your courtesy. I very much appreciate it. Dr. Ross, Dr. Powers, you have been extremely courageous in the actions which you have taken thus far and I just want to congratulate you for that. I am going to go through some of the provisions in a piece of legislation which I am introducing, the Swift Approval Full Evaluation Drug Act, that I plan to reintroduce this week with some changes and I want your opinions on whether these provisions will improve things at the FDA and if so, how.

Number 1, you have talked about the culture of scientific suppression and intimidation at FDA. The Safe Drug Act will prohibit FDA employees from directing other FDA employees to censor or suppress scientific research, analysis, opinions or recommendations, directing employees to disseminate scientific information that is known to be false or misleading. There will be penalties for any employee who engages in this conduct. Will that provision help minimize the culture of suppression and intimidation at the FDA? Dr. Ross?

Dr. ROSS. Representative Markey, yes, I believe it would. Ketek happened because there were no penalties for FDA managers who engaged in suppression of reviewers and ordered reviewers to disseminate false information to an advisory committee. This provision of the Safe Drug Act would deter, I believe, FDA managers who might be tempted to suppress reviewers either explicitly or by threatening retaliation through performance reviews.

Mr. MARKEY. Great. Dr. Powers?

Dr. POWERS. It is very hard to legislate culture, but people do things for two reasons, either to avoid pain or to gain pleasure. And if, in this case, as Dr. Ross is pointing out, someone would try to force someone to alter their review to refuse to take accountability for their own actions, and this kind of a provision would help there be some transparency and accountability.

Mr. MARKEY. Dr. Ross, in your response to Chairman Stupak, you said that you believe that if you had told the second Ketek advisory committee about the problems with Study 3014 and the FDA's questions about fraud in the study, you would have been fired. I am very concerned about the FDA's policy of censoring information going to the advisory committees. We have not only heard about this happening in your case, but we also have heard that FDA is censoring science, when Dr. Marsholder wanted to present information about the risk of suicide in children taking SSRIs. The Safe Drug Act would ensure that any FDA employee working on a matter related to an issue before an advisory committee shall be allowed an opportunity to make a presentation to the committee. This FDA employee presentation shall be separate from the time allotted to the public to comment on an issue before an advisory committee. Why is it important for all FDA employees working on a matter to have an opportunity to speak at advisory committee meetings? Would this provision help ensure that advisory committees get complete information from the FDA?

Dr. ROSS. I think it is important that advisory committees hear the full range of scientific opinions held by reviewers, not just those that are approved by management. It is a sad fact—and I am not saying it happens often, but I certainly have seen it happen, that an FDA manager can manipulate the information received by an advisory committee to get the desired the conclusion. I think that the provision that you outlined would help lessen the risk of advisory committees being manipulated by FDA managers.

Mr. MARKEY. OK. Dr. Powers, do you have a view on that?

Dr. POWERS. Yes, I think it is often said at FDA that they need to speak with one voice. I think they need to make one decision, obviously, but the scientific process isn't about speaking with one voice. It is about hearing lots of voices and then being able to make a cogent decision after that. Advisory committees usually occur before the drug is approved and that is the time to actually hear everybody's side of the story to be able to give the advisory committee the information that they need to give good advice.

Mr. MARKEY. OK. Thank you. My bill provides that, unless publication or presentation of the data is subject to national security laws or regulations or as proprietary information, FDA and FDA-sponsored authors shall have the right to publish or present their work. Have FDA employees had difficulty publishing their work in the past, how would that provision change things as they work today at the FDA?

Dr. ROSS. I have definitely witnessed this when you submit a manuscript. This did not happen at oncology. They are proud of their work there and they publish it. But in the Office of Antimicrobial Products, for example, you send a manuscript for clearance and it vanishes into a black hole. I think that this provision is important because it would allow removal of arbitrary barriers for publication. It would be important, I will say, to define proprietary information, that term, as narrowly as possible so it couldn't be used as a pretext to block a publication.

Mr. MARKEY. OK. Dr. Powers?

Dr. POWERS. I can say that I myself was reprimanded for writing a book chapter in the Premier Infectious Disease textbook 2 years after I wrote it, actually.

Mr. MARKEY. Wow.

Dr. POWERS. And even though this was not part of my work at FDA, done on my own time, I cleared it with the ethics department and I put a disclaimer at the bottom of it. So I think it is very important that FDA reviewers should be allowed to participate in the scientific discussion, not just within FDA, but with their peers outside the FDA as well. And I would actually say that the outside activity form that FDA requires you to fill out now should be for informational purposes only, that you allow the managers to know you are going to publish something, but that should not be that there needs to be a clearance process of what you are going to say.

Mr. MARKEY. OK. Thank you. You have talked about how it seems that some people within the FDA act as if they were working for the pharmaceutical industry rather than regulating it. Part of this comes from the fact that the FDA must negotiate with the industry over what they drug labels should look like. My bill would give the FDA the authority to mandate changes to drug labels instead of negotiating the label with the sponsor company. Many other Members of Congress have also proposed similar legislation. Do you think the FDA needs greater authority to mandate label changes and require specific information on the label? And do you think it will help empower the FDA to act more like a full-fledged regulatory agency?

Dr. ROSS. Yes. Under the current system, changes proposed by the FDA are frequently watered down through extensive negotiations with the sponsors and information on risks and benefits that is accurate is not communicated to providers or the public. And I think that that authority would be very helpful. The comprised language that FDA accepted in June 2006, on Ketek, with regard to myosenic gravis, is a perfect example. That should have been a contrary indication to begin with, but the company clearly didn't want it that way.

Mr. MARKEY. Dr. Powers?

Dr. POWERS. I think it would be very helpful to spell this out. One of the things I remember that I found very confusing when I got to FDA was how people talked about it in terms of labeling negotiations, and it went back and forth and back and forth. I think the drug sponsor needs to obviously be a part of that process and in fact, they are the ones who write the first draft of the label. But it should come to FDA, go back one more time, and then make a final decision. I think FDA already has that authority, they don't use it, and it would actually be very helpful to spell that out, that that is the way things should work.

Mr. MARKEY. I would like to believe that we can reform the FDA so that the FDA employees will no longer need to blow the whistle on the FDA. We need to protect whistleblowers so that they can come forward to warn the public, when necessary, without fear of retaliation. My bill will require increased protections for whistleblowers if they are retaliated against for reporting violations of laws or regulations, or a significant threat to public health and safety, to Congress, GAO, Federal agencies or their bosses. How would whistleblower protections improve the situation at the FDA?

Dr. ROSS. I think they would allow greater freedom for reviewers to inform the public about threats to public health, they would discourage the suppression of reviewer reviews, and they would help reform the culture at FDA with regard to scientific dissent.

Dr. POWERS. The hope is that if you had whistleblower legislation, that that would mean you wouldn't need to use it, actually, that that would form some transparency and openness and that people would have that as an outlet valve if they needed to, but that would form a culture at FDA where you wouldn't have to have people going outside the agency to solve the problems.

Mr. MARKEY. Thank you. Dr. Ross, Dr. Powers, Ms. Cisneros, I thank all of you for your excellent testimony today. It is a real tragedy that the FDA is losing good people with highly specialized expertise, like Dr. Powers and Dr. Ross, because they have dared to raise concerns about the safety of drugs. According to the FDA mission statement, the FDA is responsible for protecting the public health by assuring the safety, the efficacy and security of human and veterinary drugs, biological products and medical devices. If FDA's own medical reviewers are prevented from raising questions about the safety and effectiveness of drugs, the FDA cannot possibly fulfill its stated mission. Instead of suppressing dissent and preventing reviewers from asking questions about the safety of drugs, the FDA should demand careful review of the risk of drugs that they are putting on the market. You are latter day Paul Reveres trying to warn the public about the dangers in the review process at the FDA. You should be praised rather than punished. We need to act now to reverse this dangerous trend at the FDA, not only to protect public health, but also to restore the public's confidence in the FDA. A recent Harris Poll found that 80 percent of adults now say they are concerned about the FDA's ability to make independent decisions that will ensure that patients have access to safe and effective drugs and medicines. We need to turn the

FDA around now, before further dangerous decisions are made. I thank you, Mr. Chairman.

Mr. STUPAK. I thank the gentleman. Just one or two questions if I may. Ms. Cisneros, in response to Congressman Green, the last question he put to you, you responded that, due to repercussions, others would not come forward. Who are you referencing, others at PPD, Aventis, Copernicus?

Ms. CISNEROS. At PPD.

Mr. STUPAK. OK. So these would be private individuals who had a desire to come forward but were fearful of repercussions?

Ms. CISNEROS. Yes. And what was told to me is that these people were called by PPD attorneys and reminded of their confidentiality agreement and that a PPD lawyer would have to be present with them in order to talk to the agency.

Mr. STUPAK. So they chose not to talk to the agency, then?

Ms. CISNEROS. This one person did with a PPD lawyer present. It is just an intimidation factor, in my mind. They don't probably say as much as they would like to with that person present.

Mr. STUPAK. I thank you for your testimony. Dr. Powers, if I may, we have talked quite a bit about noninferiority testing in that example. But has FDA approached the problem of resistance as a safety issue, as you suggested? Could you explain that a little bit more? I just want to make sure I am clear on that?

Dr. POWERS. Unfortunately, no. I think the idea is that FDA traditionally approaches it as if somebody a drug and they get a skin rash, someone takes a drug and gets liver failure, that is the way they traditionally think about safety. But with an antibiotic, you are really not talking about just an adverse effect in one person, you are talking about population effects, which makes demonstrating effectiveness really even more important. And I think we often talk about this, safety and effectiveness, as if they are two different things. They are really parts of a scale here and when people concentrate on the side of, well, how many liver failures are there, there has got to be something on the other side of the scale to balance that. There has got to be effectiveness, otherwise even one case of liver failure is too many. But the idea here is that most antibiotics are actually used for these less serious diseases. So for instance, there are about 34 million kids who get an antibiotic a year for ear infections and there are about a 160,000 cases of hospital-acquired pneumonia. Which one is driving resistance? It is the one where people use the antibiotics the most. And some people have actually suggested that perhaps antibiotics should be regulated in a different way because of that. So for instance, in legislation that is coming up now, the Kennedy-Enzi bill says perhaps we could look at drugs for 3 years. Well, for antibiotics you are going to have to look out longer than that, because that is exactly where resistance is going to develop. The longer you use the drug, the more resistance you are going to see.

Mr. STUPAK. Thank you. Any other Members? Ms. DeGette? Well, let me thank the witnesses, then, and thank you for coming forward. It is an important issue and this committee takes it very seriously. This is the first of a number of hearings we will be having on drug safety. I think we all, on both sides of this dais, would like to see changes in the FDA. And with that, I dismiss this panel. Thank you again for your testimony and your time.

Dr. ROSS. Thank you, Mr. Chairman.

Mr. STUPAK. We will call our last panel, Dr. David Graham and Dr. Nissen. It is the policy of the subcommittee to take testimony under oath. Please be advised that witnesses have the right under rules of the House to be advised by counsel during their testimony. Do either of you desire to be advised by counsel at this time? If so, please introduce your counsel. Dr. Nissen?

Dr. NISSEN. No.

Mr. STUPAK. Dr. Graham?

Dr. GRAHAM. No.

Mr. STUPAK. OK. And as you know, we require an oath. Would you please rise and raise your right to take the oath?

[Witnesses sworn]

Mr. STUPAK. The witnesses are now under oath. Dr. Nissen, we will start with you, sir. And thank you for your time and patience in being here.

TESTIMONY OF STEVEN E. NISSEN, M.D., FACC, CHAIRMAN, DEPARTMENT OF CARDIOVASCULAR MEDICINE, CLEVELAND CLINIC FOUNDATION

Dr. NISSEN. Thank you. My name is Steven E. Nissen, MD. I am chairman of the Department of Cardiovascular Medicine at the Cleveland Clinic, and the president of the American College of Cardiology. My testimony does not reflect the views of either the Cleveland Clinic or the ACC.

We face a crisis in public confidence in the FDA, following an unprecedented series of revelations about drug and device safety. The American people no longer trust the FDA to protect their health. Unfortunately, patients are increasingly suspicious of new therapies and sometimes are reluctant to accept potentially lifesaving medications or devices. Decisive legislative action is now essential to improve the safety of drugs and medical devices and restore public confidence in this critically important agency.

I have served on many FDA advisory panels and this experience has undermined my confidence in the ability of the agency to adequately protect the public health. In 2001, I participated as a guest member of the arthritis advisory panel that recommended a warning label for cardiovascular risk for Vioxx. Under current law, the agency must negotiate with industry to make even simple changes in drug labels and FDA officials frequently make inappropriate concessions to pharmaceutical companies. Following the 2001 advisory board meeting, it took 14 months before the FDA could secure agreement from the company to accept a weakly written warning. During this period, patients and physicians were not appropriately warned about the cardiovascular hazards of Vioxx. When the label was eventually modified, the wording was so weak that it did not adequately inform physicians and patients of the potential for Vioxx to cause harm.

In 2005 another disturbing personal experience brought into sharp focus the inadequacies of the FDA in assessing a new drug application. On September 9, 2005, officials from the Endocrine and Metabolism Division presented a new diabetes drug known as muraglitazar to an advisory panel for consideration of approval. Because of a previous lawsuit by an advocacy group, Public Citizen, the FDA is required to publicly disclose the briefing materials for advisory panels. Because of my interest in this class of drugs, I reviewed the briefing documents posted on the Internet by the agency on September 8, the day before the public hearings. I observed that this investigational drug seemed to lower blood sugar, but I also noted that there was a striking excess of heart attacks, strokes and deaths in patients treated with muraglitazar compared with placebo or other diabetes drugs. Based upon this observation, I assumed that the advisory board would recommend that the agency not approve muraglitazar.

Yet, astonishingly, the following day agency reviewers presented the drug in a favorable manner, understating any concerns about cardiovascular risk. This advisory panel, that did not include any cardiologists, voted to eight to one to approve muraglitazar, ending the panel meeting at 2:00 p.m. In Cleveland I watched the news reports, complete with predictions from financial analysts that this drug would achieve annual sales exceeding $1 billion.

I felt compelled to act. My statistician and I rapidly downloaded the FDA material available from the Internet and performed our own independent analysis of the risk and benefits of this drug. We concluded that muraglitazar doubled the risk of death, heart attack, stroke and congestive heart failure. I phoned the editors of the Journal of the American Medical Association, who treated our findings as a public health emergency. Peer reviews were secured in a matter of days and JAMA posted the manuscript on their Web site October 20, just 7 weeks following the FDA advisory panel meeting. Shortly prior to our publication, the FDA issued an approvable letter to the sponsor. Following this publication, the pharmaceutical company developing muraglitazar abruptly ceased all further development. Fortunately this drug will never threaten the public health, but frankly, it was a close call.

We were able to independently analyze the risk of muraglitazar because the drug was presented to an advisory panel. For many new drugs, the agency approves them without public disclosure of the key findings in pivotal clinical trials. When drugs are presented to advisory panels, the agency frequently provides an uncritical presentation that fails to adequately inform the advisory panel members of any internal FDA concerns.

This phenomenon was very evident during a meeting of the drug safety and risk management advisory board of the FDA, which met February 9, 2006 to review drugs used to treat attention deficit hyperactivity disorder, or ADHD. I was asked to serve on this advisory panel to help evaluate the cardiovascular risks of these drugs, most of which are amphetamines or amphetamine-like agents. These drugs are closely related to methamphetamine, or speed, a major drug of abuse.

At nearly all advisory panel meetings, the FDA provides a list of questions to panel members, designed to assist in discussions and to guide the formulation of an action plan. When the advisory board briefing materials arrived, I was rather surprised by the questions that agency intended to ask. In this case, the FDA did not request the committee to consider the risks of the ADHD drugs, nor did they ask us to comment on the need to change labeling. Instead, they asked the committee to discuss how the agency might study the class of drugs. During the hearings, we learned that ADHD drugs substantially increased blood pressure and we heard reports indicating that approximately 25 children had suffered sudden cardiac death after taking these drugs occasionally after the first dose. ADHD drugs are closely related to Ephedra, a drug the FDA has sought to ban from OTC products. We also learned that 4 million Americans take ADHD drugs, including 1.5 million adults and up to 10 percent of fifth grade boys.

By mid-afternoon, I had heard enough. I departed from the FDA's carefully orchestrated agenda and introduced a motion proposing that the committee recommend a black box warning for the ADHD drugs. Surprisingly, the motion passed by an 8 to 7 vote. Agency officials looked horrified and quickly called a news conference, where they defended the safety of the drugs and sought to undermine the recommendations of the advisory committee. Some months later, the FDA actually did write new warnings, but it took a rogue advisory committee to motivate the agency to act.

It is important for the Congress to recognize that there are many fine and dedicated public servants working within the FDA, however, their concerns often fail to reach advisory committees because of the actions of their supervisors, who adopt a less courageous approach. The Congress must now fully evaluate the deficiencies within the FDA. Your engagement to investigate the problem and take decisive action can improve this agency. The 300 million Americans who rely upon drugs to stay healthy are counting on you to take action. These measures need not slow drug develop. If we improve drug safety oversight, the increased vigilance will inspire confidence and allow us to bring new medications to patients more quickly, because we will have a better safety net.

In my more extensive written testimony, I outline 10 critical initiatives needed to put the FDA back on course. I hope you will consider these ideas as you move forward, and greatly appreciate the opportunity to appear before you. Thank you very much.

[The prepared testimony of Dr. Nissen appears at the conclusion of the hearing.]

Mr. STUPAK. Thank you, doctor. Dr. Graham, your opening statement, please.

TESTIMONY OF DAVID J. GRAHAM, M.D., MPH, ASSOCIATE DIRECTOR, SCIENCE AND MEDICINE, FDA OFFICE OF SURVEILLANCE AND EPIDEMIOLOGY.

Dr. GRAHAM. Chairman Stupak and members of the subcommittee, thank you for the opportunity to speak about a subject of vital importance to all Americans. My name is David Graham and I am the Associate Director for Science and Medicine in FDA's Office of Surveillance and Epidemiology, or OSE. For more than 20 years, I have worked as an FDA physician/epidemiologist concerned with post-marketing drug safety. The statements I make today are my own. I do not represent the FDA's official view.

As we have heard from the previous panels, the Ketek story is about FDA's betrayal of the public trust. FDA ignored safety concerns raised by its own advisory committee and concealed from the committee the evidence that a crucial clinical trial was fraudulent. Subsequently, FDA issued a public health advisory that referenced the same fraudulent study as proof of Ketek's safety. FDA scientists were intimidated, suppressed and ultimately compelled to the leave the agency. CDER used post-marketing case reports from Europe and Latin America, where reporting is far worse than it is in the United States, to declare Ketek safe, rather than using clinical trials as it should have. I cannot think of a single other example where FDA used such data as the primary basis for the approval of a drug safety. OSE, ostensibly responsible for post-marketing safety issues, was relegated to the role of backseat consultant, with no power or authority.

Unfortunately, Ketek is not an anomaly. In November 2004, I testified before the Senate Finance Committee that FDA's handling of Vioxx was a profound regulatory failure and that FDA, as currently configured, was incapable of protecting America against another Vioxx. I am here to tell you that nothing has really changed. Our Nation is still at risk. Vioxx was enormous national catastrophe. Up to 60,000 Americans, most over the age of 50, died from Vioxx-related heart attacks, about as many as the number of U.S. soldiers killed during the Vietnam War. Another 80,000 suffered nonfatal, but nonetheless life-threatening heart attacks. FDA had multiple opportunities to prevent this but did nothing. To this day, FDA denies that it made any mistakes and has yet be held accountable Accompanying my testimony, I have included a table that would show that every State in this country, every congressional district in this country, had constituents who suffered heart attacks and who died of heart attacks related to Vioxx.

Sadly, Vioxx was not anomaly either. Think SSRIs and suididality in children. Think Accutane, pregnancy exposure, and the need for restricted distribution. Think Propulsid and sudden death; a drug that barely worked for nighttime heartburn was left on the market for years while it killed hundreds, including infants. The list goes on and on.

When it comes to drug safety, what is wrong with the FDA? In my view, there are four broad areas of critical FDA malfunction: (1) organizational structure; (2) organizational culture; (3) the misuse and abuse of science; and (4) suppression and intimidation of scientific staff. The most important is organizational structure. CDER's primary mission is to review and approve new drugs. Within CDER, the Office of New Drugs, or OND, has this responsibility. Post-approval, OND continues to have regulatory authority for all post-marketing safety issues that arise. This represents an inherent conflict of interest, because the same people who stamp their approval on new drugs and certify that they are safe and effective, also get to decide if a post-marketing safety issue is important and if anything needs to be done about it. There is no internal control; there is no safety net.

This organizational weakness is amplified by a massive imbalance in staffing and resources within CDER between pre- and post-market activities. Overall, roughly 90 percent of CDER staff are focused on the review and approval of new drugs. As the IOM report found, "the imbalance in formal role and authority between the review, that is OND, and surveillance/epidemiology, that is OSE, staff denotes the subservience of the safety function, and along with that, a management devaluation of the latter discipline and approach."

CDER's culture regards industry as the agency's primary client rather than as an entity in need of regulation. The agency's bias toward drug approval, noted by the IOM, is enshrined in PDUFA, which requires the FDA to negotiate with industry over how user fees shall be spent. Patients and consumers, the public, get no seat at the table.

Finally, although this is not a legislative hearing, I am compelled by conscience to make the following comments. Vioxx is the main reason why legislation to reform FDA is being considered. Hence, the litmus test by which potential legislation should be judged is whether it would have prevented the Vioxx disaster in the first place.

FDA's response to the IOM report, recently released, even if fully implemented, would not have prevented a single Vioxx death or heart attack. Vioxx was not a failure of surveillance or resources. It was a failure of institutional decision making. FDA's response to IOM would not have prevented Ketek or the SSRI antidepressant issues from unfolding the way they did. Unless post-marketing safety experts at FDA have regulatory authority over the post-marketing portion of a drug's life cycle that is separate and independent from OND and CDER, all the money and databases in the world won't change the end result.

Similarly, had the Kennedy-Enzi bill been in place when Vioxx came to market, not a single life would have been saved. This bill also would have had no effect on the way Ketek or the SSRI antidepressant issues unfolded. Why? The bill does not correct the root cause of FDA's failure to protect the public health. FDA's failure with Vioxx and the other mentioned drugs was a failure of institutional decision making, and the organizational structure giving rise to this failure has been left unchanged. Kennedy-Enzi leaves OND, the Office of New Drugs, in charge of post-marketing drug safety. Unless this is changed, we should expect more Vioxxes, more Keteks and more SSRI disasters. Sadly, Kennedy-Enzi is not fundamental FDA reform; it is fundamentally the status quo.

By contrast, the Dodd-Grassley bill in the Senate would create line authority in a post-market center within FDA, with explicit authority to protect the public from unsafe medicines. This bill also frees post-marketing from the corrupting influences of PDUFA. Had it been in place prior to Vioxx, most of the 140,000 Vioxx-related heart attack deaths and injuries would have been prevented. Likewise for Ketek and the antidepressant issues.

Thank you for your consideration of this critical subject and the opportunity to address you today.

[The testimony statement of Dr. Graham appears at the conclusion of the hearing.]

Mr. STUPAK. Thank you, Dr. Graham. Dr. Nissen, if I may. I understand that you oppose Senator Grassley's proposal to create a drug safety operation separate from the reporting line through CDER. Both you and IOM seem to think that there is a so-called culture at the FDA. Regulators are too close to those they regulate. How do we get the FDA to take or to make the best risk benefit decisions, if those with the safety expertise are still subservient to the hierarchy that believes that the industry is your primary client?

Dr. NISSEN. Well, first of all, I think there are lots of potential solutions and I don't, at least on the first pass, the Grassley approach, which is to separate the safety and efficacy assessment, has both benefits and there are risks. And by the way, I greatly respect the Senator's passion and commitment and his testimony today was compelling for all of us that have been involved in this area. But here is the problem. From my perspective, safety and efficacy are inextricably linked. If you had a drug, a new drug for lung cancer that rapidly killed 10 percent of the people that got it, but cured the other 90 percent of lung cancer, it might be a very good drug. It would save a lot of lives. It would have a huge safety problem, but it would be a drug that I might want to approve. And so I like the idea that an agency that is well run can integrate safety and efficacy into a single decision. I think the failure is a failure of leadership. I think we have had horrible leadership at the top in the FDA and at the next couple of levels down. The leadership is actually quite good at the rank and file, although, frankly, there is a streaming of talented people out of the agency now because of this culture that exists. And so I think to fix the FDA, we need new laws, but we also need new people at the top. And being very frank, I think that goes all the way to the top.

Mr. STUPAK. Could you discuss the negative publication bias issue that you raised in your written testimony?

Dr. NISSEN. This is one of the most profound problems in medicine, I think, in general and here is the issue. When companies do clinical trials, if the trials do not show a favorable result, that is either efficacy or good safety, they are simply never published. Only a small minority of clinical trials that are actually conducted are published. And so as physician/scientists, we only get to see a tiny fraction of the actual data. One example I give in my written testimony is for a class of drugs called PPARs, where there have been more than 50 drugs that are filed INDs, where the drugs have been discontinued during development due to toxicity, and not one single publication has appeared of why any of those more than 50 drugs were actually discontinued. How can we make good decisions about successor drugs, about the next generation? How can we protect people in clinical trials if we never get to see the information?

And so negative publication bias, the practice of allowing people to participate in clinical trials but we never see the results of those studies, is not scientifically acceptable. It is not acceptable in a public health sense for the citizens. And here is the principle I would like you to consider. If one of our citizens volunteers to participate in a clinical trial, the results of that trail belong in the public domain; that there is an ethical and a moral responsibility that that individual's noble commitment will translate into advancement of science. If that study is buried in a pharmaceutical company, then their commitment results in no gain for the public at all and it is just not an acceptable practice.

Mr. STUPAK. In your PPARs example, where do those studies end, phase I, phase II? Do you know?

Dr. NISSEN. Some drugs were discontinued in animal studies, but many were in phase I, many were in phase II. A few of them got to phase III. The toxicities that had been reported were extensive and bizarre; tumors in various organ systems, kidney failure, cardiac injury. And by the way, muraglitazar, the drug that I wrote about, is a member of that class.

Mr. STUPAK. Thank you. Dr. Graham, you have been subpoenaed to appear here today, correct?

Dr. GRAHAM. Correct.

Mr. STUPAK. The other witnesses—and there has been discussion about retaliation for testimony and things like that. If you have any experiences like that, please let this committee know. We appreciate your willingness to come forward. You are still an FDA employee?

Dr. GRAHAM. I am still but only because Senator Grassley prevented the retaliation from being completed that I was subject to after my Senate Finance testimony in 2004. And I must confess that I am extremely apprehensive that I will be the victim of retaliation for appearing here today.

Mr. STUPAK. Like I said, let us know. You stated in your testimony—and this is your testimony, I take it. It wasn't cleared through the FDA. This is your testimony?

Dr. GRAHAM. That is correct.

Mr. STUPAK. And this is your personal belief based upon how many years in the FDA?

Dr. GRAHAM. Twenty-three.

Mr. STUPAK. Twenty-three years. You stated in your testimony that the FDA doesn't believe it needs new regulatory authority to ensure drug safety. Why do you say that and what new regulatory authority or legal authority would you prescribe for the FDA?

Dr. GRAHAM. OK. Well, FDA has repeatedly said that it doesn't need new regulatory authority and in this and many other areas, FDA really cannot be trusted. During the hearings that were held by the IOM to investigate FDA and drug safety, senior managers were asked by the IOM committee, does the FDA need new resources and more resources to do drug safety? And categorically, all the managers who presented said no, we don't. And the staff people complained to these managers after the meeting, why are you guys lying to the IOM? What I was told was and what my colleagues were told was that the word had come from higher up that they were to state, if asked, that no resources were needed.

Now, when it comes to labeling, FDA has repeatedly also said, we don't need new authority. When all of this came out about FDA, Vioxx, labeling delays, and does FDA have the authority or don't they, FDA gave very evasive answers during the Senate Finance testimony and then subsequently, where one official was quoted as saying, no, we don't have the authority, the official FDA spokesperson came out and said, oh, we have the authority but we prefer to negotiate with companies. What is really needed, in my opinion, is explicit authority. The problem is going to be how does that authority get exercised? We heard in the last panel that you really have a management structure that is reluctant to use even the authority that it has. Giving it new authority will not mean that that authority gets used. And this, I think, it gets back to who is calling the shots. Pre-approval, making a decision about whether a drug comes on the market, and post-approval about what needs to happen safety-wise, you need to have those handled by different people and the regulatory authority needs to be separated out.

In the United Kingdom, which has, I believe—the world would probably attest to this—they have a better pharma vigilance system than we have in the United States. They are the gold standard. In their system, the baton gets passed from the pre-approval to the post-approval. The two sides talk to each, but they have separate authority and regulatory responsibility so that what happened with Vioxx, what happened with Ketek—let us say that I am the FDA, I am the pre-approval side and I want to approve cyanide. Well, cyanide is a universal poison and it will kill everybody who takes it, but I am the FDA, I am OND, and I say I am going to approve that drug. Well, right now, cyanide would stay on the market because there is no authority, if OND doesn't want it to happen, for the drug to be removed from the market. You need to deal with that.

You see, here is another thing that gets back to the culture. There is so many things. This is like a carpet, with so many different interwoven threads. The people who go in the pre-approval side of the house, they focus on these clinical trials. Basically a handful of patients, really. We are talking a few thousand patients, which really, when you talk about a drug that is going to be used by millions of people, it is a handful. Think of it as an envelope and you got a little postage stamp up in the corner. That postage stamp is the diversity of the types of patients that get studied in a clinical trial, in terms of age, gender; do you have an underlying disease; what medicines are you taking? Once the drug gets on the market in the real world, that is the rest of the envelope and FDA doesn't pay any attention to that, because that is the world I live in and that is the post-marketing world. You need to have people who know what they are doing and whose orientation is different. I come from a public health background, internal medicine and public health. My orientation is towards treating the population, treating the 300 million people who are out there. They are my patients. And that population perspective can take an adverse reaction and put it into perspective, and that doesn't happen now. Sorry I went on so long.

Mr. STUPAK. That is all right. In your time in the FDA, have you been on advisory panels?

Dr. GRAHAM. I have presented to advisory committees, but I am not a member of any of the advisory panels.

Mr. STUPAK. Have you, in presenting to the advisory panels, has your testimony been restricted or have you been forbidden to make presentation to advisory panels?

Dr. GRAHAM. Yes, I had that experience with Rezulin. Rezulin was a diabetes drug from the same class of drugs, actually, as muraglitazar. It was the original. OK. So this is the Adam and Eve of all of this class of drugs and it caused liver failure at a profoundly high rate and I thought that the drug should come off the market. There was critical data from clinical trials in which there were three different clinical trials, they were small, but in each of the clinical trials, a patient had died of acute liver failure and I wanted to present that in an advisory committee meeting that was being held on that topic. The company went ballistic when they learned that I was going to do this. I was at the meeting and they went ballistic and they actually raised their voices at the office director from OND, who was there, who then subsequently after the meeting asked me not to present that. And what I said to him was, I said, I have to present it. If I don't present it, that is scientific misconduct and it is a violation of my duty as a public health scientist. I said, if you don't want me to present, then you tell me not to present and I won't present, period. But if I present, I am presenting this information. Well, at the end, they allowed me to present.

Other people in drug safety—I could give you example after example and I will give you just a couple. Acetaminophen, used in Tylenol, the main ingredient in Tylenol, liver failure came up earlier. In the UK and other places in the world, they have done regulation of acetaminophen to reduce the possibility of unintentional or intentional overdose and liver failure from occurring. When our people wanted to present that at an advisory committee several years ago that was convened specifically to talk about this issue, they were ordered not to talk about it before the committee. The same thing happened with Lotronex, another drug. It has happened with Accutane. I could go on and on, but that is routine. That happens routinely and it is the Office of New Drugs telling the Office of Surveillance and Epidemiology that it can't talk about safety issues.

Mr. STUPAK. Thank you. My time has expired. Mr. Walden?

Mr. WALDEN. Thank you, Mr. Chairman. I am going to yield to Dr. Burgess here in just a moment because I know he has another meeting to get to. But I just wanted to comment and follow up on something you said and Dr. Graham, something you indicated and that is the threat of retaliation. And filling in for the ranking member here, I want you to understand and I want anybody at FDA to understand that this committee does not tolerate retaliation on witnesses who ask to come before this committee, or servants of the public who in some way are trying to make Government better for the American people. We don't want their supervisors, those above them, or anywhere else around them, to retaliate. We will not tolerate that. And so we want you to have that assurance from this subcommittee and this member that this is a bipartisan view, that retaliation is not going to be tolerated.

Dr. GRAHAM. I appreciate that.

Mr. WALDEN. Now Mr. Chairman.

Mr. BURGESS. I thank the chairman and I thank Mr. Walden for yielding. We have another hearing on global warming going on and it was pretty warm in here earlier, but it seems to have cooled off, so I am actually happy to stay.

Dr. NISSEN. I will try to heat it up again.

Mr. BURGESS. Dr. Graham, we heard testimony earlier, I believe, from Dr. Ross that there were many more Keteks out there that have yet to be either disclosed, elucidated or discovered. Is that your opinion also?

Dr. GRAHAM. Oh, yes, definitely.

Mr. BURGESS. Can you——

Dr. GRAHAM. Well, Dr. Ross is talking about—Ketek has some common features with the experiences that I bring and some that are more unique to the world that he lives on the pre-approval side that deal with the actual clinical trials that give rise to the approval of the drug and there being irregularities there, in addition to there being this post-marketing safety issue, where people try to sweep it under the rug. And it is on that post-approval side that I have my most familiarity. What I know on the pre-approval side, with clinical trials or fraudulent conducting of them, or the way safety problems get dealt with, is more by staff people who come and talk to me because I am such an infamous individual. When they run into difficulties in their workplace, I have become sort of a central clearinghouse, if you will, for helping them navigate through it. So the answer is yes.

Mr. BURGESS. OK. I want to get back to the clearinghouse function in just a moment, but let me ask you about the post-marketing aspect. Before coming to Congress, I was a physician, or still am a physician, and I would periodically get communications from the FDA and it was for reporting for adverse drug events. I can't honestly tell you that I ever filled one out and sent it in, but I would get them all the time and I would assume that they go somewhere within the structure of the FDA. Are those things, in fact, looked at or do most people just take the approach of I am too busy, let someone else fill it out and send it in?

Dr. GRAHAM. No. The Office of Surveillance and Epidemiology, where I work, has a large number—well, maybe not so large. It is like about 40 individuals whose full-time job it is to evaluate those case reports when they come in. We call them spontaneous or voluntary case reports, and sometimes it is referred to as med watch reports. And they review those, sort of a hands-on review of all reports that are classified as serious and unlabeled, so it is things that FDA doesn't know about. And then there is a long list of—I have lost count now of how many—50 or 100 of what we call designated medical events and these are particular serious things. I don't care if aplastic anemia is in the label for this drug. If a report of aplastic anemia for that drug comes along, an experienced human eye is going to read that, because they have this depository in their minds of what the experience with that drug and other drugs in that class is like.

Mr. BURGESS. Does that function now occur online? Again, I remember getting the pieces of paper that we would then mail out.

Dr. GRAHAM. There is a way that it can be done on line, it can be done by telephone and it can be done by paper. Most physicians and health professionals, when they report, actually end up telephoning the particular drug company if it is a name-branded drug. That is how FDA ends up getting most of its reports, is through the company.

Mr. BURGESS. And then does FDA periodically disseminate that information to clinicians?

Dr. GRAHAM. I think that the answer to that is probably not. I think there are plans, actually, for them to do some kind of newsletter, but I don't think that there is any formal mechanism in place up until this point.

Mr. BURGESS. Well, actually going on the FDA's Web site, I have found that, in fact, that sort of communication does happen and it has been going on for some time. I just never availed myself of the FDA Web site and went and looked at it. Let us talk a little bit about your being the clearinghouse. Can you tell the committee what other Keteks are out there? What are some of the other red flags that we should be watching for?

Dr. GRAHAM. Well, I will tell you a couple. I would pay careful attention to antipsychotic medications. Antipsychotic medications—and you have got what are called the typical and the atypical antipsychotic medications. The trend is the atypicals because they reputedly have a better safety profile, a lower side effect profile. The problem with these drugs: they are enormously expensive. The problem with these drugs are that we know that they are being used extensively off label in nursing homes to sedate elderly patients with dementia and other types of plot disorders. It is known that the drugs don't work in those settings. And it is off label, they just do what they want. But the fact is, is that it increases mortality perhaps by 100 percents. It doubles mortality. So I did a back-of-the-envelope calculation on this and you have probably got 15,000 elderly people in nursing homes dying each year from the off-label use of antipsychotic medications for an indication that FDA knows the drug doesn't work. This problem has been known to FDA for years and years and years and——

Mr. BURGESS. Well, let me just interrupt you. Is that the FDA's issue or is that an issue of the policing of medical practice?

Dr. GRAHAM. No, I believe that it is a public health issue and it is a public health issue because the companies are laughing all the way to the bank. With every pill that gets dispensed in a nursing home, the drug company is laughing all the way to the bank. The FDA isn't there to step in where it knows there is an—I am not talking about—there is off-label use and there is off-label use.

Mr. BURGESS. Sure.

Dr. GRAHAM. This is off-label use where we have got so many clinical trials that show you that these drugs don't work, that it is like malpractice to be using it.

Mr. BURGESS. Well, and that actually brings up another issue, but do you have another one to put on watch list?

Dr. GRAHAM. Well, I think it has been in the newspapers, in the New York Times, Zyprexa and diabetes. What has FDA been doing with this? All these clinical trials that we only learn about in the New York Times, of the weight gain from Zyprexa and the diabetes, and diabetes is a life-threatening disease. Don't kid yourself. It is responsible for more lost years of life than many, many disorders. It is a biggie and Dr. Nissen could talk to you more about it. Zyprexa, it turns out, the company knew for a long time, apparently, based on what I read in the New York Times, that there was a big problem. My question is—because I know FDA knew about too. And in talking to reviewers at FDA about FDA's approach in dealing with this safety issue, I am told it leaves much to be desired.

Mr. BURGESS. Well, let me ask, then, both of you a question because we have kind of got competing legislation with Kennedy-Enzi that apparently appeals to Dr. Nissen, and Grassley-Dodd that appears to Dr. Graham. Of both of these broad categories that have been mentioned, which bill is going to do the better job of protecting the American public? And I guess, let me ask Dr. Nissen that question first.

Dr. NISSEN. First of all, I must tell you that I don't think either of them go far enough and there are a lot of things that aren't in the bills and I tried to outline those in my written testimony. And I think we need to understand and be very clear about this, that we should not renew PDUFA. We should repeal PDUFA. PDUFA is not the solution; it is at least part of the problem. We started down the wrong pathway when we said that the regulated industry was going to pay the FDA to regulate itself. And I think that, ultimately, given the amount of money that is involved, we spend about $2 per person in America for drug regulation. That is the total expenditure. In the Federal budget it is a drop in the bucket. It is nothing. And yet we insist on industry paying that. Once you do that, then they become the stakeholders for the FDA rather than the American people. Why not come up with the money, find a way and fund the FDA independently without user fees and I think you will see improvements.

Mr. BURGESS. And that may be something that we need to explore, but it was done long before I got here.

Dr. NISSEN. Yes.

Mr. BURGESS. But it is my understanding, as a clinician at the time, was that this was a way to open up the pipeline to get things through in a more timely fashion. Because, as a practicing physician, I used to view the FDA as kind of an obstruction to getting new and timely treatments available to my patients. So anything that would move that process along more quickly, if it could be done in a safe manner, would be something that would be beneficial.

Dr. NISSEN. But we don't need PDUFA to do that. I think what PDUFA did was it set up an arbitrary deadline that you have to, by a certain date, make a decision and the problem is, is in conditions of uncertainty, when you have an agency which, at the top, is basically going to lean towards approval, what you end up doing is what happened with muraglitazar, which was you very nearly got a drug approved, because its PDUFA date was coming up very shortly, that would have been a catastrophe and I just don't think we can afford to do that.

Mr. BURGESS. I see the point you are trying to make. Let me just ask you, since you have brought it up. You say when you knew people at the top in the FDA in my short tenure here, we have had nothing but new people at the top.

Dr. NISSEN. Yes.

Mr. BURGESS. We just keep picking the wrong guy?

Dr. NISSEN. Yes. Yes, in fact we do. I think we need to move the FDA further away from the political arena and more into the public service arena. We have had some very disturbing events where it appears that, political decision making was affecting what the FDA did. We are all aware of those and I think we have to insulate the FDA from that kind of effect.

Mr. BURGESS. And actually I agree. My time has expired, but we always have to go through Senate confirmation process for our

FDA commissioner and administrator. Is that something that is an anachronism and we should no longer be doing?

Dr. NISSEN. No, but I think we have got to find people that see their role as a public health official and not as a political official.

Mr. BURGESS. Forgive me, but if you go through a Senate confirmation process, it is inherently political. You can't help but be political. You saw a rather impassioned Senator. There are 99 other of those men and women over there on the side of the capitol.

Dr. NISSEN. Yes. Let me just say I think——

Mr. BURGESS. And anyone can put hold on the commissioner for any reason.

Dr. NISSEN. I understand. But we can do better. We can have better leadership. We need better leadership at the FDA. It all comes from the top.

Mr. BURGESS. Well, and I agree, but it is just me wondering if the process itself, whereby that person has to go through a Senate conformation rather than a scientific assessment, leads us to the types of decisions that we have been seeing. Mr. Chairman, you have been indulgent. I will yield back.

Dr. NISSEN. Interesting idea.

Mr. STUPAK. Mr. Burgess, Senator Grassley did have a hold on the current FDA commissioner at approval time and it was released and he was approved.

Mr. BURGESS. Mr. Chairman, that is exactly my point. We have gone through a succession. Again, I have just been here a short period of time.

Mr. STUPAK. Sure—since you have been here.

Mr. BURGESS. Dr. McClellan, Dr. Crawford and now Dr. von Eschenbach. And it just seems to be a labor-intensive process to get one of these individuals through the Senate and I can't help but wonder if that doesn't harm the FDA to constantly have its head changed or under the microscopic scrutiny of the Senate.

Mr. STUPAK. Well, I am not too sure the confirmation of the commissioner results in what we are seeing within the FDA. We need strong leadership there, there is no doubt it. If we change every 2 years, you won't have that leadership. I would agree with that point.

Mr. BURGESS. But we have seen the same at Los Alamos with the frequent change of leadership and we have gotten no improvement with multiple hearings on that issue as well.

Mr. STUPAK. That is my second favorite subject and——

Mr. BURGESS. Again, I am going to go solve global warming. I will see you later.

Mr. STUPAK. OK. The gentlewoman from Colorado, Ms. DeGette.

Ms. DEGETTE. Thank you very much, Mr. Chairman. Dr. Nissen, the fact that the FDA commissioner needs Senate approval, that is not what you are talking about. You are talking about the PDUFA approval process and the way the fees are conducted, creating conflicts of interest within the FDA drug-approval process, correct?

Dr. NISSEN. Absolutely correct. And I just think it creates an inherent conflict of interest that is not going to get easily resolved until we repeal PDUFA.

Ms. DEGETTE. Dr. Graham, what do you think about Dr. Nissen's view that we should just scrap PDUFA and find some other way to do this?

Dr. GRAHAM. Well, in my testimony, I talk about the corrupting influence of PDUFA. PDUFA is a mistake. It was a predictable mistake. It has had consequences. I would claim and maintain that they are predictable consequences. I will give Congress the benefit of the doubt and say that they are unintended consequences, but they are consequences nonetheless.

Ms. DEGETTE. And in fact, what I was just sitting up here thinking, the reason that we enacted PDUFA is so that we could get important drugs approved more quickly, which is a good goal. But actually, if you have problems later with those drugs, then not only do you have a slow—it ends up being slower because you have to go back and review them, but you have a potential grave risk to human life.

Dr. GRAHAM. Right. Well, it is even worse than that. If you are on the pre-approval side of the house, your bonus, your awards, your promotions, really have to do more with getting the NDAs approved than anything else. And you are basically in a factory and lots of reviewers, medical officers, talk about it. You are in an NDA factory, a new drug application factory, and you have got to meet these timelines to get these things done. OK, I have got 6 months to review this application. Now some drug that got approved 3 years ago has a safety problem and I have this other review that I have got to do. Well, where are my priorities? My priorities are here. They are not on that safety issue. This is like the Office of New Drugs. It is the same group that approved that drug that has to deal with post-marketing and make all of the decisions. It is a backseat issue because it is not a priority.

Ms. DEGETTE. Right, I understand. Dr. Nissen, do you think there is some way that we could expedite approval of important new drugs without building in the inherent conflicts that we have built in through PDUFA?

Dr. NISSEN. Yes, I do. And something that has been talked about and I have talked about is the idea of conditional approval and I actually think this could work. You have a drug where you don't know enough about the drug, but you think it may benefit patients. Maybe it is a cancer drug and it looks like it is going to make a difference for people, but you would like to know more. If you gave that drug a 3-year approval that would automatically expire at the end of a period of time unless sufficient studies were done and you outline what those are, then you have got kind of club over the head of that manufacturer. One of the problems we have is that most of the post-approval studies that are promised are never performed. Why are they never performed? Because once the drug is on the market, the FDA rarely, if ever, puts the genie back in the bottle.

I am suggesting that you might want to consider the possibility of legislation allowing provisional approval that would expire unless certain information were brought to bear that could further describe the safety and efficacy of the drug.

Ms. DEGETTE. And in fact, they do that in Europe, as I understand.

Dr. NISSEN. Yes, there are countries that do that. We don't have to turn the FDA over to the pharmaceutical industry for funding in order to get drugs more quickly approved. We need better leadership. We need people that understand when you should move quickly because something is a lifesaving drug. And when it is an antibiotic used to treat trivial infections, maybe you ought to slow down a little bit. Good leadership can make these kinds of decisions if it is in place.

Ms. DEGETTE. And Dr. Graham, yes, go ahead.

Dr. GRAHAM. I just wonder if I could follow on to Dr. Nissen?

Ms. DEGETTE. Yes, please.

Dr. GRAHAM. Part of the problem with PDUFA is that we talk about—I have heard multiple different members talk about bringing lifesaving drugs to the American people, as if every drug was a breakthrough drug that was going to cure some cancer or something else. The truth is most of the drugs approved under PDUFA are not lifesaving drugs. They are what are called me too drugs; another drug to lower your blood pressure, another drug to treat diabetes, another drug to treat cholesterol. So the innovation that you are looking for—I guess what I am saying is——

Ms. DEGETTE. Well, but we did hear, for example, with respect to antibiotics, on the previous panel, how there really has been some difficulty in getting the development of some of these drugs.

Dr. GRAHAM. Well, that is true and part of the problem is the pharmaceutical industry is really risk adverse because it is so expensive to develop a drug. So most of the time they will go after the sure thing, which is a me too. Maybe creating incentives for industry, for example, to invest in the higher risk of new drugs to treat diseases in new ways would be something to explore. And make it more difficult, raise the bar.

Ms. DEGETTE. I understand. So what you are saying is give folks incentives to develop the drugs under stringent approval guidelines and maybe conditional approval, rather than going down the other path of approving drugs that haven't been adequately tested or worse.

Dr. GRAHAM. Right. And relating to PDUFA, I think that it is basically a tax. I know Congress hates to hear the word tax, but the companies are passing——

Ms. DEGETTE. I think all the Republicans left.

Dr. GRAHAM. OK. The companies are——

Mr. WALDEN. Not quite.

Ms. DEGETTE. Oh, well. OK, I guess you are one.

Dr. GRAHAM [CONTINUING.] Companies pass that cost on to consumers. If you were to charge a penny per prescription, a penny prescription surcharge, put it in the Treasury and it is not like Social Security, where you can transfer it, but it is dedicated to safety, you could have complete funding of the post-marketing aspects of drug regulation with no attachment to industry, no ownership of industry, no control of industry over it because it is coming from the people. Now it is called a tax and that is a dangerous word, but you have got to launder that money and you have got to cut the strings, because right now it is a quid pro quo. We have given you the money; now approve our drugs.

Ms. DEGETTE. I understand. Dr. Graham, you have spoken, and also I think you spoke, Dr. Nissen, about the culture over at the FDA. And one thing we have learned with this Los Alamos issue is that, once you develop a culture—at Los Alamos, the problem we have is that they keep accidentally losing top secret data and very—the last one we learned about because someone got searched for drugs in her home and lo, she had this information. We have the same problem. We feel like it is Groundhog Day up here because all of these key issues with senior level Government officials, we keep seeing these pharmaceuticals that are really threatening lives over and over again. And at Los Alamos, as Mr. Burgess pointed out, we keep changing the leadership and still these problems keep happening. The thing at the FDA and I guess—I am wondering, and we will start with you, Dr. Nissen, and then you, Dr. Graham, what can we do, aside from repealing PDUFA or not reauthorizing PDUFA, to change that culture at the senior levels of the FDA, because I am not convinced that it is just the head of the FDA. I think there is more of culture throughout the agency.

Dr. NISSEN. Well, there is clearly a cultural problem and I think that it goes far beyond PDUFA, I agree, and it does go beyond the director, but it does start at the top. And really, if we had really passionate leadership at the FDA that was strongly in favor of balancing safety and efficacy, rapidity of drug approval with protecting the public, it would at least in part trickle down. There are several cultural issues that I wished I understood completely, but let me give you one of them. There is the culture of secrecy, that everything seems to happen in kind of closed black box. Now, why was I able to publish a manuscript about muraglitazar? It is because they had an advisory panel meeting and because of a lawsuit a number of years ago, the FDA was forced to put on the Web the briefing materials that they gave to the panel members. If a drug doesn't go before a panel, you never get to see what actually happened. You don't get to actually see that raw data and science can't work effectively when you have blinders on. And so you can, with legislation, take the blinders off. You can say that clinical studies belong in the public domain. And then it kind of doesn't matter, because there is always somebody out there that will look at the data, reanalyze it, as I did for muraglitazar, and say wait a minute. We have got a problem here. So I think you can overcome some of that.

I wanted to say one more thing about this balance between speedy approval and drug safety and that is this: if we knew we had a robust post-marketing surveillance system that would pick up problems quickly, then we could have more rapid drug approval. This is an example where better safety monitoring actually speeds bringing new drugs to market, because when I sit on an advisory panel now, I have to be very cautious because I know that if I let the genie out of the bottle, that the chances are, if something bad happens, it won't get seen for 5 years and then we have hurt a lot of people. But if we had a very robust post-marketing surveillance system, and I think there are ways to do that, then we could be more bold in bringing medications to market more quickly.

Ms. DEGETTE. Thank you. Dr. Graham, briefly.

Dr. GRAHAM. Right, briefly. Culture is a difficult thing to address. What I would say is, is that the comments that Dr. Nissen has made are good, but if you really want to change the outcome, if you want Vioxx not to happen again and you want Ketek not to happen again, you need to work on the structure. You need to focus on how are decisions made. The orientation in the pre-approval people are towards getting the drugs out the door. The people in the post-marketing, who come from public health backgrounds of population, it is towards what is going on here? Is there a problem here? Is there something we need to do protect the public? It is two different mindsets. One is based on a population, the other is focused on these small, little studies. And the culture of those two organizations is remarkably different. What happens now is, is the dominant culture, the OND culture, suppresses that post-marketing safety culture and that is part of what we have. But if you want to solve the problem, you separate the organizations in terms of authority. How you do it, maybe you meld Kennedy-Enzi together with Dodd-Grassley, but you have got to separate out who is making decisions at which part of the life cycle of the drug. And what you will see is, is there is going to be a feedback loop now, because if we post-marketing people had pulled Ketek when we said it needed to be pulled, or pulled Vioxx when we said it needed to be pulled, or pulled Rezulin when we said it needed to be pulled, the pre-approval people now, they are getting feedback. Uh oh, we overlooked something, maybe. Uh oh, if we make a mistake on this drug, we are going to get embarrassed because those people are going to expose it. Right now there are no internal controls, there are no checks and balances.

Ms. DEGETTE. Thank you. Thank you very much.

Mr. STUPAK. I thank the gentlewoman.

Mr. WALDEN. Mr. Chairman, a point of personal privilege?

Mr. STUPAK. Absolutely.

Mr. WALDEN. I have the sad duty to notify you and the other members of the committee and our audience that moments ago we were notified that our friend and colleague who served on this committee since 1995, Dr. Charlie Norwood, has passed away at his home in Athens, Georgia. Our prayers are certainly with his wife, Gloria, and his family and friends. He ably and forcefully represented the people of Georgia in his district. And Mr. Chairman, if we could have a moment of silence in honor and memory of our friend and our colleague, a great American, Dr. Charlie Norwood.

Mr. STUPAK. Join us for a moment of silence.

[Moment of silence observed]

Mr. STUPAK. Thank you. Mr. Walden, you are recognized for 10 minutes.

Mr. WALDEN. Thank you, Mr. Chairman. I know that obviously throws a little curve in our hearing and our lives, but I appreciate you in that. Back to our questions, because I know Charlie would want us to pursue this issue, especially with his passion for healthcare and improving the lives of Americans. So Dr. Graham, let me start with you. In discussing Ketek, your testimony states that the FDA scientists were threatened, intimidated, suppressed, transferred and ultimately compelled to leave the agency. Who are the FDA scientists that you are referring to?

Dr. GRAHAM. You have heard them. You have heard them speak and I am sure they have colleagues. I know that there is at least one other reviewer who was involved in the Ketek review who was afraid of retaliation and who actually, no, is no longer with that particular group. He was transferred to another group to get out of that hell hole. But in any event, that is who we are talking about.

Mr. WALDEN. And you know, because I asked Dr. Ross or others about whether or not this is agency-wide or is it sort of isolated in a couple of places. This type of practice.

Dr. GRAHAM. This type of practice happens—I can tell you now for post-marketing. A drug has been approved; it now gets on the market. Now a safety issue comes up. I can tell you—and I could assemble a list later of the multiple examples where we in post-marketing bring a safety issue to the new drugs people and they do nothing or worse. I will give you just one example, because this was my introduction to FDA and the reality of what it is to have the people who approve the drugs decide what happens to them.

Mr. WALDEN. And how long ago?

Dr. GRAHAM. I came to the agency in 1987, so this would have been in 1988, 1989. OK, things have only gotten worse since then, but listen to this example. The drug is Vericet. It is a benzodiazepine. It is like Valium and it was used intravenously for conscious sedation, to make you sleepy during medical procedures such as colonoscopy. Well, the advantage of this drug was it was water soluble. Valium is oily and it doesn't—it causes the veins to get inflamed. So this is an improvement for patient comfort. Soon after approval, we got 23 reports of patients who died of respiratory arrest. They stopped breathing during their routine medical procedure. We brought these 23 case reports to the Office of New Drugs, to the division director and the office director. That office director is still there. He is now higher up in CDER. His name has already been mentioned once today at this meeting. Very high up. And they threw out all 23 cases, saying there was nothing here.

Mr. WALDEN. Why?

Dr. GRAHAM. Two examples are, particularly, that stuck in mind these years, one of them was a 63-year-old woman with breast cancer, who they said she has got breast cancer for—she has got to die sometime.

Mr. WALDEN. Did they actually say that?

Dr. GRAHAM. Yes, they actually said that. The other was a 91 or 92-year-old, some guy in his nineties, OK. He is 91 years old. He has got to die sometime. So he picked that very moment to stop breathing. Fine. We go back to our office in dismay. What are we going to do? Two years or so later, some academics do some pharmacokinetic experiments where they determine that FDA got the dose wrong. FDA had approved the dose of this drug at about 10 times what it should have been. And so in point of fact, these people were actually being killed by the drug and FDA had approved that and FDA—our post-marketing system is maligned, but it captures things like this. That is what it was designed and intended to do.

Mr. WALDEN. And you say have a whole list of these?

Dr. GRAHAM. Yes, I have got a list of other ones. Oh, yes.

Mr. WALDEN. Mr. Chairman, could I ask unanimous consent that we ask the witness to supply that list to us?

Mr. STUPAK. Sure.

Mr. WALDEN. That would be obviously helpful to the lives of Americans.

Dr. GRAHAM. Right.

Mr. STUPAK. OK, with Dr. Graham's assurance, he will provide that list to us. I know you have been to the Senate in 2004.

Dr. GRAHAM. Yes.

Mr. STUPAK. And there were about six of them then.

Dr. GRAHAM. Right. And I will provide a list.

Mr. WALDEN. This goes back to 1987, so——

Dr. GRAHAM. Right, but you see, we are talking culture attitude what happens when you are OND, you are the people who approve the drug and you are the lord and master and you control everything that happens afterwards. Now the thing—in the modern day, it has gotten even worse, because what happens is, is that all of our supervisors, for example, in my office, most of them come from the Office of New Drugs. We don't have any promotion from within into the upper ranges of drug safety.

Mr. WALDEN. So are you saying by that that they sort of protect their old turf, then?

Dr. GRAHAM. Some of them do. They are not—our office director is very good. He sees public health and that is really wonderful. The problem is, is that not everybody who has come over over the years—and we have had a lot of people come from OND over to OSE—they don't have that public health background. They are used to looking at the clinical trials and saying is the P value less than .05? And if it is, it is truth, and if it is not, we are going to forget about it, and that is not the way population medicine is practiced and that is not the way post-marketing is supposed to be done. Now the problem is—I just have to get this little sound bite in—physicians bury their mistakes one at a time. The FDA buries its mistakes in unmarked mass graves. And what I have just described, this dynamic of who is responsible for decision making pre- versus post-marketing, that is the crux of that issue.

Mr. WALDEN. Do you think that these sort of internal structural, cultural problems at FDA, do they predate the user fee program?

Dr. GRAHAM. They predate it, but PDUFA exacerbated it. What happened with PDUFA was it is kind of—you have got—we talk about logarithmic scales. PDUFA took what was a 10 and raised it to 100 and it did it in several ways. What it did is—and the IOM documents this. Basically it is like leash with a choke collar on the neck of FDA and it is being jerked and they are saying pay attention to getting these drugs out the door and get them out fast, and safety is an afterthought. Pre-approval—what happens now, pre-approval, is—yes, Dr. Gauson has said 50 percent of CDER's resources are spent on safety. I would like to see a real accounting of that, because the medical officers I have talked to say the safety review is the last thing that gets done and they don't spend nearly as much time on it. And that is where we are just talking pre-approval. I am most concerned about the post-approval. As I said before if FDA wants to produce a poison or approve a poison, well, if we have got a safety net out there to interdict it, then we have got a check and balance.

Mr. WALDEN. That is kind of what Dr. Nissen is saying.

Dr. GRAHAM. Well, yes and no.

Mr. WALDEN. Well, he is shaking yes, I think.

Dr. GRAHAM. Well, maybe Dr. Nissen and I need to talk off-line sometime so we can explore more, maybe, the similarities in the way we about it, this benefit that Dr. Nissen has talked about.

Mr. WALDEN. Right. Let me go on.

Dr. GRAHAM. OK. I am sorry.

Mr. WALDEN. No, really, you are very passionate on this and it is helpful. Did you perform a failure mode analysis in the Vioxx case?

Dr. GRAHAM. I did but FDA has not and this is one of the critical issues. When an airliner goes down, the National Transportation Safety Board is out there. Is the switched colored the wrong way? Is there some reason, then we can fix something, the engineer the solution. FDA did not look back at Vioxx. The IOM was not asked to look at Vioxx. What IOM looked at was FDA. IOM didn't put Vioxx up as an example and say, what we are recommending, would actually have dealt with these problems?

Mr. WALDEN. So explain to me how a failure mode analysis works? What is it?

Dr. GRAHAM. Well, it is used in engineering mostly, and in systems analysis, where you basically have boxes on a process chart or something like that and you can kind of see if this breaks down and what happens if this breaks down. The failure mode that I did was sort of looking at what is the evidence we had on the drug and——

Mr. WALDEN. So what did you find on Vioxx?

Dr. GRAHAM. OK, what I found is that pre-approval, we had ample evidence that Vioxx would cause heart attacks. We knew from the theoretical that it could cause heart attacks. That was known by the company and it was known by FDA. The clinical trials that were done showed a tendency, an increase in cardiovascular events, but it didn't reach statistical significance. And this is one of the problems at FDA. For safety, it assumes the drug doesn't work and then a company has to do a study and show statistically that it does work in order for it to get approved. But for safety, FDA assumes, before it gets on the market, that the drug is safe and now it is up to the company to prove that it is not. Well, what company in their right mind is going to do that? And the standard that FDA places on safety is unreasonably high.

So with Vioxx, for example, there is ample evidence. The medical officer says it right there: "Cardiovascular events are increased, but I don't have complete certainty." In other words, the P value wasn't less than 0.05. So that was my analogy in the Senate Finance. This was the analogy I was trying to make about that I have 90 bullets in a 100-bullet chamber and the gun is not loaded. Well, it is loaded, it is just not loaded enough for you to agree it is loaded. And so that is on the pre-approval. On the post-approval side, having the suspicion that—would occur in April 2000, FDA had the results of the bigger trial, which was a study that was started before the drug got approved, finished after the drug got approved, a large randomized clinical trial, and it showed that Vioxx increased the risk of heart attack by a factor of five. OK, a 500 percent increase. As a population medicine person, what FDA should have done as soon as it had those results was yank the high dose of Vioxx. There was no earthly reason for—this was a high does study—no earthly reason for the high dose. The high dose was approved for the short-term treatment of acute pain. Well, 4 million women a year give childbirth and have acute pain and there are a lot of safe pain relievers for short-term use that don't increase your risk of heart attack fivefold. FDA never did the benefit/risk analysis, because FDA has never done a benefit/risk analysis in its entire history. I have done several and each time I have done it, I have been reprimanded for doing so.

In any event, the public health perspective would have been to pull the high dose now, this thing called dose response. Maybe the low dose does it as well. We see in the clinical trials that as low a dose as 12½ milligrams increased the risk, but it wasn't statistically significant. You would have been faced with a dilemma there. Do I pull that dose or do I say to the company, go out and do a really big study, really fast, to answer the question on the low dose? And maybe we could debate what happens. Hindsight shows that the low dose did it as well and so—but you see, this is the difference of who is calling the shots pre-approval and post-approval and that is the core issue. The reviewers at the level—the reviewer who said we don't have complete certainty, I know her. We are friends. She is a very good reviewer. The reviewers at FDA are very good, but the rules the operate under, they are trained to think this way. So basically, in the pre-approval world, they are all trained to say, if the P value isn't less than 0.05, I can ignore it.

Dr. NISSEN. If I could jump in a second, not only did they not do that, but they let the company go ahead and put on television ads with skaters skating around pain free. And so what we saw here is here is a time, by 2000, by the time of the bigger——

Mr. WALDEN. They knew there was a problem.

Dr. NISSEN. And it was clear. It was clear in the manuscript that was published, it was clear in the FDA's study report, it was clear to us in February 2001 at the FDA panel, and yet they allowed the company to continue to show us people—a young skating around a ring without any pain.

Mr. WALDEN. Yes, Dorothy Hamill.

Dr. NISSEN. Yes. I wasn't going to mention her name because I am sure she was well remunerated for her time, but the point is that that drove millions of people to use the drug. Now a prudent agency would have said, OK.

Mr. WALDEN. Wait a minute.

Dr. NISSEN. Maybe we can disagree about the data, but at the very least, we ought to pull back here until we learn more. We certainly ought not let the company go ahead and promote this in this extravagant way.

Dr. GRAHAM. And the drug was promoted heavily. In fact, Vioxx was the most heavily promoted product on the Internet. It exceeded promotion for pornography on the Internet. OK. Yes, it was huge.

Mr. WALDEN. Having done a number of hearings on that issue, that would be hard to believe.

Dr. GRAHAM. Well, if I could just point out something here. Kennedy-Enzi, as I understand it, would possibly have resulted in—it was like almost this 2-year delay in FDA getting a label change done. Kennedy-Enzi would probably shorten that or deal with that, but you see, but that is not the problem. The problem was this drug shouldn't have been there in the first place. The high dose should have been gone immediately and the low dose should have been feet to the fire, prove that it is not dangerous. And Kennedy-Enzi—see, this is the mindset. So just to give you insight into the way these things work.

Mr. WALDEN. I just have to probe one other issue that is somewhat not related, but we had a hearing on this issue as well, and that is supplements, dietary supplements. We had the panel witnesses on Ephedra who, I think, the common denominator—I don't think I will get in trouble for saying this—is they had some sort of conviction for fraud and maybe a high school education and the recipe was written on the back of an envelope. This stuff is out there being marketed and people are dying from that. Do you have any counsel? That is way off our topic.

Dr. GRAHAM. Dr. Nissen, you go first.

Dr. NISSEN. In my written testimony, I actually speak to this and I am going to tell you that if we don't do anything, there will be a major catastrophe involving the dietary supplement industry. What we are doing is absolutely insane. I could go out in my backyard and I could cut up grass clippings and put it in a capsule and put it in a bottle and say promotes heart health and I could sell it at the local pharmacy for $300 a bottle and people just do that, that very thing. I recently saw a patient. There is a drug we use called niacin. Niacin is a drug that is used to raise HDL, the good cholesterol, and it is an effective drug, although it has a problem, which is it causes a lot of continuous flushing. People flush very badly when they take the drug. And so health food stores, unregulated by the FDA, have begun selling something called no-flush niacin and there is only one problem with no flush niacin: it doesn't have any effect on HDL. It is inert.

I had a patient recently that came in that had a very low HDL. I had gotten his HDL up to a very high level and he was counseled by his local health food store to go on no flush niacin. His HDL dropped. He came in with a heart attack. The patient came in with a heart attack, subsequently developed severe congestive heart failure, needed a heart transplant and died while waiting for a transplant. Now, anybody who tries to tell you that dietary supplements are harmless is out of their ever loving mind. Taking garlic rather than a real cholesterol-lowering medication is harmful. And the greatest setback to drug safety in the last 100 years was the Hatch-Richardson Act, which took away the FDA's authority to regulate dietary supplements. This has got to be dealt with if you are going to deal with drug safety.

Mr. WALDEN. Mr. Chairman, thank you for your great indulgence on the time. Thanks to our witnesses for your input. It is most helpful.

Mr. STUPAK. Thank you. Just one question, Dr. Nissen, if I may. Dr. Graham mentioned a number of drugs. He was going to provide a list to us of couple of drugs that he thought are out and approved in the marketplace that we should take a closer look at or someone should take a closer look at for safety. If you have any suggestions or would like to provide a list to the committee, we would be receptive to receiving that.

Dr. NISSEN. I will certainly think about that and I will inform you about some thoughts I have about that, but I do think there are real issues in currently marketed drugs. I don't think we have seen the end of the kind of drug safety revelations that have occurred. Something that has come up recently, if you watch the news that yesterday in the New England Journal of Medicine there were five manuscripts about the drug—which is a very hot controversy right now about whether they, in fact, are as safe and effective for the indication which the were developed. You are going to hear a lot more about that in the next couple of years. We haven't talked at all about the device side and one of the things that is not in Enzi-Kennedy that really is missing, that I hope, on the House side, something can be done about is the device world. We have had problems with defibrillators that failed. We have had a lot of safety issues on devices, heart valves, and stints are a great example. And so if you want to look at safety, it is not just pharmaceuticals, it is also devices. And if anything, the regulatory environment on the device is more like the wild west than it is on the drug side. It is actually, if anything, worse.

Mr. STUPAK. Well, it sounds like it is a great topic for this committee. As we often say, we deal with crime, drugs and sex all the time in this subcommittee and I am sure we will in the future. As I said, this was the first of many hearings we will be having on drug safety, and the three panels, the excellent panels that we had today, have suggested other areas that we will explore over the course of this Congress. Well, that concludes our questioning and I want to thank all our members, our panel members, and I think all of the Members for coming down. A little bit of bookkeeping, or health keeping, I should say. These documents found in the white pamphlet, without objection, will be in for the record.

If any Members have additional questions for the record to be answered by our relevant witnesses, we will give you 10 days to submit them to the committee clerk within the next 10 days. Please do so in electronic form. That will conclude this hearing. Thank you again for all our witnesses. Thank you for everyone for being here today.

[Whereupon, at 2:30 p.m., the subcommittee was adjourned.]

[Material submitted for inclusion in the record follows:]

TESTIMONY OF JOHN H. POWERS, M.D.

Good morning. My name is John Powers. I was a physician-scientist at the U.S. Food and Drug Administration for the last 8 years, the last 5 of which I was the Lead Medical Officer for Antimicrobial Development and Resistance Initiatives. I would like to state that I do not consider myself as having "blown a whistle", since I pointed out the very issues that I will discuss today to FDA managers up the chain of command. I chose to leave the agency to pursue other research opportunities after over half a decade of attempting to advance the science of clinical trials in infectious diseases, feeling that I could better serve the public outside the agency. There are numerous individuals in both FDA and the drug industry who work hard appropriately evaluating new medicines for people. I learned a tremendous amount at FDA and I would still be there today if I felt I could perform my job in the way it should be done.

Many of the recent discussions regarding evaluation of new drugs have focused on their safety. However, there are also important issues with the evaluation of effectiveness, especially regarding antibiotics. In 1962, the Food, Drug and Cosmetic Act was amended to state there must be substantial evidence of effectiveness from adequate and well-controlled trials in order to justify the adverse events inherent with the use of all drugs. In the absence of evidence of effectiveness, any adverse effect, no matter how rare, is not justifiable.

The drug Ketek is a symptom of much larger problem. Over the last 25 years, FDA has approved approximately 68 new drug applications for ear infections in children, sinus infections and bronchial infections in patients with underlying lung disease. All of these drugs were approved based on so-called "noninferiority" trials. While the word "noninferior" strictly means "not worse", the purpose of these trials is in fact to rule out an amount by which the new drug' effectiveness may be worse than an old drug. Therefore, noninferiority trials are really "not too much worse" trials. Showing a new drug is potentially worse than an old drug when the effectiveness of the old drug is unclear is like the Billy Preston song, "nothing from nothing leaves nothing". An evaluation of previous placebo controlled trials shows that 12 of 17 studies in sinusitis and 9 of 14 studies in bronchial infections lack evidence of a benefit for antibiotics and the situation is similar for ear infections. Based on these data, showing that Ketek may be less effective than older drugs does not provide evidence that Ketek is effective at all in sinus and bronchial infections, and this was clear at the time the drug was approved in 2004. Initiation of a noninferiority trial with Ketek in ear infections in children is inappropriate and unethical, as it exposes children to harm without the potential to clearly provide evidence of benefits.

Noninferiority trials are justifiable in serious infections where the benefits of antibiotics are large and reproducible. However, even in serious diseases the trial must be designed, performed and analyzed appropriately in order to provide meaningful results. The major problem is that many of the common safeguards in clinical trials that protect us from drawing false conclusions are less useful in noninferiority trials. For instance, if one performs a trial to evaluate a drug in patients with pneumonia, but most of the patients enrolled in the trial have the common cold, it is much easier to make two drugs appear similar when in fact this says nothing about the new drug' effectiveness in pneumonia. This is like testing a new parachute against an older proven parachute, when all the test subjects are jumping out a plane that is standing still and only two inches off the ground. Everyone will do well, but it says nothing about how the new parachute will really work in a real life situation.

Lack of effectiveness is an even larger problem with antibiotics than it is for other types of drugs. If a non-antibiotic doesn't work, it only affects the person who takes it. If an antibiotic doesn't work, it affects not only the person who takes it, but can also affect other people who don't take it by spreading resistance not only to that drug but to other related drugs as well. Antimicrobial resistance is a safety issue as lack of effectiveness can promote the very problem of antibiotic resistance we are trying to combat.

We need new antibiotics to combat the inevitable increase in antibiotic resistance, but approval of ineffective and therefore inherently unsafe antibiotics is not an incentive for drug development. After approval of numerous antibiotics whose effectiveness is unclear, we have seen no boom in antibiotic development, and in fact drug sponsors have exited this field. Developing appropriate economic incentives to promote development are the province of Congress, not the FDA.

We need to address these problems now. FDA needs to require sponsors to perform superiority trials in self-resolving diseases. Even in serious diseases, FDA needs to require appropriately designed, conducted and analyzed noninferiority trials to give clinicians the information they need to make decisions for their patients. FDA needs to address the issue of drugs that still carry approvals for self-resolving diseases without evidence of effectiveness. FDA needs to promptly publish new guidances based on appropriate scientific and regulatory principles and remove the old guidances from their Web site now, since they continue to mislead drug sponsors.

The bottom line is this is about people, not about "bad bugs". Most of us in this room have taken antibiotics or will need to take them. We must preserve this precious resource that has been one of the marvels of modern medicine by ensuring these drugs are effective, safe, and used appropriately. Thank you.

ANSWERS TO SUBMITTED QUESTIONS

1. When did the issues with noninferiority trials first become apparent to FDA managers?

These issues have been known for some time. At a recent advisory committee on September 12, 2006, a senior FDA official pointed out that drug sponsors knew about the issues with noninferiority trials and that, in his words, this was "not hot news". It was senior FDA officials who published some of the first articles in the medical literature in the early 1980' that address the problems with noninferiority trials. In 1985, wording was added to the section in FDA regulations that defines adequate and well-controlled trials to state, "If the intent of the trial is to show similarity of the test and control drugs, the report of the study should assess the ability of the study to have detected a difference between treatments. Similarity of test drug and active control can mean either that both drugs were effective or that neither was effective. The analysis of the study should explain why the drugs should be considered effective in the study, for example, by reference to results in previous placebo-controlled studies of the active control drug."

2. Did FDA managers ever enforce these regulations with antibiotics?

Over the last 8 years I can only remember one sponsor who submitted a justification for doing a noninferiority trial, and that was for an antifungal drug, not drugs like Ketek. At the September 12 advisory committee another senior FDA official pointed out that the drug sponsor had not, in his words, "done the mental exercise" needed to scientifically justify this kind of trial. Recently, after a letter from several members of Congress raised issues about noninferiority trials, the statistical team members began to send letters to drug sponsors asking for a justification for noninferiority trials. One division director expressed displeasure at them doing this. The justifications sent in by many sponsors were not scientific ones, but their reasoning was that FDA had allowed many of these trials before, so that they should be allowed to continue this practice.

3. You said that FDA managers knew that the evidence of effectiveness for Ketek was lacking at the time it was approved in 2004. Had there been prior discussions within and outside of FDA about the issues with noninferiority trials?

Yes, there had been numerous discussions. In 2000, the International Conference on Harmonization guidance E–10, titled Choice of Control Groups and Related Issues in Clinical Trials was first published. This guidance outlined many of the issues with noninferiority trials. In addition, FDA held an advisory committee in February of 2002 to specifically address the issues of noninferiority trials, held advisory committees in July of 2002 on ear infections, two workshops in November of 2002, an advisory committee on sinusitis in October of 2003, and another workshop in April of 2004, and an internal regulatory briefing in July of 2005. These issues again came up at recent advisory committees in September and December 2006.

4. What were the results of these meeting?

At all these meetings there was scientific agreement that noninferiority trials were not justifiable in self-resolving diseases. FDA statisticians did lobby hard and got a change in the FDA guidance on antibiotic development referred to as the "Points to Consider" document. However, sponsors continued to submit applications based on noninferiority trials without an accompanying scientific justification as specified in the regulations. Regarding serious diseases, at the February 2002 advisory committee on developing drugs for diseases due to resistant pathogens, the Office director at the time implied that the only thing sponsors needed to obtain approval in serious diseases due to resistant pathogens was "a few well characterized cases". This seemed to contradict FDA' own regulations about the need for adequate and well- controlled trials. FDA regulations require some comparison with a control, even if it is a comparison with a group of patients in the past who did not receive treatment in what is called a "historical" control.

5. Did ignoring the regulations occur commonly?

I can only comment on the area in which I worked. It seemed that there were other priorities other than following the scientific principles spelled out in the regulations. It' important to realize that the regulations are based in good science, and they are not just rules for rules sake. But often it was implied that the regulations were just a guide and they FDA, in the managers words, "had to be flexible". Certainly one can be flexible within what good science and the regulations allow, but there is also a point where one can go beyond what these principles allow as well. The major issue seemed to be approving drugs for less serious diseases, which are far more common, to provide an economic incentive for drug sponsors to develop drugs for more serious diseases. Some FDA managers also seemed to have the idea that FDA could not make it "too difficult" for sponsors to do studies. Of course, this depends on what you consider "difficult", which is subject to opinion, not science.

Sometimes it is challenging to do an appropriate study that is meaningful, but this is far better than exposing people to harm in a study that cannot provide useful information.

6. Did you inform senior FDA officials of there problems?

Yes. I informed several levels of senior managers over the span of 5 years that these issues were occurring.

7. Why did they not address the problem?

I was never certain as to why the issue was never resolved. At several internal meetings, senior managers pointed out that these noninferiority trials were not appropriate and yet antibiotics continued to be approved on this basis.

9. Even after these meetings, were drugs for self-resolving diseases still approved based on noninferiority trials?

Yes. There were several drugs approved since 2000 for these indications based upon noninferiority trials. At the September 2006 advisory committee, the drug sponsor pointed out that they felt ill used since other drugs were approved based on noninferiority and they felt they should be approved also. They specifically pointed to Ketek as an example of where a drug had been approved based on noninferiority trials. One of the issues is some FDA managers believe that once FDA has agreed on a trial design, it cannot be changed. Section 505(b)(5)(C) of the Food Drug and Cosmetic Act states that FDA can change the parameters of a study if "a substantial scientific issue essential to determining the safety or effectiveness of the drug has been identified after the testing has begun.

10. Do you think drug sponsors will do placebo controlled trials in these diseases?

Yes. At the November 2002 workshop we held on antimicrobial drug development, one drug company representative stated that companies would be unwilling to do these trials, but they would do them if FDA made it clear that they were a regulatory requirement. That hasn't happened. And that same person submitted an application a few years later for a drug for ear infections in children based on noninferiority trials, and few years after that submitted another application for a different drug for sinusitis and bronchitis. You almost can't blame companies if it' not made clear to them that noninferiority trials are no longer acceptable. On the other hand, however, companies clearly know these kind of trials are not substantial evidence of effectiveness, yet they continue to submit them.

11. Haven't some drug sponsors said that investigators will not enroll patients in placebo controlled trials?

There have been 8 published placebo controlled trials in sinusitis since the year 2000 and two published just last year in ear infections so clearly people are doing these trials. If an investigator does not wish to participate in these trials they are free not to participate, but that does not mean FDA should not insist on doing trials in a way that provides the necessary information to evaluate drug effectiveness and potential harms.

12. If investigators have been doing these trials, what was FDA manager' response as to why they did not insist on drug sponsors doing placebo controlled trials?

At meeting with drug sponsors, some sponsors insisted that their investigators would not enroll patients in placebo controlled trials. Of course, these investigators are free not to participate in the trials if they wish, but the publication of placebo controlled trials in medical journals shows these trials can and are being done. The companies brought in experts who insisted these trials cannot be done or would be difficult to do. But allowing expert opinion to determine which trials are done and how they are done sets us back to a time when drugs were approved based on expert opinion alone. The hearings at the time of the passage of the 1962 amendments and subsequent court cases made it quite clear that clinician opinion was not the standard upon which drug approval should be based. FDA should taking a leadership role in advancing the science and requiring trials that will answer important medical questions, such as whether the drug is effective in the first place. FDA has done so in the past in other therapeutic areas.

13. Don't we need drugs like Ketek for disease due to resistant infections?

We do need new antibiotics, but we need them in serious and life threatening diseases where resistance in a test tube has the most impact on people. If it' not clear when and where we need to use antibiotics in less serious disease, or whether we need to use them at all, the impact of resistance is also unclear. We have taken for granted that a measurement in test tube must inherently mean something for patients, but that is why we do trials, to see if what we find in the lab translates into some meaningful benefit for patients. That is still unclear in these less serious diseases. In addition, the definition of resistance is not clear for many of these diseases and it may overestimate the number of resistant organisms, making drugs look ineffective when they are not.

14. How about people who are allergic to other drugs? Wouldn't Ketek be an option for them?

For Ketek to be an option for any patient, even those who are allergic to other drugs, it still have to be proven to be effective first. It would not be useful to give an ineffective drug to someone just because they have allergies. It is important to realize that noninferiority trials do not show two drugs are equal, and even in appropriately designed and analyzed noninferiority trials, you might be giving up some effectiveness for whatever other benefits the drug might have, for instance improved safety. In the case of Ketek we just don't know what those benefits are since we don't know if the drug is effective in sinus and bronchial infections, and we probably won't know if it is effective in ear infections if it is studied in a noninferiority trial.

15. Who defines what organisms are called "resistant"?

FDA defines resistance in the labeling for a drug when it is approved. Over time, however, this definition may change as the drug is used and more resistance may develop. There have been many discussions over the last few years about how FDA will interact with other non-governmental groups as to how resistance will be defined. What is clear is that defining and monitoring resistance is an important safety issue just like other adverse events for other drugs. FDA need to approach antibiotic resistance as a safety issue and change labeling when necessary to make sure the definitions of resistance are accurate. The changes should be based on adequate evidence and not isolated case reports.

16. So when drugs organisms are called resistant when they are not, does it cause doctors to use other antibiotics instead?

Yes it does. And those antibiotics are usually newer, which means that we have less experience with them in terms of their safety, and they are usually more expensive. Taxpayers may foot the bill for more expensive drugs that are really no better than older drugs.

17. So for all these drugs approved without knowing that they are any better than placebo, the American taxpayer is still paying for these.

A. Yes, they are.

18. If noninferiority trials only rule out how much worse a new drug might be compared to an old drug, why are we doing these trials in situations where we are concerned the old drugs don't even work any more because of resistance?

That is an important point. It is illogical even in serious diseases to compare a new drug to an old drug when we have concerns the old drug is no longer effective.

19 Yesterday the label for Ketek was changed to remove the indications for sinusitis and bronchitis. What should be done about the other drugs that carry labels for these indications?

FDA needs to clearly inform clinicians and patients that the evidence of effectiveness for these drugs is insufficient. That would not mean taking all those drugs off the market, as most of those drugs are approved for other diseases like pneumonia. FDA' own labeling regulations state, "If there is a common belief that the drug may be effective for a certain use or if there is a common use of the drug for a condition, but the preponderance of evidence related to the use or condition shows that the drug is ineffective or that the therapeutic benefits of the product do not generally outweigh its risks, FDA may require that this section state that there is a lack of evidence that the drug is effective or safe for that use or condition." A statement such as this should be included in all drugs that carry indications of sinus, ear and bronchial infections as well as older drugs that include these indications under the older name of lower respiratory tract infections. This is not regulating the practice of medicine, as some have asserted as clinicians can continue to use these drugs where they see fit, but it does state a fact that there has not been substantial evidence of effectiveness for these drugs. It was concerning to hear a senior FDA official state at the December 16 advisory committee that FDA will not address these drugs unless there is a safety issue. Lack of substantial evidence of effectiveness is a requirement according to the FD&C Act, and these criteria are not meant to be applied prospectively only, as court precedent has shown. Lack of evidence of effectiveness is a safety issue, given the inevitable spread of resistance and deaths from adverse events without evidence of benefits. Since self-resolving diseases are so common, a good proportion of the adverse events with antibiotics occur in people who take them for self-resolving diseases. Many of these people don't even have a bacterial infection.

20. Why do clinicians believe these drugs to be effective in treating human disease when so many placebo controlled trials fail to show their benefits?

First, clinicians confuse mechanisms of action with outcome. Because a drug kills bacteria in a test tube or even in a person does not necessarily mean that the drug is helping the person if they get better anyway without the drug, or if the cure is worse than the disease in terms of adverse effects. Secondly, the placebo controlled trials are not designed very well, and people correctly point to those flaws, but incorrectly state the drugs are effective until proven otherwise. This goes against the basic medical premise of "first do no harm". Thirdly, some researchers have attempted to combine these studies together in what is called a meta-analysis. However, if you pool together flawed studies, you get a flawed answer. A study in the New England Journal of Medicine in 1997 shows that meta-analysis were contradicted by subsequent large randomized trials almost half the time.

21. How would we avoid another Ketek?

FDA needs to operate with transparency and with accountability. Managers need to make the final decisions on drug approvals, but they need to make those decisions based upon appropriate science and following FDA regulations. The reviews for all approvals, including any non-approvals or approvable actions for already approved drugs should be posted on FDA' Web site and linked to *clinicaltrials.gov* where the trials are registered within 7 working days of FDA taking an action. FDA needs to take action on drug when there is a safety or effectiveness issue even if sponsors do not initiate the request. And there needs to be accountability for FDA staff who do not follow the regulations or who attempt to intimidate of bully other staff. Science is a process of discussion, and some of the most momentous discoveries were made by people who did not accept the status quo. FDA needs to have an environment where those scientific discussions can take place without an emotional overlay. It would help tremendously to have a separate group evaluate drugs post-approval than the group who evaluate drugs pre-approval. This would put checks and balances into the system, and allow a fresh set up eyes, and might stimulate more rigorous decision making if people knew their decisions would be reviewed by both the public with the posted reviews and by their peers. Finally, there needs to be no more noninferiority trials in these self-resolving diseases and FDA needs to take a leadership role in advancing the science of clinical trials in infectious diseases.

TESTIMONY OF ANN MARIE CISNEROS

Good morning Mr. Chairman and members of the Committee. I am honored that you are giving me the opportunity to tell my story.

My name is Ann Marie Cisneros, I am currently an independent clinical research associate. I was trained in the United States Air Force as a Medical Technologist, have a Bachelors of Science Degree in Occupational Education from Wayland Baptist University and a Masters of Business Administration Degree from Pfieffer University.

I have worked as a clinical research associate for approximately eight years. My first three years in this industry I spent at PPDI, a Contract Research Organization, where I monitored a number of protocols that included Study 3014. At the time of the 3014 study, I was a senior clinical research associate and was tasked to assist with the monitoring of Dr. Anne Kirkman-Campbell' site.

Dr. Kirkman-Campbell is currently serving a 57-month prison sentence for fraud associated with Study 3014. In addition she was ordered by the court to pay restitution to the drug sponsor, Aventis, which had paid her $400 per patient enrolled.

Mr. Chairman, based upon what I observed and learned in monitoring the Kirkman-Campbell site, Dr. Kirkman-Campbell indeed had engaged in fraud. But what the court that sentenced her did not know is that Aventis was not a victim of this fraud. On the contrary. Let me explain.

Even before conducting the Kirkman-Campbell site visit, a number of "red flags" were apparent. I knew that Dr. Kirkman-Campbell had enrolled over 400 patients or 1 percent of the adult population of Gadsden, Alabama. (By comparison, another site in Gadsden had enrolled just twelve patients.) In a recent Quality Assurance audit by Aventis several Informed Consent issues were noted as well as a significant under-reporting of Adverse Events and no reports of Serious Adverse Events. No patients had withdrawn from the study and no patients were lost to follow up, an unusual occurrence given the number of subjects. She enrolled patients within minutes of each other and upwards of 30 patients per day. She enrolled patients at times and on days when the office was closed..

Once we started reviewing patient charts, we discovered that:

- Every informed consent had a discrepancy.
- Most of the consents looked like they had been initialed by someone other than the patient.
- A lot of the consents were dated by someone other than the subject.
- One consent was blatantly forged.
- There were date discrepancies as to when patients were enrolled in the study, had their blood drawn or signed their consent.
- Most patients diagnosed with bronchitis either had no history of the ailment or did not have a "chronic" condition.
- She enrolled her entire staff in the study.

Frankly, all Kirkman-Campbell seemed truly interested in was getting more business from Aventis as an investigator. At one point during my site visit, she told Aventis Project Manager Nadine Guenthe that I could only stay if Nadine got her other studies at Aventis. Nadine agreed. It is my understanding that when the FDA audited the Kirkman-Campbell site, she was participating in another Aventis clinical trial.

While at the site, I was so concerned about patient safety I called Copernicus Independent Review Board to express my concerns and seek guidance. An IRB, which is under contract to the drug sponsor, has as its primary purpose patient advocacy. It is allowed to contact patients directly and is duty-bound to report to the FDA any unanticipated problems involving risks to subjects and serious noncompliance with regulations. I spoke with the president of the company and was told that, while she shared my concerns, she preferred to wait and see what actions Aventis took. I never heard from the IRB again. To my knowledge Copernicus never did audit or blacklist the site, or report any irregularities to the FDA.

I e-mailed a summary of my site visit findings to Robert McCormick, head of quality assurance at PPD, and copied Aventis personnel. I also participated in a teleconference between PPD and Aventis at which I discussed issues identified in my site visit. At some point after that I understand that Aventis took site management responsibilities away from PPD because Dr. Kirkman-Campbell would not cooperate with anyone but the sponsor.

I subsequently left PPD but learned that the Kirkman-Campbell site was being audited by the FDA. In preparation for the audit, Aventis' Nadine Guenthe coached Dr. Kirkman-Campbell with leading questions on how to explain away improper conduct. Nadine would say, for example: "Is the reason you enrolled so many patients in one day because that is when your supply of the drug came in?" I was told about this by a trusted and distressed former colleague at PPD who witnessed the prepping.

In my eight years in clinical research work, this is the only instance I've come across of such bad behavior by a drug sponsor.. I feel I can speak for those who agonized over this situation when I say we are pleased that Dr. Kirkman-Campbell is serving prison time for her actions. But what brings me here today is my disbelief at Aventis' statements that it did not know that fraud was being committed. Mr. Chairman, I knew it, PPD knew it, and Aventis knew it.

Thank you for this opportunity to tell my story.

Answers to Submitted Questions

As of what date do you believe that Sanofi-Aventis (Aventis) first knew that the problems at Dr. Kirkman-Campbell' site constituted fraud?

I believe Aventis concretely knew of the fraud when their own QA auditor, Rhanjan Khosla, audited the site. That was a few weeks before my visit to the site in February 2002.

What is the basis for your belief that Aventis knew the problems at Dr. Kirkman-Campbell' site constituted fraud?

The fraud was blatant, there was no attempt by the Investigator to cover it up. Most research professionals and especially employees of a Quality Assurance department receive some level of fraud training. For Aventis to claim they didn't recognize the sort of oddities described below constituted a suspicion of fraud makes them either incompetent or not completely honest.

Please remember that Aventis was never tasked with the responsibility to prove fraud; the requirement is to report to the FDA any site where fraud is merely suspected.

Please identify the particular circumstances, problems, or events that you believe constituted fraud and of which Aventis knew?

These events individually might have equaled GCP deviations as is being claimed by Aventis. However, collectively, the evidence is overwhelming the site was committing fraud.

- The number of patients enrolled, 407 with no sub-Investigator and only 3 study coordinators.
- Forged consents.
- Every informed consent was either initialed or dated by someone other than the patient. (It is never acceptable to forge anything on an Informed Consent)
- Medical Charts consisting of one or two pages.
- Every patient completing the study, adhering to all study visits, being 100 percent compliant with study medication.
- Overwrites of dates and adding study diagnosis in different color ink than what was used for the initial visit in the medical chart.
- The office staff would not speak with the monitors.
- Enrollment of patients within minutes of each other, on times and days the office was closed and enrolling patients when the site was completely out of study drug (meaning sick patients would have to come back at a later date to pick up the study drug)
- Patients diagnosed with Acute Exacerbation of Chronic Bronchitis that had never had bronchitis or a limited history not meeting "chronic" definition.
- The first several hundred patients were enrolled with primarily Acute Sinusitis; when enrollment was closed for that indication, the Investigator' remaining hundred or so patients all had AECB. You would expect to see the enrollment pattern intermingled, not all one group and then the other.
- Significant under-reporting of Adverse Events and Serious

Adverse Events given the number of subjects. This was an indication that she was not following the patients after they started taking the study medication.

c. Please identify the Aventis employees who were on notice of the fraud you describe in response to question 1 (b).

Nadine Grethe
Rhanjan Khosla
Rhanjan' boss (head of QA department)

d. Please identify the employee of Pharmaceutical Product Development, Inc. (PPD) who were on notice of the fraud you describe in response to question 1 (b)

The following PPD employees diligently reported the fraud:
Beth Heding, CRA
Abby Wear, CRA
John Reynolds, MD
The following PPD employees were also aware of the fraud:
Stephanie Love, CRA
Robert McCormick, Head of QA
Roxann Evans, Project Manager

TESTIMONY OF STEVEN E. NISSEN, M.D.

My name is Steven E. Nissen, M.D. I am chairman of the Department of Cardiovascular Medicine at Cleveland Clinic and the President of the American College of Cardiology (ACC). My testimony does not reflect the views of either Cleveland Clinic or the ACC.

We face a crisis in public confidence in the Food and Drug Administration (FDA) following an unprecedented series of revelations about drug and device safety. The American people no longer trust the FDA to protect their health. Unfortunately, patients are increasingly suspicious of new therapies and sometimes are reluctant to accept potentially life-saving medications or devices. Decisive legislative action is now essential to improve the safety of drugs and medical devices and restore public confidence in this critically important agency.

I have served on many FDA Advisory Panels and this experience has undermined my confidence in the ability of the agency to adequately protect the public health. In 2001, I participated as a guest member of the Arthritis Advisory Panel that recommended a warning label for cardiovascular risk for Vioxx". Under current law, the Agency must "negotiate" with industry to make even simple changes in drug labels and FDA officials frequently make inappropriate concessions to pharmaceutical companies. Following the 2001 Advisory Board, it took 14 months before the FDA could secure agreement from the company to accept a weakly written warning. During this period, patients and physicians were not appropriately warned about the cardiovascular hazards of Vioxx". When the label was eventually modified, the wording was so weak that it did not adequately inform physicians and patients of the potential for Vioxx to cause harm.

In 2005, another disturbing personal experience brought into sharp focus the inadequacies of the FDA in assessing new drug applications. On September 9, 2005, officials from the Endocrine and Metabolism Division presented a new diabetes drug known as muraglitazar to an Advisory Panel for consideration of approval. Because of a previous lawsuit by the advocacy group Public Citizen, the FDA is required to publicly disclose the "briefing materials" for Advisory Panels.

Because of my interest in this class of drugs, I reviewed the briefing documents posted on the Internet by the Agency on September 8, the day before the public hearings. I observed that this investigational drug seemed to lower blood sugar, but I also noted that there was a striking excess of heart attacks, strokes, and deaths in patients treated with muraglitazar compared with placebo or other diabetes drugs. Based upon this observation, I assumed that the Advisory Board would recommend that the Agency not approve muraglitazar.

Yet astonishingly, the following day, Agency reviewers presented the drug in a favorable manner, understating any concerns about cardiovascular risk. This Advisory Panel, that did not include any cardiologists, voted 8:1 to approve muraglitazar, ending the panel meeting at 2 p.m. In Cleveland, I watched the news reports, complete with predictions from financial analysts that this drug would achieve annual sales exceeding $1 billion.

I felt compelled to act. My statistician and I rapidly downloaded the FDA material available from the Internet and performed our own independent analysis of the risks and benefits of this drug. We concluded that muraglitazar doubled the risk of death, heart attack stroke and congestive heart failure. I phoned the editors of the Journal of the American Medical Association, who treated our findings as a public health emergency. Peer reviews were secured in a matter of days, and JAMA posted the manuscript on their Web site October 20, just 7 weeks following the FDA advisory panel meeting. Shortly prior to our publication, the FDA issued an "approvable" letter to the sponsor. Following this publication, the pharmaceutical company developing muraglitazar abruptly ceased all further development. Fortunately, this drug will never threaten the public health, but frankly, it was a close call.

We were able to independently analyze the risks of muraglitazar because the drug was presented to an advisory panel. For many new drugs, the agency approves them without public disclosure of the key findings in pivotal clinical trials. When drugs are presented to Advisory Panels, the agency frequently provides an uncritical presentation that fails to adequate inform the advisory panel members of any internal FDA concerns.

This phenomenon was very evident during a meeting of Drug Safety and Risk Management Advisory Board of the FDA, which met February 9, 2006, to review drugs used to treat Attention Deficit Hyperactivity Disorder or ADHD. I was asked to serve on this Advisory Panel to help evaluate the cardiovascular risks of these drugs, most of which are amphetamines or amphetamine-like agents. These drugs are closely related to methamphetamine or "peed", a major drug of abuse.

At nearly all Advisory panel meetings, the FDA provides a list of questions to the panel members designed to assist in discussions and to guide the formulation of an action plan. When the Advisory Board briefing materials arrived, I was rather surprised by the questions that the Agency intended to ask. In this case, the FDA did not request the committee to consider the risks of the ADHD drugs, nor did they ask us to comment on the need to change labeling. Instead, they asked the committee to discuss how the Agency might study the class of drugs.

During the hearings, we learned that the ADHD drugs increase blood pressure and we heard reports indicating that approximately 25 children has suffered sudden cardiac death after taking these drugs, occasionally after he first dose. ADHD drugs are closely related to ephedra, a drug that the FDA has sought to ban from OTC products. We also learned that 4 million Americans take ADHD drugs, including 1.5 million adults, and up to 10 percent of 5th grade boys.

By mid-afternoon, I had heard enough. I departed from the FDA' carefully orchestrated agenda and introduced a motion proposing that the committee recommend a black box warning for the ADHD drugs. Surprisingly, the motion passed by an 8 to 7 vote. Agency officials looked horrified and quickly called a news conference, where they defended the safety of the drugs and sought to undermine the recommendations of the Advisory Committee.

Some months later, the FDA actually did write new warnings. But it took a rogue advisory committee to motivate the Agency to act.

What the solutions to improving the performance of the FDA?

The FDA operates in a "culture of secrecy." When studies reveal toxicity or lack of efficacy, the Agency does not release the results and the findings are often not published, thereby denying patients and physicians access to vitally important safety information.[1] This approach is antithetical to the public health and undermines good scientific practice. Free and open access to all relevant information is required to enable physicians to thoughtfully select therapies for their patients. The FDA withholds findings in deference to industry' claims that such information constitutes "trade secrets." In my view, this is misguided. When a patient volunteers to participate in a drug or device study, there is an implicit moral obligation that the patient' participation will benefit medical science and their fellow citizens.

Most relevant information on drug safety is readily available to the FDA through "study reports" routinely submitted by pharmaceutical and device companies. However, these reports are usually not widely circulated within the agency and invariably not released to the public or scientific community. It remains theoretically possible to access submitted study reports via a Freedom of Information Act (FOIA) request, but we are usually unaware of the existence of relevant studies. Accordingly, no one ever requests such information.

There are innumerable examples of drug safety information that took years to reach our attention despite reasonable knowledge of the problem within the Agency. Examples include Baycol, Ketek, Vioxx, and antidepressants risks in children. During the months to years in which safety information was not publicly available, many patients suffer complications needlessly. Often, the FDA knew there was a problem. Those of us who prescribe drugs did not.

This lack of transparency dramatically worsened after passage of the Prescription Drug User Fee Act (PDUFA) legislation. Although a well-intentioned effort to speed drug development, PDUFA has seriously undermined the effectiveness and transparency of the Agency. PDUFA makes industry, not the American public, the FDA' primary stakeholder and creates a conflict in loyalty for FDA employees. The time pressure induced by PDUFA deadlines often forces the FDA to make hurried decisions under conditions of considerable uncertainty, resulting in poor outcomes. The premature Advisory Board hearings on muraglitazar represent an excellent example of this phenomenon.[2] Good regulatory decisions are not performed in an environment where a "rush to judgment" is forced by artificial legally-mandated deadlines.

We should fund the FDA from public funds, not fees paid by the regulated industry. Virtually, every American takes one or more medications, so drug safety affects all of us. Yet the annual expenditure for drug regulation approximates only about $2 per person. We cannot expect outstanding performance for an Agency operating on an inadequate budget. The Agency needs more staff to adequate supervise a huge and complex industry. Salary levels should be adequate to attract the most skilled professional staff. The current flight of talented staff from the Agency must be reversed. It takes many years of experience to perform complex regulatory tasks in a skillful fashion. The individuals currently leaving the FDA are simply irreplaceable.

The Agency has suffered from instability in leadership extending to the highest levels. Regardless of which party holds the White House, the FDA needs a passionate and committed leader who will resist pressure to make regulatory decisions based upon political expediency, rather than scientific evidence. The successful efforts by political forces to prevent or delay approval of over-the counter sales of "Plan B", an emergency contraceptive for women, seriously undermined morale at the Agency and must not be repeated. This Agency is too important to allow political expediency to influence decisions.

We need new laws to strengthen the authority of the FDA. Currently, the Agency must "negotiate" with industry to make even simple changes in drug labels. Companies routinely make commitments to perform Phase IV studies, but never actually launch the promised clinical trials and the agency is powerless to act. The requirement for the consent of the regulated industry to change drug labels is simply bad regulatory practice. Professional staff at the Agency should decide the content of labels, not pharmaceutical and device companies.

Some industry practices have seriously undermined drug safety. This problem of "negative publication bias"—the practice of suppressing and never publishing unfavorable studies has a catastrophic effect on the drug development system.[3],[4] When drugs show serious toxicity in patients, the results are rarely published. Accordingly, other companies expose patients to closely related drugs without knowing that study of a similar agent showed significant harm. I am aware of a class of drugs where more than a dozen compounds showed serious toxicity, resulting in termination of development, but without a single publication of results. When studies are not published, we learn nothing from the experiment and make the same mistakes over and over again. This practice also significantly increases the costs of drug development (and ultimately drug prices), because companies continue to follow nonproductive routes to drug development.

The post-marketing surveillance system for drugs and devices functions poorly. Adverse event reporting is voluntary and studies show that only 1 to 10 percent of serious adverse events are ever reported to the Agency. Accordingly, the actual incidence of serious or life-threatened complications cannot be calculated accurately. There are many examples where the failure of the FDA' Averse Event Reporting System (AERS) resulted in serious harm to our citizens. Baycol" caused serious muscle toxicity at rate nearly 100 times greater than other cholesterol lowering drugs in this class.[5] Yet it was marketed for years before this hazard became known and the drug withdrawn.

I believe that Direct to Consumer (DTC) Advertising requires decisive legislative action. The standard for acceptable DTC advertising should require demonstration of a compelling public health advantage for this type of communication. Drugs with an addiction potential, such as sleeping medications, should be specifically prohibited from consumer advertising.

We must address another critical drug safety problem not addressed in this bill—the nutraceutical industry, currently not subject to regulatory scrutiny. This multibillion dollar industry sells so-called "dietary supplements" that are often worthless and sometimes harmful.6 Patients take such drugs instead of effective medications with catastrophic implications for their health. I recently saw a patient who suffered a heart attack after switching from prescription niacin, a drug that raises HDL, the good cholesterol, to "no flush" niacin, a fraudulent therapy with no favorable effects. His cholesterol levels rapidly became abnormal after switching, resulting a very bad outcome.

We need to amend or repeal the Dietary Supplement Health and Education Act (DSHEA) of 1994. By moving dietary supplement out of the regulatory scrutiny of the FDA, we are inviting a public health catastrophe.

It is important for the Congress to recognize that there are many fine and dedicated public servants working within the FDA. However, their concerns fail to reach advisory committees because of the actions of their supervisors, who adopt a less courageous approach.

The Congress must now fully evaluate the deficiencies within the FDA. Your engagement to investigate the problem and take decisive action can improve this Agency. The 300 million American who rely upon drugs to stay healthy are counting on you to take action.

My recommendations for a 10-point program to fix this vitally important agency:

(1) Insulate the FDA from political influence. Let scientific data determine the outcome of regulatory decisions, not politics.

(2) Install FDA leadership with a passion to properly balance the vital need for speedy drug approval with appropriate vigilance on safety.

(3) Create an "open access" system that allows the public and the scientific community access to study reports to enable full discussion of risks and benefits of therapies.

(4) Require all trials involving human subject to be registered and either published or publicly disclosed.

(5) Repeal PDUFA and increase public FDA funding to enable a more thorough, rapid and accurate review of new drug applications and the safety of existing drugs.

(6) Strengthen the laws to allow the FDA to unilaterally re-label drugs when issues of safety of efficacy arise.

(7) Consider stiff civil monetary penalties, and in extreme cases, criminal penalties for withholding vital safety findings from the Agency.

(8) Restructure the post-marketing surveillance system to enable better identification of emerging safety issues.

(9) Restrict DTC advertising to messages that offer a compelling public health benefit.

(10) Enable the FDA to regulate dietary supplements and nutraceuticals.

These measures need not slow drug development. If we improve drug safety oversight, the increased vigilance will inspire confidence and allow us to bring new medicines to patients more quickly, because we will have a better "safety net."

References

(1) Avorn J. Dangerous deception—hiding the evidence of adverse drug effects. N Engl J Med. 2006 Nov 23;355(21):2169–71

(2) Nissen SE, Wolski K, Topol EJ. Effect of muraglitazar on death and major adverse cardiovascular events in patients with type 2 diabetes mellitus. JAMA. 2005 Nov 23;294(20):2581–6. Epub 2005 Oct 20

(3) Smith ER.The importance of negative and neutral clinical trials. Can J Cardiol. 2004 Oct;20(12):1267–8.

(4) Hensley S, Abboud L. Medical research has 'black hole': negative results often fail to get published in journals; some blame drug industry. Wall St J (East Ed). 2004 Jun 4;:B3

(5) Staffa JA, Chang J, Green L.Cerivastatin and reports of fatal rhabdomyolysis. N Engl J Med. 2002 Feb 14;346(7):539–40.

(6) Fontanarosa PB, Rennie D, DeAngelis CD.The need for regulation of dietary supplements—lessons from ephedra.JAMA. 2003 Mar 26;289(12):1568–70. Epub 2003 Mar 10.

(7) DeAngelis CD, Drazen JM, Frizelle FA, Haug C, Hoey J, Horton R, Kotzin S, Laine C, Marusic A, Overbeke AJ, Schroeder TV, Sox HC, Van Der Weyden MB; International Committee of Medical Journal Editors.Is this clinical trial fully registered? A statement from the International Committee of Medical Journal Editors. JAMA. 2005 Jun 15;293(23):2927–9.

Statement of U.S. Senator Chuck Grassley of Iowa
"The Adequacy of FDA Efforts to Assure the Safety of the Drug Supply"
Subcommittee on Oversight and Investigations
House Committee on Energy and Commerce
February 13, 2007

Chairman Dingell, Chairman Stupak, Ranking Members Barton and Whitfield and distinguished colleagues, thank you for holding this important hearing on drug safety and the Food and Drug Administration. Thank you also for inviting me to speak today on this important subject.

During the last three years, I conducted extensive oversight of the Food and Drug Administration while I was Chairman of the Senate Finance Committee, which is responsible for Medicare and Medicaid. I view my role as working to ensure the safety and well-being of the more than 80 million Americans who are beneficiaries of these programs. The Medicare and Medicaid programs spend a lot of money on prescription drugs and medical devices, and that money should be spent on drugs and devices that are safe and effective.

In the course of my oversight of the federal bureaucracy, I have developed many good relationships with whistleblowers. And it was FDA whistleblowers and concerned FDA scientists who first drew my attention to problems at the Food and Drug Administration.

It started in early 2004 with an FDA psychiatrist named Dr. Andrew Mosholder, who realized through his work that there was a serious suicide risk for teenagers taking certain antidepressants. He wanted to make a presentation about his findings to an FDA advisory committee. But for some reason, FDA supervisors didn't want this information to get out. They canceled Dr. Mosholder's presentation and instructed him to write a script approved by his supervisors that he would use if anybody asked him why he was no longer presenting.

That Fall, I held a hearing on drug safety in the aftermath of Vioxx – the blockbuster pain medication – being pulled from the market by its manufacturer, rather than the Food and Drug Administration. The testimony at my hearing turned a bright spotlight on problems with the FDA's postmarket surveillance effort. The FDA works tirelessly, as it should, to approve new life-saving and life-enhancing drugs. But it could do a lot better job of keeping track of developments with these drugs after they're on the market. Reviewing what happened inside the FDA with Vioxx, and in working with a number of whistleblowers who bravely stuck their necks out and came to me after that landmark hearing, I've identified problems at the FDA that consistently fit into a few themes.

First, scientific dissent is discouraged, quashed, and sometimes muzzled inside the Food and Drug Administration. Second, the FDA's relationship with drug makers is too cozy. The FDA worries about smoothing things over with industry much more than it should with its regulatory responsibilities. Third, inside the FDA there's widespread fear of retaliation for speaking up about problems. And fourth, the public safety would be better served if the agency was more transparent and forthcoming about drug safety and drug risks.

These problems involve the culture of the Food and Drug Administration. They're not isolated but systemic. And they can be partly attributed to the organizational structure of the FDA.

My concerns are not isolated either. During the last year, they've been validated by the highly regarded Institute of Medicine, as well as the independent Government Accountability Office and respected medical journals. What's at stake is public safety and public confidence in our nation's world-renowned Food and Drug Administration.

My investigations of FDA issues have also revealed a deeply troubling disregard for Congress' responsibility to conduct oversight of the executive branch of government. The FDA and the Department of Health and Human Services have put up so much resistance to my effort to find out what happened inside the FDA with a relatively new antibiotic called Ketek that I can only wonder what there is to cover up.

Every excuse under the sun has been used to create roadblocks, even in the face of Congressional subpoenas requesting information and access to FDA employees.

In denying access to documents responsive to the subpoenas, the Department and FDA have claimed "prosecutorial deliberative process," "confidential communications," and "agency prerogative to determine who will be interviewed or testify before a jurisdictional committee." Yet, during my years in the Senate, my investigators have obtained access to every single one of these categories of so-called confidential information from HHS as well as other executive branch agencies.

Furthermore, I asked the Congressional Research Service to look into the Department's policies regarding this matter and CRS told me that there is "no legal basis" for the Department's executive branch assertions.

Nevertheless, the Department and FDA not only withheld documents that do not appear to be privileged, but they also won't say what has been withheld and why. The subpoenas compel a privilege log, but the Department and FDA will not provide one.

The Department and FDA say that they have been responsive to the Finance Committee's Ketek investigation because they made available millions of pages of documents to the Committee. But what they provided is quantity, not quality.

They delivered hundreds of pages simply marked, for example, "57 pages removed," or "43 pages removed." (see attachments 1-5) Other documents have whole pages, paragraphs or sentences redacted with no explanation for what has been withheld or redacted and why. (see attachment 6) In fact, the FDA redacted some of the same documents differently[1] and even redacted one of my own letters to them on a different matter (see attachment 7)

When I point out the absurdities in the Department's responses to my requests for documents and interviews related to Ketek, the Department argues it could not provide access to information and individuals related to open criminal investigations. But I didn't

---

[1] For example, FDA redacted a paragraph from one copy of an email without redacting the same paragraph in the second copy. The documents are not attached to this statement because the unredacted portions contain information related to ongoing investigations.

ask for access to open criminal investigations; I don't want to jeopardize a criminal matter. The Department and the FDA know that, yet they keep using that excuse anyway.

Even so, what I've learned about what happened with Ketek troubles me. I've learned that:

- FDA gave its advisory committee questionable data on Ketek and did not tell them about problems with that data. I sent a letter to the FDA in December regarding my findings on this matter and am awaiting a response from the agency.
- FDA approved Ketek without much safety data from the U.S.; the agency relied almost exclusively on foreign, post-marketing safety data ; and
- Ketek's sponsor in all likelihood was aware of the fact that it submitted some questionable data to the FDA regarding its large safety study; the sponsor was informed of problems with one of the study sites prior to data submission to the FDA. However, according to FDA reviewers, the sponsor never raised these problems to the FDA. FDA learned about them after its own investigators inspected the site.

I plan to continue my investigation of Ketek and issue more reports. But I am heartened to hear that FDA came to a decision yesterday that mirrors the recommendations of its internal scientists as well as its advisory committees.

During the last three years, I've also tried to work in a productive way with the Commissioners and Acting Commissioners of the FDA. It will take bold leadership to get on top of the FDA's troubles and turn the agency around. So far, the lip service has been fine. The reality a lot less so.

Last month, Senator Chris Dodd and I reintroduced two reform bills that we first proposed in 2005 to get at the safety shortcomings of the FDA. Our first bill would elevate and empower the office with the FDA that is responsible for monitoring FDA-approved drugs after they're on the market. It would make the "postmarket drug safety" function independent within the FDA, instead of under the thumb of the office and center that puts the drugs on the market in the first place, the way it is today.

Chairman Dingell, the *Wall Street Journal* has reported that you're intrigued by the idea of a drug safety center within the FDA. I appreciate that view. It doesn't make any sense that the FDA officials who are supposed to monitor the safety of a drug on the market serve only as consultants to the FDA officials who approved the drug in the first place. The officials who approved the drug would obviously be conflicted in making a judgment that approval is no longer appropriate or was a mistake in the first place. A separate center for drug safety within the FDA is a vital lynchpin when it comes to meaningful reform and improvement of the agency's postmarket surveillance work.

The second bill that Senator Dodd and I introduced would expand an existing public database by mandating the registry of all clinical trials and the results of those trials. This reform is key to establishing greater transparency regarding clinical trials, the good ones and the bad ones, and to holding drug makers and drug regulators accountable.

Both of these legislative initiatives would make drug information used by doctors and patients more complete and more accessible. American consumers should not have to second guess the safety of the pills in their medicine cabinets.

I appreciate the attention all of you are giving to this important national issue with this hearing. You will hear from some of the heroic whistleblowers who have helped my work, without whom my work wouldn't have been possible. Two of the whistleblowers have left the FDA. It's a tremendous loss for our country when an agency like the Food and Drug Administration gets so dysfunctional that specialists like these whistleblowers are forced to leave the agency to avoid retaliation. I want to work closely with you to make sure FDA whistleblowers can communicate to Congress without fear.

In addition, the existing agreement between the Inspector General for the Department of Health and Human Services and the Food and Drug Administration gives too much power to the FDA when it comes to how allegations of criminal misconduct by FDA employees are investigated. That agreement should be revisited by reform minded leaders in Congress.

I look forward to reform opportunities in the year ahead. There's no doubt that the FDA needs additional tools and resources to do its work. The FDA also needs an overhaul to make the agency more transparent, more forthcoming, and more independent-minded.

I look forward to working with this Committee and in particular with you, Chairmen Dingell and Stupak and Ranking Members Barton and Whitfield, as well as my colleagues in the Senate to enact reforms at the FDA.

Thank you. I would be happy to stay and take a few questions. Unfortunately, I have several other hearings that I must attend so I can't stay long.

United States Senate

COMMITTEE ON FINANCE
WASHINGTON, DC 20510-6200

August 24, 2005

Via Electronic Transmission
Original via USPS Mail

The Honorable Lester M. Crawford, D.V.M., Ph.D.
Commissioner
U.S. Food and Drug Administration
5600 Fishers Lane
Rockville, MD 20857

Dear Commissioner Crawford:

Thank you for the Food and Drug Administration's (FDA) timely response to my letter dated June 24, 2005. I requested that the FDA address questions and provide documents related to non-arteritic anterior ischemic optic neuropathy (NAION) and the use of drugs prescribed by physicians to treat erectile dysfunction (ED), including Viagra, Cialis and Levitra,.

In particular, I asked the FDA to describe, in detail, any actions that will be taken to ensure that patients are informed of NAION and its association with ED drugs. The FDA stated in a letter dated July 20, 2005, that Patient Information Sheets for each ED drug have been posted on the FDA's website that include information about possible vision loss and patients who may be at risk for NAION. That letter also stated that information was provided to over 50,000 individual subscribers by e-mail through MedWatch, the FDA's safety information and adverse event reporting program.

According to IMS Health, a company that monitors prescription drug sales across the nation, prescriptions for ED drugs in 2004 totaled more than [redacted] including [redacted] prescriptions for Viagra, [redacted] prescriptions for Cialis, and [redacted] for Levitra. Although there is a possibility that the 50,000 subscribers to the MedWatch e-mail list and individuals who have accessed the Patient Information Sheets may now be aware of the NAION risks associated with ED drug use, there are millions more who remain in the dark. It seems likely that many millions of men with ED drugs sitting in their medicine cabinets have not visited the FDA's website and/or seen the media reports about the risk of permanent vision loss. In addition, it is unlikely that these millions of men have followed up with the physicians who prescribed them the medication because ED drugs are typically used on an as-needed basis. Dr. Crawford, who will inform these patients and consumers of the concerns that have come to light with regard to the use of ED drugs? Has the FDA considered initiating other action(s) to inform adequately these millions of patients about NAION and its association with ED drug use? More importantly, in the future, how will the FDA attempt to inform patients who do not require regularly scheduled physician follow-up about important safety information regarding their medications?

Finally, the FDA has still not addressed two issues that concern me. Why did it take so long for the FDA to negotiate the label changes for ED drugs and to notify the public of the NAION risk associated with ED drugs? The FDA has a duty to notify the public promptly about a serious risk associated with a drug and identified in the post-market. Permanent blindness surely is such a serious risk.

In closing, I look forward to hearing from you regarding this important matter by no later than September 14, 2005. Should you have any questions regarding this letter, please do not hesitate to contact Emilia DiSanto or Tom Novelli at (202) 224-4515. All formal correspondence should be sent electronically in PDF searchable format to thomas_novelli@finance-rep.senate.gov or via facsimile to (202) 228-2131. All originally material should be sent via USPS mail.

Sincerely,

Chuck Grassley

Charles E. Grassley
Chairman

Memorandum of Understanding

Between the Food and Drug Administration

and

Office of Inspector General

Department of Health and Human Services

PURPOSE:

Recognizing the statutory mandates of both components, and their important roles, and the necessity for maintaining a capable and trained internal investigational unit to conduct internal investigations, to provide a centralized investigative liaison between the Food and Drug Administration (FDA) and the Office of Inspector General (OIG), and to support the OIG's criminal investigations that involve FDA employees, the two components enter into this Memorandum of Understanding concerning the procedures they will observe in internal investigations involving FDA employees.

THE OFFICES

A. <u>The Office of Inspector General</u>

The Inspector General Act of 1978, Public Law 95-452, as amended by Public Law 100-504, 5 U.S.C. App., established the Office of Inspector General as an independent office within the Department of Health and Human Services (HHS). A major purpose of the OIG is to "conduct and supervise audits and investigations relating to the programs and operations of [HHS]." Section 2(1) of the Inspector General Act. The Act further provides that, "in carrying out the duties and responsibilities established under this Act, each Inspector General shall report expeditiously to the Attorney General whenever the Inspector General has reasonable grounds to believe there has been a violation of Federal criminal law." Section 4(d).

D. The Office of Internal Affairs

The FDA, including its Office of Criminal Investigations (OCI), is a component of HHS and is responsible for implementing the Food, Drug, and Cosmetic Act, 21 U.S.C. § 321 et seq. and other statutes. The Office of Internal Affairs (OIA) which is staffed by special agents detailed from OCI, was authorized and established by the Secretary of HHS, within the FDA, Office of Commissioner, to conduct internal investigations of employee misconduct. 60 Fed. Reg. 4417 (January 23, 1995). The OIA Statement of Organization states that OIA "provides a centralized investigative liaison between FDA and [OIG]" and shall serve "as an FDA investigative resource to conduct internal FDA investigations and to support OIG investigations." Id.

PROCEDURES

1. FDA will continue to ensure that its Office of Internal Affairs (OIA) is properly equipped and supported and staffed with trained and experienced criminal investigators (1811-series), and will continue to refresh the OIA staff by assigning agents from FDA's Office of Criminal Investigations to the OIA for duty tours on a rotating basis.

2. The OIG will continue to staff its FDA investigations with trained and experienced criminal investigators (1811-series) and will endeavor to provide adequate resources for investigations so as to enable OIA to investigate promptly after allegations are made.

3. OIG and FDA's OIA shall have prompt access to all files and documents within the FDA relevant to their investigations, and the resulting open investigative files and documents of these investigative entities shall be disclosed outside the Department only to prosecutors and other law enforcement entities, consistent with applicable law and regulation and as necessary to accomplish the respective missions of the OIG and OIA.

4. When OIA receives an allegation of criminal misconduct or violation of the HHS standards of conduct by an HHS employee, OIA shall immediately notify the OIG in writing or by electronic mail. Similarly, when OIG receives an allegation of criminal misconduct or violation of the HHS standards of conduct by an FDA employee it shall, as appropriate with its role under the Inspector General Act, immediately notify OIA in writing or by electronic mail. This notification by the OIG should occur unless the OIG determines that the notification is inconsistent with its role under the Inspector General Act.

5. If, at any point during an investigation, OIA determines that a criminal violation has likely been committed by an FDA employee, OIA shall immediately notify the OIG in writing or by electronic mail. If at any point during an OIG investigation, OIG determines that a criminal violation by an FDA employee has likely occurred, but the OIG determines it will not investigate that violation, it will, as appropriate with OIG's role under the Inspector General Act, immediately notify the OIA in writing or by electronic mail.

6. In recognition of the availability and performance of the FDA OIA, as an existing, trained, equipped and supported investigative unit engaged in investigations of allegations of violative or illegal conduct by FDA employees, and to avoid the duplication of resources and effort that would result from dual focus on any particular investigation, both components anticipate that such investigations will be conducted expeditiously by FDA's OIA, subject to OIG's reservation

of the right in all cases to pursue a case jointly with OIA, or, after consultation with OIA, to replace OIA as the primary agency assigned to an investigation of an FDA employee. OIA will maintain an open file until it receives a final summary and disposition from the OIG on such cases. Any referral of an investigation by the OIG to the OIA will be made expeditiously, enabling OIA to begin any necessary investigation on current information. If OIA believes that its development of an investigation requires issuance of a subpoena duces tecum, it may request that the OIG pursue the case jointly with the OIA.

7. A headquarters OIG/OI supervisor will meet with the OIA Special Agent in Charge on a monthly basis for the purpose of examining all open investigations or cases, preliminary investigations, and any other informal investigative matters which in the judgment of OIA would be of interest to OIG. OIA will provide OIG with a report of all open investigations or cases, preliminary investigations, and any other informal investigative matters which in the judgment of OIA would be of interest to OIG. The outcome of all cases and investigations concluded during the course of the previous month will also be discussed at this meeting.

8. The OIA will provide reasonable notice to the OIG prior to any presentation to the Department of Justice of an investigation in order to allow OIG to participate in the presentation if OIG chooses.

This Memorandum of Understanding is entered into voluntarily by both OIG and FDA. It may be modified at any time by agreement of the parties and may be terminated upon thirty days prior written notice by either agency.

This Memorandum of Understanding shall become effective upon the date of signing by both parties and shall continue until it is modified or terminated.

Signed this 30th day of July, 1998

[signature]	[signature]
...ael A. Friedman, M.D.	June Gibbs Brown
...Deputy Commissioner	Inspector General
...and Drug Administration	

United States Senate

COMMITTEE ON FINANCE
WASHINGTON, DC 20510-6200

December 13, 2006

Via Electronic Transmission

The Honorable Andrew C. von Eschenbach, M.D.
Commissioner
U.S. Food and Drug Administration
5600 Fishers Lane
Rockville, MD 20857

Dear Commissioner von Eschenbach:

The United States Senate Committee on Finance (Committee) has exclusive jurisdiction over the Medicare and Medicaid programs. Accordingly, the Committee has a responsibility to the more than 80 million Americans who receive health care coverage under Medicare and Medicaid to oversee the proper administration of these programs, including the payment for prescription drugs regulated by the Food and Drug Administration (FDA), Department of Health and Human Services (HHS).

Last Spring, the Committee on Finance began investigating extremely troubling allegations related to, among other issues, the approval and post-market surveillance of telithromycin (Ketek) by the Food and Drug Administration. Two of the allegations brought to the attention of the Committee relate to an FDA advisory committee meeting,[1] specifically the Anti-Infective Drugs Advisory Committee (AIDAC or Advisory Committee) meeting held on January 8, 2003. On April 27, 2006, I brought to your attention allegations related to FDA management instructing FDA officials to present fraudulent data to the Advisory Committee because discussing issues regarding data integrity and the conduct of a safety study would not be "productive." The second allegation related to the FDA actually presenting fraudulent study data to the Advisory Committee. The purpose of this letter is to report the Committee's preliminary findings solely with respect to these two allegations. The Committee continues to investigate several other allegations relating to the approval and post-market surveillance of Ketek by the FDA.

---

[1] The FDA convenes expert advisory panels pursuant to the Federal Advisory Committee Act. *See* http://www.access.gpo.gov/uscode/title5a/5a_1_.html. According to the FDA, the value of an advisory committee is to provide independent expert advice, to lend credibility to the FDA's review process, and to allow for public discussion of controversial issues, among others. *See* http://www.fda.gov/oc/advisory/Presentations/NMT05/NMT05TalkShermanLinda.pps#260,20,The Value of an Advisory Committee.

This letter report presents findings and information obtained by the Committee based on the Committee's ongoing investigation to date. It is limited to those allegations related to the AIDAC meeting the FDA convened on January 8, 2003. It is based on interviews conducted by the investigative staff of the Committee (Committee Staff), letter requests to Advisory Committee members, and the Committee's review of documents and information obtained by and provided to the Committee to date. The Committee will continue to investigate all allegations related to Ketek.

The findings presented in this letter may be preliminary for several reasons. First and foremost, the FDA has yet to respond to multiple questions asked by the Committee on June 7, 2006. More than half a year later, the Committee does not have answers from the FDA related to the allegations regarding the AIDAC meeting. In addition, last May the Committee subpoenaed documents and information related to Ketek. To date, HHS and FDA have failed to comply fully with the two congressional subpoenas issued seven months ago. For months, HHS and FDA have failed to take good faith steps toward complying with the Committee's subpoenas.

I also am fully aware that relevant documents and information have been "overlooked" or purposefully withheld from the Committee. Throughout this investigation the Committee has sought and received assurance from FDA that all relevant FDA officials who worked on Ketek matters were notified to produce documents responsive to the Committee's subpoenas. However, the Committee confirmed that at least three FDA officials, who played integral roles in the FDA's review of Ketek, were never asked to review their files and turn over relevant documents in their possession. Therefore, the findings and conclusions in this report to you may be limited in some respects.

To summarize, the Committee Staff reviewed documents and information obtained and received from the FDA and sanofi-aventis,[2] the manufacturer of Ketek, and found the following:

- FDA management knew or should have known that a multitude of questions and concerns regarding serious data integrity problems with a large safety study, Study 3014, were unresolved. Nevertheless, FDA management instructed FDA officials to present that data to the Anti-Infective Drugs Advisory Committee and the public. About two months prior to the Advisory Committee meeting, the study site with the largest number of enrolled subjects was under investigation by FDA's Office of Criminal Investigations. The FDA also inspected the second and third highest enrolling sites and found them to have similarly violated the protocol for Study 3014. In addition, 72 other sites raised red flags for FDA officials and investigators, including nonadherence to the study protocol, which recommended between 4 and 50 study subjects per site. 72 sites enrolled more than 50 subjects and 30 sites enrolled more than 80 subjects. FDA officials also questioned how quickly more than 24,000 patients were enrolled in the study.

- The FDA presented data from Study 3014 to the Advisory Committee, including study data from one study investigator whom the FDA's Office of Criminal

---

[2] Sanofi-Synthélabo merged with Aventis Pharmaceuticals in 2004, forming sanofi-aventis.

Investigations, Division of Scientific Investigations, and the local United States Attorney's Office all believed had falsified and fraudulently submitted clinical trial data. Based in part on data from Study 3014, a majority of the Advisory Committee voted in favor of approving Ketek for the indications of community-acquired pneumonia, acute bacterial sinusitis, and acute exacerbation of chronic bronchitis. Many of the Advisory Committee members were not aware until this past spring of the serious data integrity problems with Study 3014 and that the FDA did not use Study 3014 in approving Ketek.

- The FDA did not ensure that the Advisory Committee had all of the accurate, science-based information it needed to provide the FDA with informed recommendations and advice regarding Ketek. Despite reaching the conclusion that data from the site under criminal investigation should be censored, the FDA did not censor the suspect data before the Advisory Committee meeting. Some of the Advisory Committee members stated that the FDA should have informed them of significant issues or problems related to Study 3014, in a confidential manner if necessary, and that knowledge of the data integrity problems might have affected their actions at the Advisory Committee meeting.

I. Background

On December 13, 2002, the FDA published in the Federal Register a notice for a meeting of the AIDAC. The agenda for the meeting read: "On January 8, 2003, the committee will discuss new drug application (NDA) 21-144, KETEK (telithromycin), Aventis Pharmaceuticals, Inc., proposed for treatment of community-acquired pneumonia [CAP], acute exacerbation of chronic bronchitis [AECB], and acute maxillary sinusitis."[3]

Aventis Pharmaceuticals, Inc., (Aventis) originally submitted its Ketek NDA to the FDA on February 28, 2000. The Ketek NDA was assigned for review to the FDA's Division of Anti-Infective Drug Products (Review Division), Office of Drug Evaluation IV (ODE 4, now Office of Antimicrobial Products), Center for Drug Evaluation and Research (CDER). Accordingly, supervisory authority of the Ketek NDA review was held by the Director of the Review Division, and the Director of ODE 4, who supervised the Division Director.

The AIDAC meeting convened by the FDA on January 8, 2003, was the second meeting of the Advisory Committee to consider the Ketek NDA. Previously, the FDA convened the AIDAC in April 2001. At the first meeting of the AIDAC, the Advisory Committee members recommended that Aventis obtain additional safety data from a large sample of patients before Ketek could be approved for acute bacterial sinusitis (ABS) and AECB.

After consideration of the Ketek NDA by the Review Division, as well as the recommendations made by the AIDAC, the FDA issued an "approvable letter" to Aventis on June 1, 2001, for the indications of CAP, ABS, and AECB.[4] The FDA's approvable

---

[3] http://www.fda.gov/ohrms/dockets/98fr/02-31443.htm.

[4] According to a Medical Officer Review on hepatic adverse events of special interest, dated July 24, 2002, "During the review of that [Ketek] application and in subsequent discussion by the Anti-Infective Drugs Advisory Committee on April 26, 2001, safety concerns, including potential for hepatotoxicity, were

letter requested that Aventis perform a large safety study of patients in a usual care setting to examine the potential toxicities of Ketek with regard to cardiac, hepatic (liver), visual, and vascular safety. The FDA's approvable letter stated:

> It would be helpful to conduct a Phase III study of CAP/AECB/ABS to assess further adverse events associated with telithromycin, particularly in patients at increased risk for potential drug-related toxicity. Such a study should be randomized, with at least 35% of the recruited study population consisting of patients 50 years of age and older. Exclusion criteria regarding concomitant medications should be minimized. Recruitment of patients with renal and/or hepatic impairment is encouraged. This study should include the monitoring and analysis of all adverse events, with particular attention to hepatic, visual, cardiovascular, and vasculitic adverse events.

In response to the FDA's June 2001 approvable letter, Aventis submitted an amendment to the Ketek NDA on July 24, 2002, containing the large safety study requested by the FDA to evaluate adverse events in the usual care setting (Study 3014).[5] Aventis conducted Study 3014 primarily to address the request for a large safety study to examine adverse events of special interest (cardiac, hepatic, visual, and vasculitic) and to better characterize the hepatic risk profile of Ketek in a usual care setting.[6]

Pursuant to the FDA's Bioresearch Monitoring (BIMO) Program,[7] the FDA inspected the highest enrolling investigation center for Study 3014—Dr. Marie "Anne" Kirkman-Campbell, who enrolled 407 subjects—in mid-October 2002. Shortly thereafter, the FDA field investigator reported to the FDA's Office of Criminal Investigations (OCI), within the Office of Regulatory Affairs (ORA)[8] that the regulatory inspection of Dr. Kirkman-

---

raised...there were two serious hepatic adverse events plausibly associated with telithromycin administration...These cases factored into the recommendation by the AIDAC and the Division's decision to require a larger safety study prior to drug approval. Study 3014 was designed to examine adverse events of special interest, including hepatic events, in a large population of patients with acute community-acquired respiratory infections...The study was powered to detect with 95% confidence adverse events occurring at rates of at least 1 in 4,000."

[5] Randomized, Open-Label, Multicenter Trial of the Safety and Effectiveness of Oral Telithromycin (Ketek®) and Amoxicillin/Clavulanic Acid (Augmentin®) In Outpatients With Respiratory Tract Infections in Usual Care Settings, HMR3647A/3014, Telithromycin.

[6] At the request of the Committee, Aventis prepared and submitted a "Ketek® Study 3014 Timeline" in October 2006. Aventis completed design of the protocol for Study 3014 on September 27, 2001, and officially submitted it to the FDA on October 17, 2001. According to the clinical study protocol, the duration of the study was expected to be five to eight months. Aventis enrolled the first subject on October 19, 2001, and the last on January 29, 2002. Over 24,000 patients were enrolled at 1824 investigation centers in less than four months.

[7] According to the FDA, the BIMO Program is a comprehensive program of on-site inspections and data audits designed to monitor all aspects of the conduct and reporting of FDA-regulated research. The BIMO Program was established to assure the quality and integrity of data submitted to the agency in support of new product approvals, as well as, to provide for protection of the rights and welfare of the thousands of human subjects involved in FDA-regulated research. It has become a cornerstone of the FDA pre-approval process for new medicines, medical devices, food and color additives, and veterinary products introduced to the U.S. consumer. See http://www.fda.gov/ora/compliance_ref/bimo/background.html.

[8] According to the FDA website, the Office of Criminal Investigations "has the primary responsibility for all criminal investigations conducted by the FDA, including suspected tampering incidents and suspected counterfeit products." OCI investigates criminal activities that violate the Federal Food, Drug, and

Campbell "identified numerous regulatory deficiencies along with possible criminal violations."[9] At the end of October, OCI reported the preliminary results of its investigation to the United States Attorney: "it is believed Dr. Campbell falsified clinical trial results … ."[10] By mid-November 2002, OCI notified the Review Division that a criminal investigation of Dr. Kirkman-Campbell had been initiated.[11] By then the Review Division had also requested additional BIMO inspections of the second and third highest enrolling sites.[12]

While the DSI inspections and OCI investigation related to Study 3014 were ongoing, the Review Division continued its preparations for the second AIDAC meeting to be held on January 8, 2003. Data from Study 3014, as well as foreign post-marketing data, were prepared for presentation to the AIDAC. On January 8, 2003, the FDA asked the Advisory Committee members to address four questions[13]:

1. Do the safety and effectiveness data presented support the use of Ketek for CAP, ABS and/or AECB? If yes, are there any special caveats that should be included in the label? If no, what other information would be required?
2. Do the safety and effectiveness data presented support the use of Ketek for the treatment of penicillin-resistant *S. pneumoniae* for CAP and/or ABS? If yes, are there any special caveats that should be included in the label? If no, what other information would be required?
3. Do the safety and effectiveness data presented support the use of Ketek for the treatment of macrolide-resistant *S. pneumoniae* for CAP and ABS? Please consider in your discussion the public health impact of macrolide-resistant *S. pneumoniae*. If yes, are there any special caveats that should be included in the label? If no, what other information would be required?
4. Are there any additional studies of Ketek you would recommend?

For question 1, 11 members voted yes and 1 member voted no for the indications of CAP and ABS; 8 voted yes and 4 voted no for AECB. For question 2, 7 members voted yes and 5 members voted no for both indications. Similarly, for question 3, 7 members voted yes and 5 members voted no for both indications.

Two weeks after the Advisory Committee meeting, DSI provided the Review Division with its findings and recommendations to date regarding data from the three highest enrolling investigation sites. In its memorandum dated January 21, 2003, DSI recommended that the Review Division consider excluding specific data from one site and not use any data from another in support of the Ketek NDA until outstanding issues

---

Cosmetic Act, including schemes to defraud the Medicare and Medicaid programs that involve FDA-regulated products. OCI often collaborates with other federal and state law enforcement agencies.
[9] FDA, OCI, Report of Investigation submitted by Special Agent Robert West on November 29, 2002.
[10] Letter to United States Attorney Alice Waters from Mr. R. Bradenbaugh, Acting Special Agent in Charge, FDA Office of Criminal Investigations, dated October 30, 2002.
[11] Email from OCI to Review Division and DSI, dated November 14, 2002.
[12] "DSI Consult: Request for Clinical Inspections," dated November 13, 2002.
[13] http://www.fda.gov/ohrms/dockets/ac/03/questions/3919Q1.htm.

were investigated and resolved. Several days later, on January 24, 2003, the FDA issued an approvable letter to Aventis.[14]

II. FDA Management Instructed FDA Officials to Present Highly Suspect Study Data to an Advisory Committee; FDA Presented Study Data to an Advisory Committee Despite Numerous "Red Flags" About the Integrity of the Study Data

Prior to the Advisory Committee meeting on January 8, 2003, FDA management, the Office Director and Division Director, should have been fully aware that a multitude of questions, concerns, and red flags regarding serious data integrity problems with Study 3014 were unresolved. In fact, nearly two months before the Advisory Committee meeting, OCI notified the Review Division and DSI that a criminal investigation was underway involving Study 3014. In November 2002, OCI communicated to the Review Division that the site under investigation might affect "the overall 'approvability' of this [Ketek] NDA." Communications between DSI and the Review Division in early December also suggest that "the [Ketek] NDA should be placed on hold until the matters are resolved."

Six days before the AIDAC meeting, the team leader for the Ketek NDA emailed the Office Director and copied the Division Director seeking to talk about "the extent to which we should communicate to or discuss with the committee issues regarding data integrity and study conduct for Study 3014":

> DSI has sent us the 483 for the second highest enrolling site (Dr. Lang) for the large Ketek safety study (Study 3014); they identified some (although not all) of the same GCP problems seen in the highest enrolling site (Dr. Kirkman-Campbell), including:
>
> - Patient enrollment far in excess of limits recommended by the IRB
> - Enrollment of clinic staff in the study
> - Enrollment of patients who should have been excluded (patients with drug allergy or who were nursing)
> - Failure to obtain baseline LFTs in >two dozen patients (~10% of total) or on-therapy LFTs in a dozen patients.
> - Significant discrepancies between source documentation and clinical investigator memos.
>
> Dr. Kirkman-Campbell had similar GCP issues; in addition, she enrolled a substantial number of patients who presented to her clinic for weight control, and were not seeking medical attention for a respiratory tract infection. DSI has recommended exclusion of data from her site, has referred her case to the Office of Criminal Investigations, and is considering an official action such as disqualification.

---

[14] A timeline of major events related to the approval and post-market surveillance of Ketek is attached to this letter (Attachment 1). An approvable letter means the NDA substantially meets the requirements of the Food and Drug Administration's regulations on the approval of new drugs (Part 314 of Title 21 of the Code of Federal Regulations), and the agency believes that it can approve the application if specific additional information or material is submitted or the applicant agrees to specific conditions.

> The third largest enroller, Dr. Salerno, did not have signficant [sic] GCP violations, but had been placed on probation by the state of California for poor record-keeping at the [time] that he was involved in the study; three months after the last patient was enrolled at his site, he was arrested on weapons and drug use charges.
>
> We do not know how pervasive these problems are at this point. Since we will be asking the AC to make recommendations on the basis of the data presented to them, Janice and I would like to talk with you about the extent to which we should communicate to or discuss with the committee issues regarding data integrity and study conduct for Study 3014. Is there any time this afternoon that would work for you?

The Office Director replied: "In general I don't believe spending time on these issues in front of the AC [Advisory Committee] wil [sic] be productive. I do feel that having the company make the best possible presentation of their PM [foreign post-marketing] data focusing on information from countries where we have confidence in reporting will be useful."

However, at least as early as November 19, 2002, the Review Division reached the conclusion that data from the highest enrolling site, which was under criminal investigation, would have to be censored from Study 3014. Despite reaching this conclusion nearly two months before, several Review Division officials informed Committee staff that data from this site was not censored after all. Data from all sites submitted by Aventis was included in the FDA's and Aventis' presentations to the Advisory Committee on January 8, 2003. FDA officials stated that there was not enough time to remove the data and re-analyze Study 3014 before the meeting. Other FDA staff stated that removing the data from the site under criminal investigation, or data from any other site under for-cause inspection related to data integrity problems, would raise questions from Advisory Committee members and potentially jeopardize ongoing investigations.

A. Criminal Investigation of Highest Enrolling Study Site—Dr. Kirkman Campbell

Two months before the AIDAC meeting, the FDA's Office of Criminal Investigations initiated an investigation of the highest enrolling site in Study 3014. The principal investigator at this site, Dr. Kirkman-Campbell, enrolled 407 patients in the study, eight times more than the recommended maximum enrollment specified in the study protocol and approved by the institutional review board.

According to Committee interviews with FDA officials, the number of enrolled patients, as well as how rapidly Dr. Kirkman-Campbell reached those numbers, raised red flags within the Review Division. The Division of Scientific Investigations conducted its inspection of Dr. Kirkman-Campbell's site in September 2002,[15] and referred its

[15] A "DSI Consult: Request for Clinical Inspections," dated September 11, 2002, shows the Review Division Director requested that inspections be performed and Inspection Summary Results be provided for Dr. Kirkman-Campbell by December 17, 2002.

inspection findings to OCI for criminal investigation in October 2002[16] On November 1, 2002, DSI notified the Review Division about "major documentation problems" found at Dr. Kirkman-Campbell's site.[17]

OCI began investigating Dr. Kirkman-Campbell in October 2002. On November 14, 2002, OCI notified the Review Division and DSI about its investigation:

> As I have stated, OCI has initiated a criminal investigation of Dr. Kirkman-Campbell. There is good reason to believe that Dr. Kirkman-Campbell falsified a lot of the patient data on this study . . . It is my understanding that the advisory committee will convene on 01/08/2003 to review this NDA for approval. I would encourage a careful consideration of the impact Dr. Kirkman-Campbell's data might have on the overall 'approvability' of this NDA.

According to an email written by the Regulatory Project Manager responsible for the Ketek NDA, dated November 19, 2002, the Review Division reached the conclusion that Dr. Kirkman-Campbell's data would have to be censored from Study 3014:

> We have an advisory committee meeting on January 8, 2003, and the action date is January 24, 2003. But do not despair yet!!! The Division already decided to take Dr. Kirkman-Campbell's data out of the database.

The conclusion that Dr. Kirkman-Campbell's data would be censored from Study 3014 is also supported by an email exchange within OCI, dated November 25, 2002: "My contact at CDER advised that Campbell's data has been removed from the NDA database."

---

[16] According to a summary of a Regulatory Briefing held on February 19, 2003, DSI referred Dr. Kirkman-Campbell to OCI based on the following findings as well as communications with PPD, the contract research organization (CRO) hired by Aventis to monitor the study: "Enrollment of patients who were being seen for weight loss therapy, rather than the conditions specified in the protocol," "Documentation of patients as having completed courses of therapy despite statements from patients that they had not received medication," "Enrollment of patients in numbers far in excess of those approved by the local IRB, without IRB review," and "Enrollment of patients documented as being ineligible for the study on the basis of drug allergies." Other findings of concern were enrollment of the investigator's family and staff and the absence of any reported adverse events for the first 100 patients enrolled at the site. According to the Regulatory Briefing Summary, the investigator did not begin reporting adverse events until confronted by PPD.

[17] Email sent from DSI to Review Division on November 1, 2002: "This is an update to you all in regards to our inspection of Dr. Kirkman-Campbell at Gadsden, AL site. DSI has not received the EIR yet. But, the field has issued a 483 to Dr. Campbell. It appears that the site has major documentation problems. One of the items on 483 stated 'subjects were routinely enrolled in the study that were seen by the PI for reasons other than the conditions under study (AS, AECB, CAP) i.e., as part of a weight loss program. Many subjects were not seeking treatment for the study conditions nor were reporting the study conditions as a reason for the visit to the clinic. Several subjects were enrolled with questionable diagnoses or lack of documentation of history of chronic bronchitis.' The field investigator also noticed that the site enrollment did not seem to include subjects with pneumonia. Dr. Campbell told her that that would require chest X-ray. The other items cited that the IRB approved protocol was to enroll 4 to 50 subjects per site and this site enrolled over 400 subjects including her study coordinator and two staff members in the study. I will inform you all with more information upon our review of the EIR and exhibits when received. Thanks."

The Honorable Andrew C. von Eschenbach, M.D.
Page 9 of 20

By early December, officials within the Review Division were greatly concerned about Study 3014. An email exchange within the Review Division on December 10, 2002, highlighted the level of concern:

> Official 1: "read these [DSI] messages. The validity of 3014 is growing more suspect by the day."
>
> Official 2: "I think [the Division Director] agrees with us. While it might not go in the briefing document, it will eventually come back to haunt all parties involved—us if we do nothing, the public if the data is not trustworthy, and the sponsor for not having disclosed these findings to us."

On December 19, 2002, the Review Division discussed its concerns during a meeting with Aventis to prepare for and discuss the agenda for the upcoming AIDAC meeting. According to the minutes of that meeting:

> Aventis indicated that they had reviewed the Division's briefing package for the upcoming AC and having identified some areas of disagreement, they would like to discuss them. These areas are related to the conduct of study #3014 . . . The Division is concerned about the integrity of the data for this study based on recent Division of Scientific Invetigations [sic] (DSI) inspection. At the Division's request, Aventis described the monitoring process they used during the conduct of the study. They pointed to difficulties with follow-up on reported irregularities, considering the fast enrollment achieved during this trial. The following investigators were mentioned specifically: [FDA REDACTION] Anne Kirkman-Campbell, M.D. (largest enroller)- DSI issued a 483 form to this investigator. Aventis indicated that when they became aware of irregularities at this site, her participation was discontinued. The sponsor indicated that they did not identify other investigators with the same degree of irregularities as Dr. Kirkman-Campbell. [FDA REDACTION] Egisto Salerno, M.D. (third largest enroller). Aventis indicated that a 483 form was issued to Dr. Salerno the same day of this meeting and that they were unaware that Dr. Salerno was on probation [FDA REDACTION] at the time the study was conducted.

An email exchange between officials in the Review Division on December 23, 2002, highlighted the frustration of one official coming out of this meeting:

> Famous quote for future reference "There are no other Kirkman-Campbells in this NDA." - said by Aventis at Thursday's meeting. I suppose technically speaking they are correct, since there is only one Kirkman-Campbell. I just wish we could find even a single credible large-enrolling site in 3014.

B. Inspections of Second and Third Highest Enrolling Sites in Study 3014—Drs. Lang and Salerno

According to DSI officials interviewed by the Committee staff, it is relatively routine for DSI to inspect several of the highest enrolling sites as part of FDA's review of an NDA. A number of Review Division officials also stated that it was common for there to be isolated data integrity problems in clinical studies, especially in a large study, conducted in a usual-care setting. The Office Director described Study 3014 as an "experiment."

After the data integrity concerns identified at Dr. Kirkman-Campbell's high-enrolling site, the Review Division submitted requests to DSI on November 13, 2002, for inspections of the second and third highest enrolling sites prior to the AIDAC meeting. The Division Director requested that inspections be performed and Inspection Summary Results be provided for Dr. Carl Lang, who enrolled 251 subjects, and Dr. Egisto Salerno, who enrolled 214. Based on the Committee Staff's review of emails, there appeared to be a sense of urgency among DSI staff to get these additional inspections completed before the AIDAC meeting. The day after the Review Division submitted the request, DSI sent it to the regional field investigators, setting a deadline of December 20, 2002, for completion of the inspections.

The FDA's inspection of the second highest enrolling site was completed prior to the AIDAC meeting, and the investigators found some of the same GCP problems that were seen at Dr. Kirkman-Campbell's site. On December 23, 2002, a DSI official notified two Review Division officials regarding its inspection of the second highest enrolling site:

> The 483 for Dr. Lang is being drafted and will be issued 12/30. The inspector is seeing some similar problems found at Kirkman Campbell. The issues were 251 subjects enrolled over the the [sic] max 50 recommended, enrolling study coordinator and his family, inadequate documentation that subjects were not hypersensitive to beta-lactam and macrolide antibiotics, some records lacked documentation of negative pregnancy test results for wocbp, and drug accountability log entries were not concurrent. Also the site shipped laboratory samples incorrectly, and numerous laboratory samples were beyond stability. When we receive the 483, [DSI will] fax it to you . . . .

Shortly thereafter, the email was circulated within the Review Division, including to the Division Director and the Office Director, with the message:

> As you may recall, Dr. Lang is the second largest enroller in study # 3014, with 251 patients. The first enroller was Dr. Kirkman-Campbell with 407 patients, and a 483 was issued to her too. The third enroller (214 patients) was Dr. Salerno, who had his license suspended at the time of the study, as per the California Medical Licensing Board. This brings the total of 872 patients (3.5%) with questionable data."

The FDA ran into some difficulties with the inspection of the third highest enrolling site. An email exchange between a DSI official and Review Division officials, dated December 4, 2002, identified problems encountered in attempting to inspect the third highest enrolling site:

> FDA Investigator [] is trying to arrange the inspection with Dr. Salerno . . . he is out on medical leave, for brain tumor, until January. Due to the pending advisory meeting and PDUFA due date, we have asked . . . to see if the study coordinator could provide access to the records earlier. Meanwhile, [the field investigator] emailed me the following "interesting reading" on Dr. Salerno. It appears that there may be problems with his study site too, even before starting the inspection.

According to the "interesting reading," in June 2001, Dr. Salerno had been disciplined by his state Medical Board for gross negligence and failing to maintain adequate and accurate medical records. He was placed on 2 years probation. In May 2002, a state judge also ordered the temporary suspension of his medical license.

An email from a DSI official to an FDA field investigator, dated December 10, 2002, stated, "....With the new findings (see below) and your 'interesting reading' on Dr. Salerno, the review division feels it is very important to look at the quality of his data and have a report before the Advisory Committee meeting on January 8, 2003."

Aside from communicating this information regarding Dr. Salerno, DSI did not provide a report to the Review Division prior to the AIDAC meeting. However, according to a DSI memorandum to the Review Division dated January 21, 2003, DSI received the observational findings from the field investigation of Dr. Salerno on December 19, 2002 three weeks before the Advisory Committee meeting.

C. FDA Officials Aware of Red Flags Regarding Study 3014 prior to Advisory Committee Meeting

In addition to the criminal investigation of Dr. Kirkman-Campbell, the FDA had several additional red flags regarding Study 3014. Even before Aventis submitted Study 3014, FDA received at least one complaint from a study subject in Study 3014. As early as January 2002, FDA investigators interviewed a study subject enrolled in Study 3014, who "reported that following her completion of the study she complained of abdominal pain, headaches, and dry mouth. Four days later she had chills, fever (108°) and cough . . . the subject alleges that the investigator may not have reported adverse event(s)." In May 2002, DSI requested that an FDA field investigator initiate a directed inspection of this site to determine if adverse event reports were adequately documented and if the Clinical Investigator's overall conduct of the study was in compliance with federal regulations and good clinical practices.[18]

Also, in June 2002, Aventis notified FDA that data from two low-enrolling study sites, the fourth and fifth questionable sites, "cannot be confirmed or corrected, and therefore will not be included in the study."[19] Pursuant to notification from Aventis, DSI issued a request for a "for cause" inspection of one of these study sites in October 2002.

Review Division officials interviewed by the Committee Staff stated that "red flags" were apparent as soon as Aventis submitted Study 3014 in July 2002. One official stated that he recognized potential data integrity issues with Study 3014 and recalled that more than 100 centers did not adhere to the study protocol, which recommended enrollment between 4 and 50 subjects per site. Another red flag for this official was how quickly Aventis enrolled more than 24,000 patients. This official wanted to look at the study data closely because the study was conducted in a "usual care setting" where one would

---

[18] By letter dated May 8, 2003, the FDA notified this study site's clinical investigator that: "You did not maintain adequate and accurate records [21 CFR 312.629(b)] in that you did not document a past medical history of chronic bronchitis for subjects [4 out of 30 subjects] to support the diagnosis of acute exacerbation of chronic bronchitis; and you did not document that a visit 1 pregnancy test was performed for [a] subject."

[19] *See* footnote 4.

expect to see less rigor. On August 4, 2002, this Review Division official sent an email under the subject "Ketek – Statistical Issues" to colleagues in the Review Division, and wrote:

> When I began to look at the report it appears we have a significant under reporting of AE in the big study 3014 approx 23% while in the phase III studies about 50%. The number [Aventis] gave at our pre-NDA meeting of 50% is not true for the big study. I think more care should be given to what we want to achieve.

Several FDA officials told Committee Staff that the sponsor's past behavior on the Ketek NDA was also a red flag. As a result, these FDA reviewers and investigators stated that they were raising questions and concerns about the completeness and timeliness of the information submitted by the sponsor after FDA received the sponsor's resubmission of the Ketek NDA in July 2002. As summarized in his email dated February 19, 2006, an FDA official in the Review Division stated, "[Aventis'] 'cultural' problem is something that has been a consistent recurrent theme throughout the history of the NDA and its something that we've just had to work around."

A series of emails between FDA officials also highlight the scrutiny being given to high-enrolling sites in Study 3014. These emails between officials in OCI, DSI, ORA, and the Review Division show that a fourth high-enrolling study site in Study 3014 had problems. In fact, ORA raised to the Review Division placing a hold on the Ketek NDA. By email dated December 9, 2002, the FDA field investigator who inspected Dr. Kirkman-Campbell's site reported similar problems at a fourth study site:

> We just learned (from a source) of another [site] that should be inspected on the Ketek study . . . The town is smaller than Gadsden, AL & [the site] enrolled 99 patients . . . [including] staff and [] family members. There were scant study records & numerous informed consent violations. It looks like there were many other sites with numerous [informed consent form] violations, small towns w/large enrollment, & sites that enrolled their won [sic] staff, etc. . . . It looks like the NDA should be placed on hold until the matters are resolved.

DSI forwarded this email to the Review Division and stated:

> [The FDA investigator for Dr. Kirkman-Campbell] has unearthed more troubling news on the Ketek study. It is too late to issue an assignment now though we could certainly inspect the site post-PDUFA. I will let you know as soon as I hear any findings on Lang and Salerno.

An email dated December 23, 2002, stated:

> One thing that all three of these investigators have in common is that they enrolled a total number of patients that was in excess of the allowable amount (which was 50, I believe). I looked through the rest of the sites and there are a total of 72 sites that enrolled over 50 patients. The total number of patients at sites in which an excess of 50 patients were enrolled comes to 6,459. I'm not sure what this means. Is it common for companies to allow centers to enroll beyond the allowable amount? Is this viewed as acceptable? Obviously, the

company is sending the investigators additional ketek to cover the additional patients, so they must be aware of this.

An email exchange on December 14, 20002, between Review Division officials, which copied the Division Director, related to the subject "High Enrollers in 3014 – food for thought":

> Official 1: "I looked at enrollment patterns for all sites in 3014 that randomized 80 patients or more; there were 30 such sites. Of these, 9/30 (30%) enrolled 1% or more of the adult population of the city or town in which they are located (based on 2000 census figures). This is equivalent to a site in Montgomery County enrolling over 6500 patients in a 3 month period. While for some sites high enrollment can be explained by the size of the catchment area, this is not true for all such sites. . . . Another point to keep in mind is that the incidences of the respiratory tract infections studied in 3014 probably don't exceed 1% in this country; thus, for those sites where high enrollment figures cannot be explained by the size of the surrounding catchment, virtually *every* patient seeking medical attention for a community-acquired RTI would have had to be enrolled for the figures to be real.
>
> Official 2: "that's very interesting and very concerning. It certainly adds further doubt as to the veracity of the study results. It seems a little unusual for a study to have so many questionable sites and it certainly raises alarms as to the way in which the study was conducted."
>
> A third official responded in early January: "I agree with your thinking on this--I would like to look at how census and CDC reporting data may help us locate fraudulent sites in NDA databases. I am not sure why so many are classified as 'Unknown Race' not Caucasian, Asian/oriental or black---could be Hispanic?? but that should have been a known category. When race and age are missing data fields it often suggests the subjects are made up. I guess without DSI's help it is very difficult to know."

Contemporaneously with the scrutiny of the high-enrolling sites, including Drs. Campbell, Lang, and Salerno, in November and December 2002, the FDA conducted an investigation of a seventh site in Study 3014 and also found objectionable observations.[20]

In his memorandum dated November 6, 2003, the Medical Team Leader summarized other red flags regarding the conduct of Study 3014. Specifically, he stated:

> The settings in which high enrollment occurred also raised concern over data integrity. Of the top 30 enrollers, 8 enrolled 1% or more of the adult population of the cities in which they were located. Although in a few sites high enrollment may be explained by proximity to large urban areas, for others the actual

---

[20] By letter dated February 11, 2003, FDA concluded this site "did not adhere to applicable statutory requirements and FDA regulations governing the conduct of clinical investigations . . . includ[ing] your failure to maintain completed informed consents and case report forms for study subjects, and your failure to sign the return shipment form for investigational product [21 C.F.R. 312.62 (a) and (b)]."

> enrollment is inconsistent with the enrollment predicted on the basis of the catchment population. Given the incidences of the respiratory tract infections under study and the investigational nature of this drug, this finding raises further concerns over data integrity in this study. . . . None of these issues regarding data integrity were presented at the January 2003 AIDAC meeting.

During his interview with Committee Staff, the Review Division official charged with presenting Study 3014 at the AIDAC meeting stated that he was not satisfied with what he knew about the integrity of Study 3014 and he was against presenting it at all. When asked why he presented a study he knew to have data integrity problems, the official replied that he was asked directly by the Division Director to present Study 3014 during a team meeting. He said he viewed this as a verbal instruction. He said he proposed a closed session to discuss the agency's "significant concerns" with Study 3014 with the Advisory Committee members, but was told by his Division Director that FDA could not disclose information related to an ongoing FDA investigation. The official who presented Study 3014 stated to the Committee, "[the FDA] should never have a role in deceiving the public," and added, "[a]ll of us will have a consequence for this."

Many FDA officials interviewed acknowledged that, at a minimum, Dr. Kirkman-Campbell's data should have been censored. Several officials acknowledged that, with hindsight, the AIDAC meeting should have been postponed or canceled.

II. Anti-Infective Drugs Advisory Committee Member's Comments

In October, the Committee sought comments from 11 voting members[21] of the Advisory Committee present at the January 8, 2003, meeting.[22] The Committee provided copies of two letters the Committee sent to the FDA in April and June of 2006, which outlined the allegations and concerns brought to the attention of the Committee regarding the FDA's approval and post-market surveillance of Ketek. Since October, seven Advisory Committee members have provided comments to the Committee.

The October letter to the AIDAC members requested their response to a series of questions regarding their knowledge of the data integrity problems of Study 3014 and their participation in the January 8, 2003, meeting. A table of the AIDAC members' responses is attached to this letter (Attachment 3). Information that could identify the respondents directly or indirectly has been redacted. Also redacted are references to products other than Ketek.

The data integrity problems with Study 3014 were intentionally withheld from the AIDAC members during the January 8, 2003, meeting. However, the Review Division Director stated to Committee staff that she advised members of the advisory committee of the data integrity problems with Study 3014 during a closed session of the AIDAC on March 6, 2003. Given that participation of advisory committee members may vary from meeting to meeting, the Committee asked the members who attended the January 8, 2003, meeting, "Did you attend a closed meeting of the AIDAC on March 6, 2003? If yes, do

---

[21] The Committee was not able to obtain contact information for one of the voting members of the January 8, 2003 Anti-Infective Drugs Advisory Committee.
[22] *See* Attachment 2

you recall whether or not the FDA discussed data integrity problems with Study 3014?" Five of the seven members who responded to the Committee's letter did not attend that meeting, and one of the two respondents who may have attended stated that Study 3014 data integrity problems were not discussed at that meeting. Therefore, even if the AIDAC did receive a status report on Study 3014 in March 2003, it appears that the FDA was not updating all of the appropriate members of the advisory committee—the members who actually voted on Ketek and recommended approval in a public forum.

Since the AIDAC voted on Ketek based, in part, on Study 3014 data, which FDA ultimately did not consider in its decision to approve Ketek, the Committee asked the AIDAC members, "If you did not attend the AIDAC meeting on March 6, 2003, when do you first recall learning about data integrity problems with Study 3014?" Five out of the 7 respondents were not aware of the data integrity problems until this year. One did not provide a response and another was not sure when he/she first became aware of the problems. Two members stated that they were not aware of the data integrity problems associated with Study 3014 until they read a report in the media regarding Ketek. Two other members first learned of the data integrity problems associated with Study 3014 when they received the Committee's letter.

A copy of DSI's March 2004 memorandum, which outlined DSI's findings and recommendations regarding the data integrity of Study 3014, was provided to the AIDAC members as an attachment to the Committee's October letter. The AIDAC members were asked about their awareness of the extent of data integrity problems associated with the conduct of Study 3014 prior to reviewing the DSI memorandum, and none of the respondents stated that they had been aware of the extent of the problems. For example, one AIDAC member stated, "I was not aware of the extent of data integrity problems until I received a letter dated July 7, 2006, from the FDA that included Senator Grassley's letter dated June 7, 2006, and subsequent materials from Senator Grassley's office dated October 27, 2006." Another stated, "I was certainly not aware that FDA had decided to withdraw any consideration of Study 3014 in their decision but there was discussion, limited, at the 2nd Advisory Committee meeting concerning the availability and validity of the EU data."

Several AIDAC members also responded that knowledge of the data integrity problems might have affected their vote. The Committee asked each member "Do you believe your vote and recommendations regarding the risk-benefit profile of Ketek would have changed if the FDA had disclosed that Study 3014 had some data integrity problems and that the FDA was still reviewing the extent of the problems?" Two members stated their votes would have changed, and one of those individuals added that had the information been revealed to the advisory committee, "the meeting might well have gone a different way." Another AIDAC member said that he/she would have recommended postponing the decision on Ketek "until the extent and significance of the data integrity problems were better defined," while another said he/she would have sought more information about the nature and extent of the problems.

Furthermore, several AIDAC members did not share the Office Director's opinion that it would not have been "productive" to spend time on issues regarding data integrity and the conduct of Study 3014. While some of them responded that there are conditions under which known data integrity problems could be withheld from an advisory committee, such as information associated with an ongoing investigation or minimal or trivial data integrity issues, others felt that the advisory committee should have been informed of the problems with Study 3014. For example, one respondent stated, "I believe that all information of note or with significant ramifications should be made available to the committee." One of the respondents who commented that it would be appropriate to withhold trivial information from the advisory committee noted that "study 3014 appears to be riddled with problems and these should have been disclosed to the subcommittee (in a confidential manner if necessary)." Five of the respondents also answered that FDA should have disclosed data integrity problems to the AIDAC, especially when the problems are "as extensive and potentially significant as the problems evident with Study 3014" or "problems that may have affected the validity of the data."

In addition to specific questions related to Study 3014 and the Janaury 8, 2003 AIDAC meeting, the Committee's October letter asked the AIDAC members to provide any additional comments or concerns regarding Ketek or any other matter. One respondent's comments raised further questions about FDA's decision to present Study 3014 to the advisory committee on January 8, 2003. During his interview with Committee staff, the Office Director stated that he decided to proceed with the AIDAC meeting because he wanted the advisory committee's input on all of the data to be assessed (animal and human trials, Study 3014, and foreign post-marketing data). He added that based on the data that he saw, there was a reasonable chance that the advisory committee would raise concerns about Study 3014.

However, it appears that the Review Division Director spoke so positively at the AIDAC meeting about the data in support of Ketek's approval that it is not surprising that the advisory committee did not raise concerns about Study 3014. One AIDAC member wrote specifically, "...the Ketek case represents an error of commission, allowing the hearings to go forth under false circumstances. [The Review Division Director's] initial introduction to the 2nd Advisory Committee meeting is glowingly positive, which may indicate that she was not aware of any glitches in the data; if she was aware of these issues, she gave no indication that this drug should be anything but fast track approved that day."

III. Further Findings and Conclusions

When Aventis submitted Study 3014 to the FDA in July 2002, its title page included a "GCP Statement: This study was conducted in accordance with good clinical practice and Aventis standard operating procedures for clinical investigation and documentation." Aventis also provided verbal assurances to the FDA regarding the integrity of Study 3014 during a meeting held in late December 2002 to discuss the AIDAC meeting agenda, including the assurance, according to several FDA officials, that there were "no more Kirkman Campbells in Study 3014." Aside from these written and verbal assurances to the FDA regarding the integrity of Study 3014, the vast majority of documents and information available to the Committee suggest that the FDA had sufficient information to determine that Study 3014 had serious data integrity issues, which were not isolated to Dr. Kirkman-Campbell. In fact, serious questions had been raised with respect to at least

7 study sites, both high-enrolling and low-enrolling, in Study 3014. The Review Division Director and the ODE 4 Director knew, or should have known, about the extent of the concerns, questions, and problems with the data integrity of Study 3014.

Several Review Division officials indicated to the Committee that the timing of events and decisions regarding the Ketek NDA generally, and presenting Study 3014 at the AIDAC meeting specifically, were driven by concern for meeting the deadlines imposed under the Prescription Drug User Fee Act. The FDA began planning for the AIDAC meeting to review the Ketek NDA and Study 3014 within weeks after Aventis resubmitted the Ketek NDA in July 2002. The Office Director stated that ultimately it was his decision to hold the AIDAC meeting and present Study 3014 in January 2003. Further, he stated he did not consult anyone else in reaching his decision. The Division Director stated that she consulted with the FDA's Associate Director, Office of Regulatory Affairs, and the Executive Secretary of the Advisory Committee prior to deciding the Review Division should present Study 3014 at the AIDAC meeting. Both the Division Director and Office Director said that the conclusions drawn from the ongoing criminal investigation and inspections of high-enrolling study sites in Study 3014 were preliminary. The Division Director stated she did not receive a draft consultation memorandum from DSI regarding the three highest enrolling sites until after the AIDAC meeting. Therefore, she believed that issues of fraud and serious data integrity problems with Study 3014 were isolated to Dr. Kirkman Campbell's site.

Last June, the former Division Director for DSI, who is no longer at the FDA, wrote to the FDA's Director of Medical Policy to share several thoughts regarding the FDA's approval of Ketek and the Committee's investigation of these matters. With regard to the AIDAC meeting, the DSI Division Director wrote:

> It is quite unfair to say that the FDA failed to disclose the ongoing investigations to the Advisory committee. As you know, OSI and OCI never publicly reveal conclusions from an investigation until the evidence from an investigation until the evidence has been fully evaluated at headquarters, the case closed and appropriate action taken. Since most of the FDA Ketek investigations were quite complex, and often involved multiple simultaneous investigations by different authorities, I do not believe any information could have been released from OCI or DSI at the time of the Advisory committee meeting. The release of raw and unverified investigation outcomes to the Advisory committee, in the absence of a determination that a regulatory violation had occurred, would not only have been unprecedented and a violation of due process, but also would not have provided any meaningful context for Committee consideration.

Both the Division Director and Office Director confirmed to the Committee that it was their belief that they could not disclose what they knew about data integrity issues with Study 3014 at the AIDAC meeting because of an ongoing criminal investigation. Several FDA officials stated to the Committee that disclosing what the FDA knew about data integrity problems with Study 3014 during a closed session of the AIDAC meeting was not an option under FDA regulations, which limit when and how a closed session of an advisory committee may be held. The Office Director stated that it was reasonable to present Study 3014 because its findings were "consistent with other data in the Ketek NDA." He reasoned that it would be valuable for the FDA to have the AIDAC consider the Ketek NDA despite the concerns with Study 3014. The Office Director expected that Advisory Committee members would raise more concerns regarding the Ketek NDA and that the AIDAC would come down more negatively on the drug than it did. Both the Division Director and Office Director concluded that proceeding with the AIDAC meeting was the right thing to do. Both appeared to believe that postponing or canceling the AIDAC meeting, rather than present Study 3014, was out of the question.

Consequently, the Division Director instructed a Review Division official to present Study 3014 at the AIDAC meeting despite not having a reasonable assurance of the data integrity of Study 3014. The documentary record and interviews conducted by the Committee, suggest that officials within OCI, DSI, and the Review Division raised and communicated sufficient data integrity issues regarding Study 3014 in the months preceding the AIDAC meeting to call into question the decision and judgment of the ~~Division Director and Office Director to convene the AIDAC meeting for FDA to present~~ Study 3014 findings publicly.

Furthermore, the aforementioned statement made by the Director of DSI with the benefit of hindsight underscores the rationale that appeared to hold sway at FDA. Despite "doubt as to the veracity of the study results," "alarms as to the way the in which the study was conducted," and concerns that "the validity of 3014 is growing more suspect by the day," "it will come back to haunt all parties involved—us if we do nothing, the public if the data is not trustworthy, and the sponsor for not having disclosed these findings to us," and, finally, "just wish we could find even a single credible large-enrolling site in 3014,"—all concerns expressed by staff within the Review Division—supervisory officials at the FDA continued to believe it was neither an option to disclose data integrity problems nor would it be "productive."

In sum, the FDA did not ensure that the public received accurate, science-based information regarding the Ketek NDA. Advisory Committee members and the public who relied on the FDA's presentation of Study 3014 were misled because not all of the relevant findings and conclusions regarding the Ketek NDA were presented. If the FDA could not find a way to present only accurate, science-based information, the FDA should not have presented Study 3014 publicly or, alternatively, should have postponed or canceled the AIDAC meeting.

Many of the FDA officials involved with the Ketek NDA are highly accomplished professionals with graduate degrees—either an M.D. or Ph.D. or both—and with numerous published works to their name. During interviews conducted by the Committee, the question was posed to a number of them: "Would you submit your work product for peer review and publishing, if you had any reason to believe your data was suspect or potentially had data integrity problems?" No official answered affirmatively.

Commissioner von Eschenbach, I appreciated the comments you made by email to all FDA staff following your confirmation. Specifically, you avowed:

> We will be a science-led regulatory agency. We will look closely at how we do business and make improvements where appropriate, and we will do this in an atmosphere of openness and with mutual respect for others' opinions. I will be

expecting much of you, but I expect even more of myself and of FDA's leadership.

In light of your recent avowal to FDA staff and the findings presented in this letter to you today, I respectfully request answers to the allegations and questions I brought to your attention more than 6 months ago:

1. What regulations and/or policies govern withholding relevant information and/or data from an FDA advisory committee?

2. What categories of information may be withheld from an advisory committee that otherwise would be considered relevant information necessary to fulfill its advisory function?

3. Describe in detail the basis and rationale for withholding potentially detrimental information related to a safety study while presenting beneficial information from that same safety study. For example, if a matter regarding data integrity has been identified in a study and is under investigation by the Office of Criminal Investigations and/or under review by the Division of Scientific Investigations, why would it be appropriate to present study data when there are unresolved concerns about the integrity of the study data?

4. How many times since January 1, 2000, has the FDA presented study information and/or data to an advisory committee when unresolved integrity concerns existed? For instance, the data integrity concerns were the subject of an internal FDA investigation and/or review, by the Office of Criminal Investigations, the Division of Scientific Investigations, and/or an Application Integrity Policy Committee at the time of presentation?

In addition, I request answers to the following questions:

5. What is your opinion of the comments the Advisory Committee members provided to the Committee? Do you share their concerns?

6. What steps, if any, has FDA taken since the allegations regarding the January 8, 2003, AIDAC meeting were brought to your attention?

7. Given the explanation provided by the Division Director and Office Director as to why data integrity issues with Study 3014 were not shared with the Advisory Committee members, *i.e.*, ongoing criminal investigation and a closed session of the AIDAC meeting was not an option under FDA regulations, will you reconsider how FDA will handle such matters in the future? Under what conditions, if any, do you believe known serious data integrity problems and/or other information that would be relevant to an advisory committee discussion should be withheld from an advisory committee by the FDA?

I look forward to hearing from you regarding the allegations, concerns, and questions set forth in this letter by no later than January 17, 2007. If you anticipate any difficulty in complying with the deadline, please immediately contact my Committee Staff. Any questions or concerns should be directed to . All formal correspondence should be sent via electronic transmission in PDF format or via facsimile to and original by U.S. mail.

Sincerely,

Charles E. Grassley
Chairman

Attachments

Senate Finance Timeline

ATTACHMENT 1

Timeline of Major Events Related to FDA's Approval and Post-market Surveillance of Ketek

Date	Event
February 28, 2000	Aventis submits New Drug Application (NDA) for Ketek to FDA
April 26, 2001	First Anti-Infective Drugs Advisory Committee (AIDAC) meeting on Ketek – committee recommends that Aventis obtain additional safety information from a large sample of patients
June 1, 2001	FDA sends Aventis an approvable letter for the indications of community-acquired pneumonia, acute bacterial sinusitis, and acute exacerbation of chronic bronchitis and requests a large safety study to evaluate hepatic, cardiac, visual and vasculitic effects
	FDA sends non-approval letter for Ketek for the indication of tonsillopharyngitis
July 2001	Ketek is approved for marketing in Europe
September 27, 2001	Aventis completes design of the protocol for Study 3014, a large usual care study
October 19, 2001	Aventis enrolls the first subject in Study 3014
January 29, 2002	Aventis enrolls the last subject in Study 3014; more than 24,000 patients are enrolled at 1824 sites
October 2001-June 2002	PPD, the contract research organization selected by Aventis to monitor Study 3014, conducts on-site and phone monitoring of the study sites
June 25, 2002	Aventis notifies FDA that data from two low-enrolling study sites could not be confirmed or corrected and thus would not be included in the study
July 24, 2002	Aventis resubmits NDA to FDA with data from Study 3014 and foreign post-marketing safety data from first million prescriptions
September 27, 2002	FDA's Division of Scientific Investigations (DSI) issues inspection assignment on the highest enrolling site of Study 3014, the site of Dr. Marie "Anne" Kirkman-Campbell
October 15-24, 2002	FDA investigators inspect Dr. Kirkman-Campbell's site and find study protocol violations and concerns regarding the conduct of the study, including enrollment of patients who should have been excluded, e.g., for drug allergies, documentation of patients having completed the course of therapy even though those patients stated that they did not receive the medication, and absence of any reported adverse events for the first 100 patients enrolled
October 31, 2002	FDA's Office of Criminal Investigations formally initiates investigation of Dr. Kirkman-Campbell
November 14, 2002	DSI issues inspection assignments on the second and third highest

ATTACHMENT 1

Date	Event
	enrolling sites of Study 3014, the sites of Dr. Carl Lang and Dr. Egisto Salerno
December 19, 2002	DSI receives observational findings from the inspection of Dr. Salerno's site; Dr. Salerno was disciplined by his state Medical Board for gross negligence and failing to maintain adequate and accurate medical records, and was on probation at the time of his participation in Study 3014
December 30, 2002	DSI receives observational findings of inspection of Dr. Lang's site; field investigators identified Good Clinical Practices violations, including enrollment of patients who should have been excluded and significant documentation discrepancies
January 8, 2003	Second AIDAC meeting on Ketek; data from Study 3014 and foreign post-marketing data are presented to the advisory committee; majority of AIDAC members votes for approval of Ketek for CAP, ABS, and AECB
January 21, 2003	DSI provides its Clinical Inspection Summary of the site inspections of Drs. Kirkman-Campbell, Lang, and Salerno to the Division of Anti-Infective Drug Products, the division responsible for review of the Ketek NDA
January 24, 2003	FDA sends approvable letter to Aventis requesting further information on Study 3014 and additional foreign post-marketing safety data
April 2, 2003	FDA inspects Aventis to assess sponsor's oversight of Study 3014
October 17, 2003	Aventis resubmits NDA to FDA
October 23, 2003	Dr. Kirkman-Campbell pleads guilty to fraud
March 25, 2004	DSI concludes that data from Study 3014 is unreliable
April 1, 2004	FDA approves Ketek for the treatment of community-acquired pneumonia, acute sinusitis, and acute exacerbation of chronic bronchitis
January 20, 2006	FDA issues public health advisory on Ketek
January 26, 2006	*Annals of Internal Medicine* releases article on three cases of liver damage in North Carolina patients who took Ketek
May 1, 2006	*Wall Street Journal* article on fraud associated with Study 3014
June 8, 2006	Sanofi-aventis voluntarily pauses enrollment in pediatric trials of Ketek
June 29, 2006	Sanofi-aventis revises Ketek labeling to include additional warnings about the risk of liver toxicity as well as strengthening warnings for patients with myasthenia gravis

U.S. SENATE COMMITTEE ON

Finance

SENATOR CHUCK GRASSLEY, OF IOWA - CHAIRMAN

http://finance.senate.gov

Floor Statement of U.S. Senator Chuck Grassley of Iowa
Pre-Cloture Vote on Nomination of Dr. Andrew von Eschenbach
to be Commissioner of the Food and Drug Administration
Thursday, December 7, 2006

Thank you Mr. President for the opportunity to speak today on the cloture vote that this body will take later today to bring up the nomination of Dr. Andrew von Eschenbach to be Commissioner of the Food and Drug Administration. I intend to vote against cloture for several reasons.

I have serious concerns about what this cloture vote means for congressional oversight of the executive branch now and in the future and what it means for members like me who placed a hold on this nominee.

I am voting against cloture and I ask my colleagues to join me because I believe we need to send a message to the executive branch that it's not okay to impede congressional investigations. It's not okay to limit the Senate's access to documents, information and employees of the executive branch.

In his book, Congressional Government, Woodrow Wilson wrote in 1885, "Quite as important as lawmaking is vigilant oversight of administration."

Our work as lawmakers does not end with the passage of legislation. This body has a responsibility to the American people to make sure the laws work and they're being implemented effectively, efficiently, and economically. Congressional oversight serves very important goals, and we should not lose sight of them. They include: (1) reviewing actions taken and regulations adopted by executive agencies to make sure the agencies are executing the laws according to the intent of Congress; (2) ensuring that the federal government is not wasting taxpayer dollars. Our oversight work allows us to evaluate the ability of agencies and their managers to carry out program objectives and to improve the efficiency, effectiveness and economy of government programs; (3) ensuring that executive policies reflect the public interest; and (4) protecting the rights and liberties of the American people.

Woodrow Wilson also said in his book, "It is the proper duty of a representative body to look diligently into every affair of government and to talk much about what it sees. It is meant to be the eyes and the voice, and to embody the wisdom and will of its constituents."

Throughout history, Congress has engaged in oversight of the executive branch. For example, the right to Congressional oversight has been asserted in the early days of our republic. As early as 1792, the House of Representatives invoked its authority to conduct oversight when it appointed a committee to investigate the defeat of General St. Clair and his army by the Indians in the Northwest and empowered it to "call for such persons, papers, and records, as may be necessary for their inquiries."

In fact, the Constitution grants Congress extensive authority to oversee and investigate executive branch activities. Congressional oversight was also recognized explicitly in the passage of the Legislative Reorganization Act of 1946, which required the standing committees of Congress to exercise "continuous watchfulness" over programs and agencies in their jurisdiction.

Numerous Supreme Court decisions all support the precedent for Congress to oversee all aspects of the federal government. In 1927, in the case of McGrain v. Daugherty, the Supreme Court upheld Congressional authority to conduct oversight in the Teapot Dome scandal. Justice van Devanter writing for the unanimous court stated, "We are of the opinion that the power of inquiry - with the process to enforce it - is an essential and appropriate auxiliary to the legislative function."

To do oversight, Congress needs access to information and people in the executive branch, and that is what I did not and still am not getting from the FDA under the leadership of Dr. von Eschenbach. So I take exception to the statement made in support of the cloture motion that "Dr. Andrew von Eschenbach has done a superb job in the position he is currently occupying."

Before you cast your vote in favor of cloture consider what's at stake.

In my interactions with the Department of Health and Human Services and the FDA these last eight months, I have seen a complete and utter disrespect for congressional authority and the law. The Department and the FDA have repeatedly failed to act in good faith in responding to congressional investigations.

Under Dr. von Eschenbach's leadership, the FDA has failed to fully comply with two congressional subpoenas that were issued seven months ago.

Efforts to accommodate the agency's concerns fall on deaf ears and I wonder if I am dealing with "dysfunction by design." Not only has FDA withheld documents that do not appear to be privileged, but it also won't say what has been withheld and why. The subpoenas compel a privilege log, but FDA has not provided one.

What is the agency's explanation? FDA has said that so many documents have been withheld that it is unduly burdensome to provide a privilege log. Even the FDA General Counsel, as recently as Tuesday of this week, could not see why the agency needed to comply with the law and the terms of the subpoenas issued by the Finance Committee.

In denying the Committee access to documents responsive to the subpoenas, the Department and FDA have claimed quote "prosecutorial deliberative process," "confidential communications," and "agency prerogative to determine who will be interviewed or testify before a jurisdictional committee."

This past summer, I asked the Congressional Research Service to look into the Department's policies regarding this matter, and CRS told me that there is "no legal basis" for the Department's executive branch assertions. The legal analysis provided by CRS supports the Committee's position that these executive agency claims have been consistently rejected and compliance with Congressional requests in the past has been forthcoming.

CRS cites numerous court cases which establish and support Congress's power to engage in oversight and investigation activities and its access to executive branch personnel and documents in carrying out this power.

The Department and FDA says it has been responsive because the agency made available hundreds of thousands, even millions, of pages of documents to the Finance Committee in response to the subpoenas. But the agency can give me all the books and documents housed at the Library of Congress and it won't matter if it's not what I asked for.

If this is the type of cooperation I am getting from the FDA under Dr. von Eschenbach, I am very concerned about the cooperation, if any, we will have once he becomes the permanent Commissioner. And every Member of Congress should be equally concerned if they take their constitutional duty of conducting oversight of the executive branch seriously.

I cannot emphasize this enough-but a vote for cloture today is a vote against oversight and that is not what this Senate should be doing and it is not what the American people sent us here to do. We need to step up Congressional oversight to protect our nation's system of checks and balances and not reward those who seek to impede our constitutional authority.

This body should not walk hand-in-hand with the executive branch and sit idly by as instances of fraud, waste and abuse continue to endanger the health and safety of the American people. This Senate needs to make it clear to the executive branch that Congress takes its oversight responsibilities seriously and vote against cloture.

Floor Statement of U.S. Senator Chuck Grassley of Iowa
Post-Cloture Vote on the Nomination of Dr. Andrew von Eschenbach
***to* be Commissioner of the Food and Drug Administration**
Thursday, December 7, 2006

Mr. President, I rise again to raise issues with the nomination of Dr. Andrew von Eschenbach. I placed a hold on this nominee and voted against cloture because I take my constitutional duty to conduct oversight very seriously.

I spend a great deal of my time in the Senate trying to make government work. I charge my staff to conduct oversight rigorously and to investigate any areas where the federal government is failing to be transparent, accountable and effective. In other words, if it fails the sniff test, I'll blow the whistle on it.

Today, I'm blowing the whistle on this nominee. In good conscience, I placed a hold on this nomination and I will not vote in favor of him today. A vote for this nominee would be an endorsement of the stonewalling and disrespect he has shown for Congressional oversight. I can say this not only because of his actions but because his words are on the record.

In response to a nomination question, I asked this nominee if he would cooperate with Congressional oversight and Dr. von Eschenbach identified a number of "executive branch interests" as a basis for not complying with Congressional requests, including "matters pending before the Agency," "pre-decisional, deliberative process information" and "open investigation information."

Dr. von Eschenbach was not well-served by whomever counseled him on these matters. He should know that during my years in the Senate, my investigators have obtained access to every single one of these categories of so-called confidential information.

His answer is at odds with my belief that Congressional oversight is one of the best ways to shake things up at a government agency and expose the truth. I say this is not just about the FDA, it's true of any government agency.

If an agency is not doing the right thing, typically behind it there's an effort to keep information suppressed. An effort to keep people from doing what they think ought to be done. An effort to keep people from doing what their job requires them to do and to not let that information out.

The muzzling of dissent and information is too common throughout our government. Things that should be transparent in government just aren't. And under Dr. von Eschenbach, the FDA has not only avoided transparency but it also has threatened those who are trying desperately to expose the truth.

I met with this nominee after the White House sent his nomination to the Senate last March. I hoped he would provide the kind of strong, permanent leadership the FDA needs. Over the next nine months, this nominee showed me that he is unlikely to provide that kind of leadership.

My belief is what you see is what you get. I fear what we will get from this nominee is what we got from him as Acting Commissioner. Let me tell you why with a few examples.

First, the doctor failed to live up to his word. In our meeting, he said he respected and understood the important role Congress plays as an equal branch of government. It didn't take long after that meeting before the first red flags appeared.

In April the Committee began its investigation of the FDA's approval and post-market surveillance of Ketek. Ketek is an antibiotic that came under renewed scrutiny last January. It looks like it is another drug where the FDA was caught flat-footed again. The Finance Committee issued two subpoenas in May after the FDA refused to provide documents related to Ketek.

During this time, the FDA also refused access to some FDA officials. The Finance

Committee was forced to issue a subpoena to a special agent in the FDA's Office of Criminal Investigations. The FDA refused to allow my staff to speak to this federal employee, citing a policy against providing access to line agents.

Yet only months before, my staff interviewed two line agents from FDA in another case. Apparently, the policy abruptly changed. I've seen it change over the years with other investigations. This "policy" is not law and it is typically enforced when the stakes are at their highest and there's something to hide.

I took this matter seriously enough that I went myself to the Department of Health and Human Services to meet with this agent. I was told that if this agent wanted to speak to me he would have to assert his status as a whistleblower under federal law.

I ask you today what I asked that day: Why does this government employee have to become a whistleblower to talk to me or anyone in Congress? Is that acceptable to the Members of this Senate?

Also, this government employee's supervisors put him in a no-win situation, and because of that, he risks being in contempt of Congress. This is an agent who put a doctor in jail for fraud in a Ketek study, he did the right thing, it's a closed case, we want to talk to him about a closed case, and FDA says no -- what does the FDA have to hide or cover up?

Under this Acting Commissioner, the FDA has also attempted to hide and cover-up documents.

The Finance Committee has received hundreds of pages that say, "57 pages removed," or "43 pages removed."

Other documents have whole pages, paragraphs or sentences redacted with no explanation as to why. Sometimes documents are marked redacted; other times they are not marked, even when it is evident that information is missing.

There is no explanation for what documents have been withheld or redacted. It is incomprehensible and looks like the work of the Keystone cops rather than an agency responsible for drugs and devices.

One of the FDA's most incompetent and absurd moments was when it sent one of my own request letters back to me with information redacted out of it. On top of such nonsense, the FDA has produced versions of the same document redacted different ways.

Recently, I wrote Secretary Leavitt and Attorney General Gonzales to explain the basis for some redactions. Again, two copies of the same document were redacted differently. It called into question the good faith basis for the redaction altogether. I could go on and on with examples showing the stonewalling and withholding of information from legitimate Congressional requests.

What it boils down to is that this nominee has demonstrated that he doesn't understand that government truly is the people's business. He doesn't seem to understand that the people who finance it have a right to know what their government is doing and how it is spending their money.

I will give you one final example. I have long been a champion of whistleblowers. I was the lead Senate sponsor of the 1986 whistleblower amendments to the False Claims Act. Back then we were interested in dismantling a too cozy relationship between defense contractors and the Pentagon. Today, whistleblowers are once again the key to dismantling the cozy relationship between some drug companies and the Food and Drug Administration.

In June Dr. von Eschenbach held a meeting with FDA staff involved with Ketek. FDA employees present say he used a lot of sports metaphors regarding being "team players" and keeping opinions "inside the locker room." Basically he said to not criticize the FDA "outside the locker room." Apparently, he stated that anyone who spoke outside the locker room might find themselves "off the team."

This nominee held this meeting in the midst of an ongoing congressional investigation of Ketek. He called the meeting after a number of critical reports in the media about the FDA's handling of Ketek.

A number of FDA employees interviewed by the Committee were offended by his comments, found them highly questionable, inappropriate, and potentially threatening. I agree with them.

The leader of an agency should not hold a meeting to suggest that dissenters will be kicked off the team. This is the type of action that shows the true stripes of this nominee. He broke his word that he respected whistleblowers and would not raise even the appearance of retaliation.

When it comes to health care and public safety, we need to empower whistleblowers more than ever. They demonstrate extraordinary courage in the face of extraordinary adversity. It's extremely difficult to be a whistleblower. As I like to say, they are about as welcome as a skunk at a picnic. Yet, it is whistleblowers in government who put their job security on the line to come forward and expose fraud or wrongdoing for the public good.

My Finance Committee staff has been investigating serious allegations raised by whistleblowers at FDA for more than three years. Many of these allegations are very serious and call into question whether the FDA is fulfilling its mission to protect the health and safety of Americans.

The way the FDA under this nominee has handled the investigation of Ketek shows the agency would like to keep its business secret. It doesn't want these issues made public or subjected to the scrutiny. The culture at FDA has been we will let the public know what we think they need to know.

The American people don't want the government making decisions about what's good for them behind closed doors.

The goal of the Finance Committee's oversight has been straightforward. As chairman, I wanted to bring out in the open the decisions made by the FDA. For too long the agency has been making its decisions behind closed doors.

This nominee is not likely to serve well because he just doesn't seem to get it. He has placed media relations over the mission of FDA. First and foremost, he is supposed to do the right thing on behalf of Americans. Dr. von Eschenbach has other interests to serve and they are not always the interests of John Q. Public.

Now I hear from time to time from other agencies that particular documents are especially sensitive, or that the release of certain documents could jeopardize a criminal investigation - I understand that. But in those circumstances, I have reached accommodations. Unfortunately, in this case, my efforts to work with Dr. von Eschenbach and his subordinates have been all but summarily dismissed.

In closing, I intend to keep pressing the FDA for greater transparency and openness. As I continue with my Constitutional duties to conduct oversight, I look forward to working with my colleagues to ensure transparency, accountability, and effective governance by the executive branch. The bottom line is that Congress needs to stay committed to oversight of the executive branch. The public depends on Congress to fulfill its duty and hold executive agency leadership accountable.

Testimony of Dr. David Graham
Before the House Committee on Energy and Commerce
Subcommittee on Oversight and Investigations
February 13, 2007

Chairman Stupak and members of the subcommittee, thank you for the opportunity to speak about a subject of vital importance to all Americans. My name is David Graham and I am the Associate Director for Science and Medicine in FDA's Office of Surveillance and Epidemiology (OSE). For more than 20 years, I have worked as an FDA physician-epidemiologist concerned with post-marketing drug safety. The statements I make today are my own. I do not represent the FDA's official view.

As we've heard from the previous panels, the Ketek story is about FDA's betrayal of the public trust. FDA ignored safety concerns raised by its own advisory committee and concealed from the committee the evidence that a crucial clinical trial was fraudulent. Subsequently, FDA issued a Public Health Advisory that referenced this same fraudulent study as proof of Ketek's safety. FDA scientists were intimidated, suppressed, and ultimately compelled to leave the Agency. CDER used postmarketing case reports from Europe and Latin America to declare Ketek safe. I cannot think of a single other example where FDA used such data as the primary basis for approval of a drug's safety. OSE, ostensibly responsible for postmarketing safety issues, was relegated to the role of back seat "consultant," with no power or authority.

Unfortunately, Ketek is not an anomaly. In November 2004, I testified before the Senate Finance Committee that FDA's handling of Vioxx was "a profound regulatory failure," and that "FDA, as currently configured, is incapable of protecting America against another Vioxx." I am here today to tell you that our nation is still at risk.

Vioxx was an enormous national catastrophe. Up to 60,000 Americans, most over the age of 50, died from Vioxx-related heart attacks, about as many as the number of US soldiers killed during the Viet Nam War. Another 80,000 suffered non-fatal, but nonetheless life-threatening, heart attacks. FDA had multiple opportunities to prevent this but did nothing. To this day, FDA denies that it made any mistakes and is yet to be held accountable. (I've included a table showing the estimated number of patients by State who were harmed or killed by Vioxx-associated heart attacks. Every Congressional district in the US suffered fatalities).

Sadly, Vioxx was not an anomaly either. Think SSRIs and suicidality in children. Think Accutane, pregnancy exposure, and the need for restricted distribution. Think Propulsid and sudden death-a drug that barely worked for night time heartburn was left on the market for years while it killed hundreds, including infants. The list goes on and on.

When it comes to drug safety, what's wrong with the FDA? In my view, there are four broad areas of critical FDA malfunction: 1) organizational structure; 2) organizational culture; 3) the misuse and abuse of science; and 4) suppression and intimidation of scientific staff.

~~The most important is organizational structure. CDER's primary mission is to~~ review and approve new drugs. Within CDER, the Office of New Drugs (OND) has this responsibility. Post-approval, OND continues to have regulatory authority for all postmarketing safety issues that arise. This represents an inherent conflict of interest because the same people who stamp their approval on new drugs and certify that they are safe and effective also decide if a postmarketing safety issue is important and if anything needs to be done about it.

This organizational weakness is amplified by a massive imbalance in staffing and resources within CDER between pre- and postmarket activities. Overall, roughly 90% of CDER staff are focused on review and approval of new drugs. As the IOM report found: "the imbalance in formal role and authority between the review (OND) and surveillance/epidemiology (ODS/OSE) staff denotes the subservience of the safety function, and along with that, a management devaluation of the latter discipline and approach."

CDER's culture regards industry as the Agency's primary client rather than as an entity in need of regulation. The Agency's bias toward drug approval noted by IOM is enshrined in

PDUFA, which requires FDA to negotiate with industry over how user fees shall be spent; patients and consumers, the public, get no seat at the PDUFA table.

Finally, although this is not a legislative hearing, I am compelled by conscience to make the following comments. Vioxx is the main reason why legislation to reform FDA is being considered. Hence, the litmus test by which potential legislation should be judged is whether it would have prevented the Vioxx disaster.

FDA's response to the IOM report, even if fully implemented, would not have prevented a single Vioxx heart attack or death. Vioxx was not a failure of surveillance or resources. It was a failure of institutional decision-making. FDA's response to IOM would not have prevented Ketek, or the SSRI antidepressant issue from unfolding the way they did. Unless the postmarketing safety experts at FDA have regulatory authority over the postmarketing portion of a drug's life cycle that is separate from and independent of OND and CDER, all the money and databases in the world won't change the end result.

Similarly, had the proposed Kennedy-Enzi bill been in place when Vioxx came to market, not a single life would have been saved. Similarly, Kennedy-Enzi would have had no effect on the way Ketek or the SSRI antidepressant issues unfolded. By requiring that FDA reach "mutual agreement" with industry before any labeling change or other regulatory action takes place, Kennedy-Enzi places industry in the driver's seat. Within FDA, it leaves all power in the hands of those who approve drugs and who view industry as their main client. This is not FDA reform; it is the status quo.

By contrast, the Dodd-Grassley bill in the Senate, would create line authority in a postmarket center within FDA, with explicit authority to protect the public from unsafe medicines. This bill also frees postmarketing from the corrupting influence of PDUFA. Had it been in place prior to Vioxx, most of the 140,000 Vioxx-related heart attack deaths and injuries would have been prevented.

Thank you for your consideration of this critical subject and for the opportunity to address you today.

Table. Estimated excess number of fatal, non-fatal, and total acute myocardial infarctions (heart attacks) attributable to US Vioxx use.

	State	Fatal heart attacks	Non-fatal heart attacks	Total
1.	AK	133	176	309
2.	AL	926	1232	2158
3.	AR	568	756	1324
4.	AZ	1074	1428	2502
5.	CA	7116	9464	1658
6.	CO	905	1204	2109
7.	CT	716	952	1668
8.	DC	120	160	280
9.	DE	164	218	383
10.	FL	3368	4480	7848
11.	GA	1726	2296	4022
12.	HI	253	336	589
13.	IA	611	812	1423
14.	ID	274	364	638
15.	IL	2611	3472	6083
16.	IN	1284	1708	2992
17.	KS	568	756	1324
18.	KY	842	1120	1962
19.	LA	947	1260	2207
20.	MA	1326	1764	3090
21.	MD	1116	1484	2600
22.	ME	274	364	638
23.	MI	2084	2772	4856
24.	MN	1032	1372	2404
25.	MO	1179	1568	2747
26.	MS	589	784	1373
27.	MT	189	252	441
28.	NC	1684	2240	3924
29.	ND	135	179	314
30.	NE	358	476	834
31.	NH	253	336	589
32.	NJ	1768	2352	4120
33.	NM	379	504	883
34.	NV	421	560	981
35.	NY	4000	5320	9320
36.	OH	2400	3192	5592
37.	OK	737	980	1717
38.	OR	716	952	1668

39.	PA	2589	3444	6033
40.	RI	211	280	491
41.	SC	842	1120	1962
42.	SD	158	210	368
43.	TN	1200	1596	2796
44.	TX	4400	5852	10252
45.	UT	463	616	1079
46.	VA	1495	1988	3483
47.	VT	128	171	299
48.	WA	1242	1652	2894
49.	WI	1137	1512	2649
50.	WV	379	504	883
51.	WY	103	137	240

Summary of testimony by
David B. Ross, M.D., Ph.D.
before the
House Energy and Commerce Subcommittee on Oversight and Investigations
February 13, 2007

The antibiotic Ketek has been linked to dozens of cases of severe liver injury, some of them fatal, as well as to deaths due to other causes. These events could have been prevented if FDA managers had taken into account the concerns of scientific reviewers at the Agency. Instead, during the course of the review of the Ketek application, FDA managers:

- Ignored written warnings from reviewers and criminal investigators regarding fraud in a pivotal safety study
- Concealed evidence of fraud in the study from a Federal advisory committee that relied on the study data to make critical recommendations to the Agency
- Used unreliable side effect reports from overseas to try to prove Ketek's safety, an unprecedented and invalid approach to pre-market safety assessment
- Suppressed reviewer concerns over fraud and Ketek's potential to cause serious liver injury
- Approved Ketek despite lack of evidence from adequate and well-controlled trials that it is safe and effective
- Repeatedly cited the fraudulent study in an attempt to reassure the public after media reports of Ketek's link to liver damage
- Allowed the drug's manufacturer to experiment with Ketek on children over reviewer protests.

Without reforms in FDA and how it assesses drug safety, a recurrence of the Ketek tragedy is inevitable.

Testimony of David B. Ross, M.D., Ph.D.
before the
House Energy and Commerce Committee's
Subcommittee on Oversight and Investigations

"The Adequacy of FDA Efforts to Assure the Safety of the Drug Supply"

Tuesday, February 13, 2007

Good morning, Mr. Chairman and Members of the Committee. Thank you for the opportunity to speak before this committee. I am here today to speak about the drug Ketek.

My name is David Ross. For purposes of identification only, I am currently National Director of Clinical Public Health Programs for the US Department of Veterans Affairs; I am here today as a private citizen. I was trained as a medical doctor at New York University and Yale and am board certified in internal medicine and infectious diseases. I take care of patients at my local VA hospital and teach medical students and residents.

I served for ten years at the FDA in positions ranging from a primary medical reviewer of New Drug Applications to a member of the Senior Leadership Team of FDA's Office of New Drugs[1]. I served as both the primary safety reviewer and safety team leader for Ketek[2].

FDA approved Ketek despite knowing that it could kill people from liver damage[3] and that tens of millions of people would be exposed to it[4]; despite FDA knowing that the drug's maker submitted fabricated data[5]; and despite knowing that Ketek is no better than other antibiotics, and may not even work[6].

Why does Ketek matter? Because FDA broke its own rules and allowed Ketek on the market[7]; because dozens of patients have died or suffered needlessly[8]; because FDA allowed Ketek's maker to experiment with it on children over reviewers' protests[9]; because FDA ignored warnings about fraud[10]; and because FDA used data it knew was false to reassure the public about Ketek's safety[11].

In March 2000, when Ketek was submitted to FDA, reviewers were alarmed over a patient treated with Ketek who had developed severe liver damage, an event that could mean hundreds or thousands of deaths every year[12]. In April 2001, a Federal Advisory Committee was so concerned about Ketek's potential to kill patients that it required a large safety study before the drug could be approved[13]. In October 2002, FDA reviewers examining the safety study found serious and pervasive misconduct pointing at fraud[14]. In December 2002, Ketek's manufacturer admitted that it had known about "issues" at its largest enroller – but hadn't told the FDA[15]. The company claimed that there were no other "issues" with the study – even though every study site inspected by FDA turned out to have major problems, an unprecedented situation[16]. In January 2003 – over reviewers' protests[17] – FDA managers hid[18] the evidence of fraud and misconduct from the Advisory Committee, which was fooled into voting for approval[19]. Starting the same month, FDA managers also pushed to use uncontrolled, unreliable side effect reports from overseas[20] – supplied by the drug's manufacturer without independent checking by FDA – as proof of Ketek's safety, something that had never been done before[21].

In April 2003, in response to a fraud investigation, the company turned over records the FDA – with most of the text blacked out. FDA managers did nothing.

In July 2003, FDA managers were warned by criminal investigators about possible fraud by the drug company with Ketek[22]. They did nothing.

In October 2003, FDA received records from the company that raised further concerns about fraud – FDA managers didn't even review them[23].

In March 2004, FDA's own Division of Scientific Investigations concluded that none of the safety study data was reliable[24]. One week later, FDA managers approved Ketek. Although FDA managers publicly deny it, internal correspondence shows that they used the safety study[25], and repeatedly cited it as evidence of Ketek's safety[26].

In February 2005 – seven months after Ketek's launch - FDA managers received the first reports of fatal Ketek-related liver failure[27]. They did nothing.

In February 2006[28], I and other reviewers warned senior FDA managers in writing about the problems with Ketek, including reviewers being pressured to change their opinions. The managers did nothing.

In March 2006, FDA managers received new warnings from criminal investigators[29]. They did nothing.

In May 2006, FDA managers received warnings from safety reviewers that Ketek was much more dangerous than comparable antibiotics[30]. They did nothing.

Only after Congressional subpoenas – which FDA resisted - and stories in the news media about Ketek and fraud, did FDA managers finally do anything – they reworded the label[31].

In late June of 2006, FDA reviewers, including myself, were summoned to a meeting with Commissioner von Eschenbach, in which he compared the FDA to a football team, and told reviewers that if they told anyone outside the FDA about the problems with Ketek, they'd be "traded from the team[32]." Rather than be silenced, I chose to move on to my current position.

How did this happen? The FDA reviewers did their job. This is not their fault. Ketek can be laid directly at the door of senior FDA managers[33] who knew better – because they were told repeatedly by reviewers and criminal investigators – but chose to look the other way. Their behavior was worse than being in a state of denial. FDA managers were so bent on approving Ketek that they suppressed evidence of fraud and pressured reviewers – including myself[34] – to change their reviews.

What's the bottom line? An unsafe drug got past the system despite warning after warning about fraud, liver damage, and death because FDA managers at the highest levels refused to listen.

Will this happen again? Yes. Without significant changes in our drug safety system and FDA[35], we are certain to see more Keteks[36]. Thank you. The views presented here are my own. I would be happy to answer any questions.

---

[1] The Senior Leadership Team I of the Office of New Drugs is composed of Office of Drug Evaluation (ODE) directors and deputy directors. From April 2004 to October 2005 I served as deputy director of ODE 6, and subsequently as associate office director in the Office of Oncology Drug Products.

---

[2] I served as the primary safety reviewer for Ketek during the first review cycle (from approximately November 2000 to April 2001), and the safety team team leader during the second review cycle (July 2002 to August 2003).

[3] Prior to approval, FDA managers were aware of a Ketek-related treated patient who developed severe liver injury; the histopathology of the liver injury was similar to that of trovafloxacin, an antibiotic implicated in dozens of deaths from liver failure in the 1990s. The nominal incidence rate of this adverse event in the original Ketek safety database was 1/3265 (0.03%).

[4] Over 120 million Americans receive antibiotics in an outpatient setting annually (McCaig LF *et al.* Emerg Infec Dis 2003; **9**:432-7), generally for respiratory tract infections of the type Ketek was approved for.

[5] FDA managers were aware as early as October 2002 – 18 months before they approved Ketek – that there were serious misconduct problems in a large Ketek safety study called Study 3014.

[6] Ketek's efficacy was determined entirely using noninferiority studies, which only show that a new product is no worse than a control drug; the FDA's own director of medical policy, Dr. Robert Temple, has written about the risk that such studies may falsely conclude that a product works when it does not (Temple R and Ellenberg SS. Ann Intern Med 2000; **133**:455-63, 464-70.). This is particularly true when a drug has only a small therapeutic effect, as is the case for antibiotics in bacterial sinusitis or acute exacerbation of chronic bronchitis. Ketek's "advantages" for resistant pathogens in respiratory tract infections have not been demonstrated in a clinical trial; for example, there is no

statistically significant difference between response rates in patients with community-acquired pneumonia due to macrolide-resistant *Streptococcus pneumoniae* treated with Ketek or with a macrolide. Furthermore, there is no clinical evidence that antimicrobial resistance plays a role in outcome in patients with sinusitis or bronchitis. Finally, it should be noted that Ketek is an oral medication approved for treatment of outpatients, a population at very low risk of complications from community-acquired pneumonia. The manufacturer of Ketek is not developing an intravenous form of the drug that would be useful in seriously ill patients with pneumonia due to resistant pathogens.

[7] The FDA violated the Food, Drug, and Cosmetic Act (21 USC 355) and implementing regulations when it approved Ketek. It approved Ketek based on a study that its own investigators said was worthless, breaking the rule about needing adequate and well-controlled trials; it used uncontrolled foreign safety reports to answer a critical safety question that should have been answered by an adequate and well-controlled trial; it failed to assess the overall integrity of the Ketek application despite warnings about potential systematic fraud; it failed to verify the integrity of foreign data submitted to it before approving Ketek; it allowed FDA managers to violate federal regulations at 21 CFR 10.70 by coercing reviewers into removing disagreements from the administrative record. Finally, by failing to take action against Institutional Review Boards that had not carried out their responsibilities, the FDA violated its responsibilities to enforce the provisions of 21 CFR 50 and 56.

[8] As of May 16, 2006, FDA reviewers had identified 12 patients who had suffered liver failure after taking Ketek (4 with fatal outcomes), and 23 patients with acute severe liver injury. Since most cases of drug-induced liver injury are never reported through passive

reporting systems (Sgro C *et al.* Hepatology 2002; **36**:451-5.), these are likely only a small fraction of patients with Ketek-associated liver injury.

[9] Pediatric trials of Ketek included a study in tonsillopharyngitis – an indication FDA had already rejected for Ketek in adults, and acute otitis media, another infection in which there is only a small benefit at best from antibiotics (Spiro DM *et al.* J Am Med Assoc 2006; **296**:1235-41). Both trials were noninferiority studies. The trials were suspended voluntarily by the sponsor after unfavorable publicity. FDA failed to place a clinical hold on the studies as outlined in 21 CFR 314.42; a clinical hold would have required the Agency to prepare a written review outlining deficiencies, the sponsor to respond to the deficiencies and the Agency to prepare a written review of the sponsor's response. The absence of a clinical hold means there is no administrative record of potential safety issues with these studies.

[10] See note 5. FDA managers received verbal and written warnings about fraud in the Ketek application from both reviewers and criminal investigators, starting in October 2002, and continuing until at least March 2006.

[11] In a Public Health Advisory issued January 20, 2006, the FDA cited Study 3014 (as "a large safety study") as evidence it had had prior to approval of Ketek's safety. See http://www.fda.gov/cder/drug/advisory/telithromycin.htm. The director of the FDA's Office of New Drugs (OND), Dr. John Jenkins, admitted citing Study 3014 in an interview with the *Wall Street Journal* published May 1, 2006, going on to admit that the FDA probably shouldn't have cited the study. The Qs and As accompanying the PHA originally referred to 3014 as a large safety study with 25,000 patients; this reference was

removed after Senator Charles Grassley complained to the Agency about posting of misleading information on its Web site.

[12] See notes 3 and 4. The nominal incidence rate for Ketek-associated severe liver injury was 0.03%, with a 95% confidence interval of 0.007% - 0.17%. Assuming Ketek acquired 10% of the market share for antibiotic prescriptions (a reasonable assumption given its manufacturer's premarket predictions of $1B US in revenues from this product), the number of liver injury cases annually could be as high as 12,000,000 x 0.17% = 20,400. Assuming a 10% mortality, this would translate into 2000 deaths annually.

[13] The advisory committee meeting minutes are available at http://www.fda.gov/ohrms/dockets/ac/01/transcripts/3746t1.html.

[14] The largest enroller was convicted of fraud. The second and third largest enrollers had significant violations of procedure that called into question the reliability of data from those sites. Of note, the third largest enroller was arrested shortly after the study on cocaine and weapons possession charges – not the type of study physician FDA likes to see conducting trials. Of ten sites inspected, every single one was found to have significant violations in what are called "Good Clinical Practices" – the rulebook for conducting clinical trials. Four of the ten were referred for criminal investigation – an astounding proportion.

One doctor was convicted of fraud. A second doctor refused to turn over his records, and FDA dropped the case. A third doctor was still under investigation as of March 2006. A fourth doctor had very suspicious findings (the doctor supposedly enrolled 90 patients in a town of about 190 adults), but there was not enough evidence to prosecute.

The doctor convicted of fraud was never disqualified from conducting clinical trials. FDA didn't even start the process to do that until Ketek hit the news, three years after the fraud was discovered. As of right now, if this doctor wasn't in jail, she could still conduct clinical trials.

[15] See http://www.fda.gov/cder/foi/nda/2004/21-144_Ketek_Admindocs_P1.pdf, p. 42 of 61. The company did not provide any explanation for retaining the largest enroller in the study, or for not informing the FDA.

[16] See note 14.

[17] On January 3, 2003 I e-mailed the FDA manager responsible for Ketek (Dr. Mark Goldberger) about extremely serious data integrity concerns known to the review division, FDA's Division of Scientific Investigations, and FDA's Office of Criminal Investigations, and copied the review division director. I asked about presenting these possible fraud issues to this Committee. His response was that it wouldn't be productive to present the data integrity issues. What would be useful, he said, would be for Aventis to make their best presentation possible using post-marketing data.

The statistical reviewer for the study protested about presenting the results as well; he was instructed by the review division director to present them without mentioning the fraud. A description of this may be found at http://www.consumersunion.org/pdf/FDA-12-06.pdf, p. 14 of 53.

[18] FDA managers from OAP have manipulated Advisory Committee votes on other occasions as well. For example, in March 2006, OAP managers deleted negative information about a pivotal study from an Advisory Committee briefing package, and

interrupted a Committee vote that appeared to be heading towards a negative recommendation.

[19] A drug company official told the Advisory Committee that they had virtually complete follow-up on the Study 3014 patients – even though many of them had never existed. Senior FDA managers were present for this assertion and did not contradict it. The Advisory Committee voted to recommend approval for all three indications. The meeting minutes for this meeting can be found at http://www.fda.gov/ohrms/dockets/ac/03/transcripts/3919T1.pdf; the assertion by the drug company is on page 106 of 289.

[20] FDA managers were warned in writing about the poor quality of the pharmacovigilance systems in the countries from which many of these reports were obtained.

[21] Although drug companies are required to submit all post-marketing reports, including those from abroad, as part of a drug application, these are always supplementary to the safety data from adequate and well-controlled trials. This is the first time that I am aware of that reports from passive voluntary surveillance have been used as the <u>primary</u> data source for answering a critical safety question prior to approval.

[22] On the morning of July 28, 2003, representatives from the Office of Criminal Investigation (OCI) briefed the director and deputy director of the Office of Antimicrobial Products (OAP), and the director of the Division of Anti-Infective Drug Products (DAIDP; now the Division of Anti-Infective and Ophthalmologic Drug Products (DAIOP)). They were told that the only way to determine if the drug company

had committed fraud with Ketek was to form a multidisciplinary, multi-jurisdictional task force to begin a wide-ranging investigation. The decision on whether or not to do this rested with CDER officials. An e-mail documenting this briefing has been turned over to the Senate Finance Committee.

[23] The records had been requested by FDA in an approvable letter of January 24, 2003. Although there were extensive meetings between FDA and the drug company between January and October 2003 to discuss these records and the format for submitting them, the primary medical reviewer for Ketek during the third and final review cycle has stated that he was instructed not to review them. No written FDA review was ever prepared for these records, even though many of them clearly show Aventis was well aware of data integrity concerns in Study 3014.

[24] DSI concluded that "the integrity of data from all sites involved in study 3014 cannot be assured with any degree of confidence." DSI also stated there had been multiple instances of fraud found in Study 3014.

[25] In an e-mail dated March 21, 2006, the deputy director of OND, Dr. Sandra Kweder, stated, "In speaking with the division about this, they did not completely ignore the data from the 3014 study, but assessed those AEs that were identified to qualitatively assess patterns of toxicity."

[26] See note 11.

[27] The death was that of a 26-year-old man previously in good health who received Ketek for an upper respiratory tract infection. Two other patients with Ketek-associated liver failure presented to the same medical center as this patient during the spring of 2005.

FDA never followed up with the reporting physician for the fatal case; had it done so, it might have discovered the cluster of cases that was to be reported in the *Annals of Internal Medicine* almost a year later. The failure to follow up on this case should be in the context of clear signals seen in the premarket review regarding hepatotoxicity.

[28] I met with the director and deputy director of OND, Drs. John Jenkins and Dr. Sandra Kweder, on February 17, 2006, I briefed them on the data, application, and review integrity issues involved with this application. During the meeting I also outlined more broadly problems in the Office of Antimicrobial Products, which regulates Ketek. The OAP issues included a general perception that product approval is being emphasized over scientific and regulatory considerations. The meeting was also attended by a medical officer who was formerly a reviewer in OAP.

The issues with Ketek were described in detail, and I emphasized to both Drs. Jenkin and Kweder that I thought that the sponsor may have willfully and intentionally engaged in fraud in connection with this application. I indicated that even if this was not the case, I did not understand why the question of Application Integrity Policy (AIP; http://www.fda.gov/ora/compliance_ref/aip_page.html) had not been referred for consideration by the AIP Committee and why fabricated data from a critical study had been presented to a Federal advisory committee without notifying the AC of the data integrity issues. I also indicated that the director of the review division, Dr. Janice Soreth, had pressured me to change my review on Ketek (in violation of 21 CFR 10.70 and CDER MAPP 5141.1), and that she routinely pressured reviewers to change review conclusions with which she disagrees, in violation of CDER policy and Federal regulations. I provided documentation on this issue to Drs. Jenkin and Kweder, as well as a list of data, application, and review integrity issues with Ketek.

We indicated that we felt that lack of response on these global issues with OAP, including Ketek, was a systemic problem in OAP, and that the problem originated with the OAP Immediate Office, headed by Dr. Mark Goldberger, director of OAP. We provided a written analysis of the problems in OAP.

We called for a global reassessment of integrity issues associated with Ketek; because of my concern that a fragmented investigation that did not draw on the pooled knowledge of all the review staff aware of these issues, I recommended that all relevant review staff, as well as DSI, OCI, and OCC, be involved in this reassessment. We also called for a survey of reviewers in OAP to determine the extent of reviewer coercion as well as education of managers in OAP regarding improper practices. The call for a global reassessment of Ketek integrity issues was repeated in an e-mail to Drs. Jenkins and Kweder that I sent on February 27, 2006.

On February 24, 2006, at the request of Dr. Kweder, I met with Dr. Goldberger, the director of OAP, and discussed my concerns over Ketek, including the fact that I had been pressured in fall of 2004 to change my review conclusions in connection with this application; I informed him that I had sent a contemporaneous e-mail documenting this to the Associate Director for Regulatory Affairs. Other issues I raised were:

* the presentation of study 3014 data to a Federal advisory committee in January 2003 without mentioning the data integrity issues connected with this study.

* the lack of follow-up with OCI prior to approval of Ketek in April 2004.

* the mention of study 3014 as supporting data for the NDA (despite multiple reviews, including one signed by Dr. Goldberger, saying that the study could not be relied on) in a Public Health Advisory issued on January 20, 2006 that was reviewed by Dr. Goldberger.

* the possibility that because the company might have been involved in fraud with study 3014, the Agency might not be able to rely on post-marketing data submitted through the company; the post-marketing data had been critical in approval of the drug. (Of note, on February 1, 2006, I had raised the issues with inclusion of data from study 3014 in the PHA with Dr. Kweder; she dismissed my concerns, saying, "It's ok - we've talked about it."). Dr. Goldberger attempted to rebut my arguments that there were application integrity issues for Ketek, but did not directly address any of the issues I had raised. I provided him with documentation with regard to the episode in which I was pressured to change my review, as well as names of three reviewers who could provide more information on the wide-spread use of intimidation in that review division to get reviewers to change their reviews. I documented my conversation with Dr. Goldberger in another e-mail to Drs. Jenkin and Kweder sent on February 27, 2006.

29. On March 5, 2006, Drs. Jenkins and Kweder were informed by e-mail of an OCI interview with the lead enroller in Study 3014 in which the physician implicated Aventis in fraud. Dr. Kweder forwarded the e-mail to CDER's Office of Compliance, asking if therewais anything other than the OCI agent's suspicions that the drug company was involved in fraud that FDA should be concerned about. She did not make the Office of

Compliance officials aware of the briefing and e-mails she had had from me, or the list of known Ketek integrity issues I had provided to her and Dr. Jenkins.

[30] An Office of Drug Safety consult dated May 16, 2006 concluded that the reporting rate for acute liver failure for Ketek (23 cases/10 million prescriptions) was 3-4 times higher than that for comparable antimicrobials. Of note, the reporting rate for trovafloxacin (see note 3) at the time of its essential market withdrawal for liver failure was 58 cases/10 million prescriptions. The incidence density (a measure of the incidence as a function of time) of acute liver failure with Ketek was as much as 167 times the background rate in the population. While these rates may seem low, it should be remembered that there are many alternatives to Ketek, and that it has not been shown to have any advantages clinically over other antimicrobials.

[31] FDA changed the label without preparing a written review to document its decision-making process, a violation of both Federal regulations and written CDER policies.

[32] Commissioner Von Eschenbach has admitted making this statement.

[33] OND managers involved included Dr. John Jenkins (director, OND); Dr. Sandra Kweder (deputy director, OND), Dr. Mark Goldberger (director, OAP); Dr. Edward Cox (deputy director, OAP); Mr. David Roeder (associate director, OAP); Dr. Janice Soreth (director, DAIOP).

[34] The second approvable letter for Ketek was issued on January 24, 2003. I had to wait to write my review documenting the basis for that letter until I finished a priority review on another drug. The review reflected the state of knowledge and my assessments as of the application as of January 24, 2003. I sent my Ketek review to the DAIDP director,

Dr. Janice Soreth in September 2003. Sometime in the next few weeks, she called me into her office, and asked me, "If I could soften my review to give Mark [Goldberger] and Ed [Cox] [her supervisors] wiggle room?" I talked to a number of colleagues, who predicted retaliation if I did not comply. I modified the last paragraph of my review to change my recommendation from nonapprovability for sinusitis and acute exacerbation of chronic bronchitis, and sent it back to her in November 2003. She waited three months and then signed it on February 16, 2004.

On February 8, 2004 – prior to Dr. Soreth's signing of my review – I sent an e-mail to Dr. Goldberger's Associate Director, Mr. David Roeder, detailing Dr. Soreth's actions. Before the drug was approved, I also placed my original review in an electronic FDA archive with a note about what happened, in case there was any question later on about what happened. Although she has denied pressuring me, Dr. Soreth has never explained the existence of my contemporaneous e-mail and review documentation.

[35] In its January 30, 2007 response to the 2006 Institute of Medicine report on drug safety, FDA rejected key recommendations of the IOM report, particularly the need to give regulatory authority to the post-marketing review divisions within CDER's Office of Surveillance and Epidemiology and to post FDA reviews of efficacy supplements and of post-marketing safety assessments. Both of these recommendations were aimed at improving the scientific decision-making ability and accountability of the Agency.

[36] In the OND workload model adopted in 2004 (used for tracking division productivity and allocating resources), there is no separate category for post-marketing safety assessments. The category that most closely resembles such a classification is that of

labeling supplement; this is given a weight of 1/20 that of a review of a New Drug Application. Thus, OND has explicitly instructed review division directors to de-emphasize post-market assessments.

ANSWERS TO SUBMITTED QUESTIONS FOR DAVID B. ROSS, M.D.

1. Why was liver damage in a single patient in the Ketek clinical trials so alarming?

First, the damage in this patient appeared very similar to that caused by another antibiotic called Trovan that was linked to dozens of deaths due to liver failure in the 1990' (and which was essentially withdrawn from the market). Reviewers were very concerned that we might be looking at a reprise of the Trovan situation with Ketek, in a setting where Ketek did not appear to have dramatic life-saving effects.

Second, there' a statistical rule of thumb that if a side effect occurs in 1 patient out of a thousand, you need 3000 patients to be sure of finding it. There were roughly 3000 patients in the original Ketek trials, and one developed severe liver damage. So, the true rate might be as high as 1 case out of every 1000 patients exposed. There are roughly 100 million antibiotic prescriptions written every year in this country for respiratory tract infections. If Ketek had 10 percent of the share for that market, that side effect would translate into 10,000 cases a year of severe liver damage, and potentially hundreds or thousands deaths a year.

2. What is the risk of liver failure with Ketek?

A. It is difficult to say with great certainty because of the poor quality of the data available, but the FDA' Office of Drug Safety estimated in May 2006 that the reporting rate (the number of cases reported divided by the number of prescriptions) is 23 reports/10 million prescriptions. By comparison, Trovan was associated with 58 reports/10 million prescriptions, while the next most riskiest drug compared to Ketek in the ODS analysis, had a rate of 6.6 reports/10 million.

If we use the rule of thumb that only one out of ten cases of severe liver injury is reported (an underreporting rate of 90 percent; the true underreporting rate is probably higher, based on a French population-based study by Sgro et al. published in 2002 in the journal Hepatology, as well as the FDA' own estimates of how often adverse events are reported), the incidence rate of acute liver failure with Ketek would be about 1 case out of every 43,000 prescriptions. According to Dr. Peter Honig, a former ODS director quoted in the May 2001 issue of FDA Consumer, a rate of about 1/50,000 is the usual cut-off for withdrawing a drug from the market or severely limiting its use.

3. Why the concern over liver failure with Ketek if other drugs such as acetaminophen are more common causes of liver failure?

Acetaminophen causes about half of all cases of drug-induced liver failure in this country, but the vast majority of these cases happen because of overdoses of acetaminophen or taking it with alcohol. Avoiding this situation greatly lessens the risk of liver failure with acetaminophen. Ketek can cause severe liver injury just with a single dose even in patients with no previous liver problems. There is no way to lessen the risk with Ketek. Second, acetaminophen is used much more than is Ketek, leading to many more opportunities for acetaminophen poisoning. Thus, the risk of liver failure with Ketek (when used as directed) is much higher than the risk with acetaminophen (when used as directed)

4. What exactly was the misconduct found in the safety study?

The largest enroller was convicted of fraud. The second and third largest enrollers had significant violations of procedure that called into question the reliability of data from those sights. Of note, the third largest enroller was arrested shortly after the study on cocaine and weapons possession charges—not the type of study physician FDA likes to see conducting trials.

5. What happened to the criminal investigations?

One doctor was convicted of fraud. From what I've been told, a second doctor refused to turn over his records, and FDA dropped the case. A third doctor was still under investigation the last I was aware. A fourth doctor had very suspicious findings (the doctor supposedly enrolled 90 patients in a town of about 190 adults), but there was not enough evidence to prosecute.

6. At the December 2006 Advisory Committee meeting, Aventis said that the fraud by this doctor had been "sophisticated." Was that true?

No. This was a blatant act of fraud that should have been evident to Aventis' clinical trial team.

7. What reason is there to think the company might have known of and been covering up fraud?

PPD warned Aventis about its lead enroller, both in terms of suspicious behavior and a statistical analysis that showed splitting of clinical samples. Aventis took over the statistical analysis, and dismissed the problems; the project manager who did this was the overall project manager for the study. There was another study site in the same town as the lead enroller that followed all the rules—this site only enrolled 12 patients, compared to over 400 at the lead enroller. It would have been impossible for Aventis to miss the contrast between the two. Aventis failed to tell FDA about the problems at the site until five months after they resubmitted their NDA.

8. What kind of warnings did FDA managers get about possible fraud on the part of the company?

In fall 2002, there were multiple warnings about fraud on the part of individual doctors in the study. In December 2002, the company admitted not telling the FDA about knowing of "problems" at the site of the physician who was convicted. In April 2003, FDA managers were told that when FDA investigators had demanded records from the company, the company had supplied them with much of the text blacked out. Finally, in July 2003, FDA managers received a briefing from FDA criminal investigators about their suspicions about the company, and recommending a task force to investigate the possibility of systematic fraud.

9. Did the FDA start that investigation?

No. It did not start an investigation until Ketek hit the news in 2006, at which it assigned an investigation to a "task force" consisting of a single agent.

10. What is the current status of the FDA investigation into Ketek?

Essentially dead. FDA had one agent, who was new to FDA and had no experience in clinical trial fraud, working on the case along with many others he was responsible for. He left the FDA recently and to the best of my knowledge, no one has been reassigned to it.

11. Do you know if the line agent whom Senator Grassley is seeking to interview is willing to talk to Congress?

Yes, he is, but FDA won't let him.

12. Is it true that the FDA couldn't tell the advisory committee about the problems because there was an open investigation?

No. First, by their own admission, FDA managers did tell the committee 8 weeks later in a closed session, when there was still an open investigation; if FDA told the committee then, FDA could have told them in January—before the committee voted. Second, all the members of the committee were Special Government Employees and were cleared to hear this information. Third, people in OCI have told me that the investigation would not have been compromised by telling members of the AC in closed session.

13. Did FDA officials mislead the advisory committee that just heard about Ketek in December?

Yes. First, they told the committee that they had stumbled on the fraud as a result of routine inspections—only the first one could be seen as routine (and even then there were suspicions before the site was inspected). Second, they told the 2006 committee that they couldn't have told the 2003 committee about the misconduct issues. That was untrue.

14. Were other reviewers pressured?

Yes. According to Sen. Grassley' report, the statistical reviewer on the safety study was instructed to present the results publicly even though he protested and thought the committee needed to be told about the misconduct issues. The primary medical reviewer who ended up recommending approval told me that he had been instructed not to look at records from the company that it was required to submit as part of the fraud investigation, even though that was supposed to be part of his review.

15. Did anyone else on the review team review those records and prepare a written report?

To the best of my knowledge, no. I had the necessary authorization to look at them myself, and did, but I was not asked to be part of the review team and so couldn't prepare a review.

16. What has happened to the FDA managers who were involved with Ketek?

My division director is still in her position. Her supervisor, who decided to allow the safety study to be presented without mentioning concerns over fraud, and who approved Ketek, was promoted last year to be director of pandemic influenza planning for the FDA. His supervisors are still in their positions.

17. Why was the liver failure death important in February 2005 if only one patient had died?

First, studies have shown that most adverse events are never reported, so that a report of one fatal case probably means there are many others that haven't been reported. Second, the appearance of this case so soon after the drug launch is very concerning— it's completely consistent with a relatively high risk of liver damage from Ketek. Third, the fact that the case occurred in an otherwise healthy young man is not only tragic, but suggests that Ketek is dangerous to people with normal livers. Finally, appropriate follow-up would have revealed that there were multiple cases of Ketek-induced liver failure at the same medical center; the occurrence of a cluster like that would be a tip-off that there may be many unreported cases.

18. Why do you say that Ketek is much more dangerous than other antibiotics?

A consult from FDA' Office of Drug Safety in May 2006 found that Ketek had a reported rate of acute liver failure 4–11 times that of comparable antibiotics.

19. Aren't those from post-marketing reports that are unreliable?

The magnitude of these differences is so huge that it would be difficult to explain by differences in things other than the drugs' relative risks. A randomized controlled trial would be better—but that was supposed to be the point of doing the original safety study.

20. Would you prescribe Ketek?

No. I do not believe it offers any advantages over other antibiotics for the same infections, I don't believe that it has acceptable risks, and given the unresolved fraud issues with this application, I do not believe that its efficacy and safety have been established.

21. A recent opinion piece by a former FDA reviewer in the Wall Street Journal of February 12 claimed that physicians attempting to obtain access to investigational drugs for patients with life-threatening diseases such as cancer have to go through hurdles with regard to manufacturing, statistical, and clinical questions that are akin to an IRS audit. Is this true?

A. No. This claim is flatly incorrect. Physicians seeking approval of emergency or single-patient Investigational New Drug Applications (IND) for individual patients typically piggy-back their request onto an existing IND from a commercial drug sponsor. The FDA' Oncology Office alone approves hundreds of such requests every year; the typical request is granted in 24 hours. In fields such as infectious diseases where such requests are made in the setting of acute disease, the approval time typically takes an hour or less; I personally approved dozens of such requests, and never turned one down. Situations where such requests are turned down are unusual and generally involve situations where a physician is requesting an investigational therapy when standard therapies known to be safe and effective are available and have not been tried.

22. How would you fix the problems with the FDA that Ketek revealed?

A. (1) Mandate (and fully fund) the use of reliable post-marketing safety data sources, such as observational data bases by FDA, (2) Remove the line authority for post-marketing regulation from the Office of New Drugs and give it to an Office of Drug Safety, either formed as a new center, or based on the current Office of Surveillance and Epidemiology. Just as OND now regulates pre- marketing with consults from OSE, ODS should regulate post-marketing with a consult from OND.,

(3) Make FDA managers criminally liable for coercion of reviewers, and make senior managers liable for failure to appropriately investigate and discipline managers who commit coercion, and (4) Mandate (and fully fund) posting of all FDA reviews immediately after a regulatory action is taken. Reviews should not be redacted except for proprietary manufacturing information. 11

ANSWERS TO SUBMITTED QUESTIONS FROM MR. BARTON TO DAVID ROSS, M.D.

1. Does the FDA hold periodic meetings called regulatory briefings?

a. If yes, please describe these briefings.

These are internal meetings held to discuss a regulatory question of current interest, with the goal of obtaining guidance from FDA managers; usually the topic is a specific New Drug Application (NDA) or Biologic Licensing Application (BLA) that is under review (or a supplement to such an application). In the Center for Drug

Evaluation and Research (CDER, regulatory) briefings are called at the discretion of the division or Office of Drug Evaluation (ODE) in which the submission is being reviewed. In CDER' Office of New Drugs (OND), the audience typically consists of the review team and upper management in the review division and ODE, along with office and division directors from OND; occasionally, management from other CDER Offices (e.g., Office of Biostatistics) will attend. The meeting is generally chaired by the director or deputy director of OND, although in some instances the director or deputy director of CDER will chair the meeting. Materials for the briefing will consist of a slide presentation and a briefing document or documents, which are distributed by e-mail in advance of the meeting. The format is generally a presentation of the relevant regulatory and scientific background, ending with key questions. The regulatory issues are then discussed. A project manager will prepare written minutes, summarizing any conclusions; these are distributed to attendees.

b. Do you believe regulatory briefings serve as an opportunity for different views or questions to be heard on drug safety?

In my experience, upper management (division directors and above) appears to feel free to offer their views at these briefings. I do not believe the environment is one that encourages primary reviewers or team leaders to speak freely, although there is no formal bar to their doing so. The best illustration I know of this is a regulatory briefing held in April 2006 on an supplemental NDA for daptomycin (Cubicin), for which the primary review team had recommended nonapproval, and division and office management were exerting pressure to approve the application. (Of note, the managers involved were the same as on the Ketek NDA). In order to encourage free discussion by the primary review team, the director of OND, Dr. John Jenkins, had to make explicit statements that any attendee who wished to speak could do so; Dr. Jenkins cited this event in an e-mail to me sent in May 2006. The need for an explicit statement that reviewers should feel free to speak up at an internal meeting suggests strongly that there is a culture at CDER that discourages free exchange of views by reviewers when they are aware that management holds a different opinion.

2. Do you agree with the Food and Drug Administration (FDA) Advisory Committee recommendation of December 15,2006, to limit Ketek's approved indication to community acquired pneumonia?

I agree with that recommendation, and I feel the Committee did an outstanding job of weighing the scientific evidence presented to it by the Applicant and the FDA. However, I will note that their recommendation was made without consideration of the questions of data and application integrity that exist for this NDA; a consideration of these issues might have led to a recommendation that marketing of Ketek be suspended until the validity of data presented to the Committee had been determined. It should be noted that the FDA permitted the Applicant to present data to the Committee that had not been submitted to or reviewed by the FDA; the Committee' vote to recommend continued marketing of Ketek for community-acquired pneumonia may have been influenced by presentation of this unvetted data.

3. Do you agree with FDA's announced labeling change of February 12, 2007, for Ketek?

No. First, the Agency has not publicly provided any scientific rationale for its label change, such as a posted review. Second, the Agency disregarded the Committee' explicit recommendation to add a Black Box warning regarding visual adverse events. Third, and most importantly, the unresolved fraud issues surrounding this application make any current determination of risk and benefit for Ketek invalid; rather than relabel the drug, the Agency should suspend its marketing until such time as the application integrity issues for this NDA have been resolved.

4. In your written testimony, you stated that FDA managers ignored warnings that Ketek was more dangerous than comparable antibiotics. In a May 1, 2006, Wall Street Journal article (attached), Dr. John Jenkins of the FDA stated that Ketek's liver-related problems look "not all that different than we would see for other antibiotics' for similar infections." Do you agree with Dr. Jenkins' statement?

No. In the same month that he gave this interview, CDER' Office of Office of Surveillance and Epidemiology (OSE) found that the reporting rate for acute liver failure associated with Ketek ranged from 3.5—11.5 times that of other antibiotics used for similar infections; the rate for Ketek was 23 cases of ALF/10 million exposures, while for Avelox' (moxifloxacin) it was 6.6 cases/10 million, and for Levaquin (levofloxacin), it was 2.1 cases/10 million; for the macrolide class that Ketek was supposed to replace, the rates were 4.2 cases/10 million (clarithromycin; Biaxin) and 3.7 cases/10 million (azithromycin; Zithromax). While there are uncertainties surrounding these estimates, differences in adverse event rates adjusted for usage and severity of infection that are greater than 3-fold generally are due to true differences in incidence rate, rather than unknown factors that bias the estimates. By way of comparison, the ALF reporting rate for trovafloxacin, an antibiotic removed from the market in the 1990's for ALF, was 58 cases/10 million, only 2.5 times that of Ketek.

Dr. Jenkins has never provided a detailed scientific explanation of the rationale for his statement. I am unclear as to how a rate of 23 is "not all that different" from a rate of 6.6.

5. To your knowledge, what is the best estimate of the actual incidence rate of liver toxicity in the patient population using Ketek and why do you consider it to be a credible estimate?

It is important to remember that most liver adverse events are never reported (please see attached paper by Sgro et al. (Hepatology 2002; 36:451–5, which found that only one out of every 16 liver adverse events was reported in a population-based survey). The OSE consult mentioned above found a total of 35 serious adverse events reported in 5.3 million exposures, a rate of 1 event/150,000 exposures. If one makes the conservative assumption that serious events are twice as likely to be reported as routine adverse events, so that for every one reported event, there are eight actual events, the incidence rate of serious liver toxicity with Ketek is approximately 1 event/20,000 exposures. This is in agreement with an estimate by Dr. William Lee, one of the world' leading authorities of drug-induced liver injury, a consultant to the FDA, and a participant in the December 2006 Advisory Committee meeting on Ketek. Dr. Lee gave as his estimate of the incidence rate of Ketek-associated liver toxicity leading to hospitalization as 1/20,000–1/30,000 at the meeting (see *www.fda.gov/ohrms/dockets/ac/06/transcripts/2006-4266t1-part4.pdf*, p. 400 (browser document p. 100 of 147)). Dr. Lee is Meredith Mosle Distinguished Professor in Liver Disease at the University of Texas Southwestern Medical Center; his address is UT Southwestern Medical Center at Dallas, 5323 Harry Hines Blvd, Dallas, Texas 75390–8887; his telephone number is (214) 648–3323; and his e-mail address is william.lee@utsouthwestern.edu.

FDA Timeline

Ketek™ (telithromycin)
Regulatory History

Janice Soreth, M.D.
Director
Division of Anti-Infective & Ophthalmology Products
CDER/FDA

Joint Meeting of Anti-Infective Drugs &
Drug Safety and Risk Management Advisory Committees
December 14-15, 2006

Ketek Regulatory History: Outline

- US Submissions: 1998-2004
  - 3 Review Cycles
- Two Advisory Committees:
  - April, 2001; January, 2003
- Division of Scientific Investigation Reports
- Efficacy & Safety Data

Joint Meeting of Anti-Infective Drugs &
Drug Safety and Risk Management Advisory Committees
December 14-15, 2006

2

Ketek Regulatory History: First Cycle 1998-2001

- 1998: clinical trials for phase 3 program discussed with FDA
  - community-acquired pneumonia, acute bacterial sinusitis, acute exacerbation of chronic bronchitis, tonsillopharyngitis
- FDA advice to sponsor on specific trial design based upon then current (1998) updated guidance
- 2000: NDA 21-144 filed
- 2001: Advisory Committee held

Joint Meeting of Anti-infective Drugs & Drug Safety and Risk Management Advisory Committees December 14-15, 2006

3

Ketek Regulatory History: First Cycle

At April 2001 Advisory Committee, four indications were discussed:

- community-acquired pneumonia*
- acute exacerbations of chronic bronchitis*
- acute sinusitis*
- tonsillopharyngitis

* including penicillin- and erythromycin-resistant *Streptococcus pneumoniae*

Joint Meeting of Anti-infective Drugs & Drug Safety and Risk Management Advisory Committees December 14-15, 2006

4

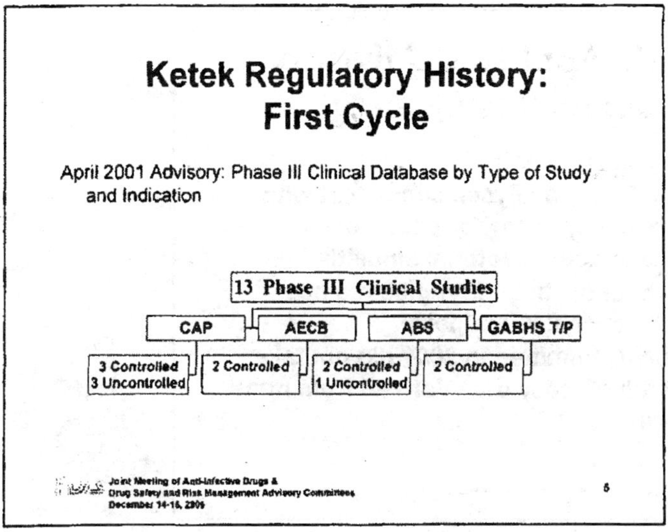
Ketek Regulatory History:
First Cycle
April 2001 Advisory: Phase III Clinical Database by Type of Study and Indication
13 Phase III Clinical Studies
CAP
AECB
ABS
GABHS T/P
3 Controlled
3 Uncontrolled
2 Controlled
2 Controlled
1 Uncontrolled
2 Controlled
Joint Meeting of Anti-Infective Drugs & Drug Safety and Risk Management Advisory Committees
December 14-15, 2006
5

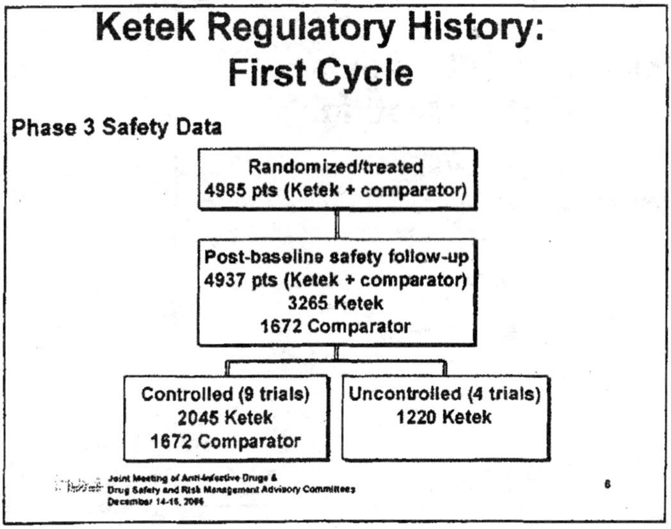
Ketek Regulatory History:
First Cycle
Phase 3 Safety Data
Randomized/treated
4985 pts (Ketek + comparator)
Post-baseline safety follow-up
4937 pts (Ketek + comparator)
3265 Ketek
1672 Comparator
Controlled (9 trials)
2045 Ketek
1672 Comparator
Uncontrolled (4 trials)
1220 Ketek
Joint Meeting of Anti-Infective Drugs & Drug Safety and Risk Management Advisory Committees
December 14-15, 2006
6

Ketek- April 2001 Advisory Committee Meeting

- Focus on safety data
- FDA's efficacy analyses consistent with those of the sponsor for pneumonia, AECB, and acute bacterial sinusitis
- Study in tonsillitis/pharyngitis did not meet pre-specified endpoint
- Advisory Committee in 2001 did not take issue with efficacy data derived from non-inferiority trials

Joint Meeting of Anti-Infective Drugs & Drug Safety and Risk Management Advisory Committees December 14-15, 2006

7

Ketek - April 2001 Advisory Committee Meeting

Chief safety concerns:

- Cardiac
- Hepatic
- Visual

Joint Meeting of Anti-Infective Drugs & Drug Safety and Risk Management Advisory Committees December 14-15, 2006

8

Ketek- April 2001
Advisory Committee Vote

- Do the efficacy and safety data presented support the use of Ketek in
  - community-acquired pneumonia 7 yes 3 no
  - AECB 0 yes 10 no
  - acute bacterial sinusitis 2 yes 8 no

- Are the data sufficient for a claim of pneumonia due to pen-resistant *S. pneumoniae*? 3 yes 7 no

Joint Meeting of Anti-Infective Drugs & Drug Safety and Risk Management Advisory Committees December 14-15, 2006

9

Ketek - April 2001
Advisory Committee Vote

Recommendations for additional Ketek studies:

- Safety
  - Larger number of patients need to be studied to determine safety
  - Special populations should be targeted (elderly, patients with hepatic impairment, renal impairment); more PK
  - Drug interactions should be evaluated
- Efficacy
  - More data requested in patients with drug-resistant *S. pneumoniae* (including bacteremia), *H. influenzae*

Joint Meeting of Anti-Infective Drugs & Drug Safety and Risk Management Advisory Committees December 14-15, 2006

10

Ketek Regulatory History: First Cycle Approvable Letter June 2001

- Ketek approvable for pneumonia, bronchitis, and sinusitis.
- Additional safety and efficacy data requested to assess risks/benefits
  - large safety trial in respiratory tract infections
  - PK studies, special populations
  - additional experience with drug-resistant *S. pneumoniae, H. influenzae,* bacteremia

Joint Meeting of Anti-Infective Drugs & Drug Safety and Risk Management Advisory Committees December 14-15, 2006 11

Ketek Regulatory History: Second Cycle

- July 24, 2002- resubmission included Study 3014 (24,000 patients, 1800 investigators), data from additional efficacy studies (CAP, AECB), PK studies, and some postmarketing data
- January 8, 2003: second Advisory meeting

Joint Meeting of Anti-Infective Drugs & Drug Safety and Risk Management Advisory Committees December 14-15, 2006 12

Ketek Regulatory History: Second Cycle January 8, 2003 Advisory

- Additional efficacy and safety data discussed: focus on study 3014, in addition to PK studies and community-acquired pneumonia targeting resistant *S. pneumoniae*
- Advisory Committee judged that safety and efficacy for the 3 requested indications had been demonstrated, in large measure on the safety data in study 3014
- DSI report of January 21, 2003: 3 clinical sites in study 3014 inspected; concerns raised about data integrity.

Joint Meeting of Anti-Infective Drugs & Drug Safety and Risk Management Advisory Committees December 14-15, 2006 13

Ketek Regulatory History: Second Cycle Approvable Letter Jan 23, 2003

- Safety could not be fully assessed
  - questions of data integrity raised by the conduct of study 3014
  - incomplete postmarketing safety data submitted from foreign marketing experience
- Requested additional information
  - on auditing, monitoring, and irregularities or violations of Good Clinical Practices in order to further evaluate data integrity in study 3014
  - complete reports (original and follow-up) and analyses of foreign postmarketing safety information

Joint Meeting of Anti-Infective Drugs & Drug Safety and Risk Management Advisory Committees December 14-15, 2006 14

**Ketek Regulatory History:
Third Cycle
CDER Regulatory Briefing February 19, 2003**

- "Issues of data integrity with Study 3014 are of concern and should be resolved before an approval action (if warranted) can be taken.
- Additional sites should be identified for future DSI inspections.
- If data provided by study 3014 cannot be used to support safety of Ketek, the Division might be able to rely on post-marketing data from those countries where Ketek has already been approved."

Joint Meeting of Anti-infective Drugs & Drug Safety and Risk Management Advisory Committees December 14-15, 2006 15

**Ketek Regulatory History:
Third Cycle
March 6, 2003 Closed Advisory Meeting**

- Closed AC meeting held to update the Anti-infective Advisory Committee on other development programs in the division.
- Committee was apprised of data integrity issues concerning study 3014 that precluded approval action.

Joint Meeting of Anti-infective Drugs & Drug Safety and Risk Management Advisory Committees December 14-15, 2006 16

Ketek Regulatory History: Third Cycle

- October 2003: Sponsor submitted analyses of foreign postmarketing data.
- Additional DSI inspections requested to provide an overall assessment of data integrity in study 3014.
- March 2004 DSI findings: Monitoring of study sites by sponsor failed to detect problems found by FDA inspections. Hence, integrity of data from all 1800 sites could not be assured with any degree of confidence.

Joint Meeting of Anti-Infective Drugs &
Drug Safety and Risk Management Advisory Committees
December 14-15, 2006 17

Ketek Regulatory History: Third Cycle

Clinical Review Summary

- Safety information included post-marketing adverse event reports generated from an estimated 3.7 million uses in foreign countries (2.2 million in France and Germany).
- All available safety data led to conclusion that Ketek appeared similar to other antibiotics in terms of hepatic and cardiac toxicity. Life-threatening exacerbation of myasthenia gravis noted in foreign use.
- Review of all available safety data supported approval of Ketek in April, 2004.

Joint Meeting of Anti-Infective Drugs &
Drug Safety and Risk Management Advisory Committees
December 14-15, 2006 18

Ketek Regulatory History: Approval April 1, 2004

The data that provided substantial evidence of safety and efficacy for Ketek (telithromycin) at the time approval included:

- Multiple comparative studies of community-acquired pneumonia (CAP), acute bacterial sinusitis (ABS), acute exacerbation of chronic bronchitis (AECB):
- These comparative studies were the basis for efficacy claims in CAP, ABS, and AECB. The studies also served as the basis for safety claims, providing information on the rates of adverse effects seen with Ketek compared to other antibiotics used for these indications.

Joint Meeting of Anti-Infective Drugs & Drug Safety and Risk Management Advisory Committees
December 14-15, 2006

19

Ketek Regulatory History: Approval April 1, 2004 (continued)

- Non-comparative studies of CAP with Ketek: In addition to the comparative CAP studies, these studies of CAP provided additional data on outcomes in patients with CAP due to multi-drug resistant *Streptococcus pneumoniae*.

- These non-comparative studies also provide safety data on the use of Ketek in the treatment of CAP.

Joint Meeting of Anti-Infective Drugs & Drug Safety and Risk Management Advisory Committees
December 14-15, 2006

20

Ketek Regulatory History: Approval April 1, 2004 (continued)

- **Phase 1 Visual study: This study of high-doses of telithromycin was performed to study the mechanism of the visual effects of Ketek.**
- **Multiple other phase 1 studies evaluating the pharmacokinetics of Ketek. These studies included food effect studies, drug interaction studies, QT prolongation, and studies of the pharmacokinetics of Ketek in patients with renal or hepatic impairment.**

Joint Meeting of Anti-Infective Drugs & Drug Safety and Risk Management Advisory Committees December 14-15, 2006

21

Ketek Regulatory History: Approval April 1, 2004 (continued)

Foreign post-marketing data in 3.7 million exposures were evaluated as part of the assessment of safety to identify uncommon serious adverse effects of Ketek (hepatic, visual, cardiac) based upon post-marketing reports from France, Germany, other European countries, and Latin America where Ketek was already approved.

Joint Meeting of Anti-Infective Drugs & Drug Safety and Risk Management Advisory Committees December 14-15, 2006

22

Sanofi-Aventis Timeline

February 5, 2007

Ketek® Study 3014 Timeline (Summary)

February 28, 2000	Ketek® NDA submitted to FDA containing pivotal Phase III safety and effectiveness studies and other supporting data.
April 26, 2001	FDA Anti-Infective Drugs Advisory Committee meeting to review Ketek® NDA. Committee recommends that Aventis obtain additional safety data from a large sample of patients.
May 23, 2001	Aventis meets with FDA with initial proposal for a large safety study to evaluate infrequently-occurring adverse events in the usual care setting.
June 1, 2001	FDA Approvable Letter calls for a large safety study with a patient population typical of actual use to evaluate potential adverse effects of special interest (AESIs) (hepatic, cardiac, visual and vasculate).
June 2001-August 2001	Aventis assesses candidates for contract research organization (CRO), contract laboratory, clinical investigator trainer and other Study 3014 functions.
August 2001 - September 2001	Aventis /FDA meetings and teleconferences on the design of Study 3014 -- the first pre-approval actual use study ever conducted for an anti-infective drug.
	Aventis submits draft protocol and monitoring plan to FDA for review and comment. Process for collection, review and statistical analysis of AESIs also submitted to FDA for review and comment.
September 11, 2001	Aventis meets with study contractors to review coordination and communication processes. Twice-a-week teleconferences between Aventis, PPD and other contractors begin on September 18, 2001.
September 27, 2001	Final study protocol, reflecting final FDA comments, completed by Aventis; officially submitted to FDA on October 17, 2001.
September 2001 - October 2001	PPD, the selected CRO, and Dimensional Health Care (DHC), the training contractor, begin the selection, qualification and training of doctors to be study investigators.
October 19, 2001	First subject enrolled in Study 3014. Enrollment continues through January 29, 2002. Over 24,000 study patients are enrolled at over 1,800 investigator sites.
October 2001 - June 2002	PPD monitors the conduct of the study through on-site monitoring visits, weekly scripted calls to study investigators and other contacts. These contacts track study progress, respond to inquiries and resolve any PPD or Aventis questions about data in case report forms and adverse event reports. On average, each site receives approximately 50 calls from PPD.

November 2001 - April 2002	PPD and Aventis monitoring visits and audits of Dr. Kirkman-Campbell Study 3014 site reveals non-conformances with good clinical practice. She was instructed to undertake corrective measures.
November 2001 - June 2002	PPD and Aventis review and assess initial reports of adverse events from investigation sites and obtain additional information to determine if any AESIs may have been unrecognized or otherwise missed. Outside consultant experts "adjudicate" AESIs to determine which ones appear to be caused by either Ketek® or Augmentin.
June 25, 2002	Aventis notifies FDA that data from two Study 3014 investigators cannot be confirmed or corrected, and therefore will not be included in the study. (Drs. Sharkar and Barber)
July 24, 2002	Study 3014 study report submitted to FDA. AESI safety data consistent with results from other clinical trials in the Ketek® NDA.
August 20, 2002	FDA letter to Aventis that July 24 submission constitutes a complete response to FDA's Approvable Letter.
October 15-24, 2002	FDA inspects Dr. Kirkman-Campbell. Inspection identifies deficiencies similar to those observed by PPD and Aventis.
December 9, 2002	FDA inspects Dr. Salerno in connection with Study 3014. List of observations identifies deviations from Study 3014 protocol and GCPs.
December 16. 2002	FDA inspects Dr. Lang in connection with Study 3014. List of observations identify deviations from Study 3014 protocol and GCPs.
December 19, 2002	Aventis/FDA meet in anticipation of the second Advisory Committee meeting on Ketek® NDA scheduled for January 2003.
January 8, 2003	Second meeting of FDA Advisory Committee on Study 3014. Committee votes to recommend approval of Ketek®.
January 24, 2003	Contrary to the Advisory Committee recommendations, FDA issues a second Approvable Letter calling for an additional assessment of Study 3014.
February 28, 2003	FDA/Aventis meeting at which FDA expresses concerns about data from some Study 3014 investigator sites, primarily Kirkman-Campbell. Aventis offers to remove data from study report for any site where fraud in study data is substantiated.
February 2003-July 2003	Aventis/FDA meetings and teleconferences to agree on analyses Aventis will conduct and data it should submit to FDA in response to FDA's January 24 Approvable Letter. FDA accepts Aventis proposal that outside experts perform an audit

	of data from a sample of Study 3014 investigators, including the Kirkman-Campbell site.
April 2, 2003	FDA inspects Aventis to assess the company's oversight of Study 3014. No objectionable observations were reported.
March 2003 - July 2003	Outside experts conduct and complete their "5-site review" pursuant to protocol based on FDA comments on issues to be addressed. The review finds that at four of the sites non-conformances were satisfactorily resolved and/or did not significantly compromise the overall integrity of the study or the reliability of the AESIs reported. The review finds that non-conformances at the Kirkman-Campbell site were not satisfactorily resolved, that those AESIs submitted by Dr. Kirkman-Campbell are reliable but that her overall AESI data set may be incomplete and the integrity of her study data may have been significantly compromised.
July 3, 2003	Aventis submits analysis of Study 3014 as agreed with FDA. The materials identify Study 3014 sites where there were significant GCP deficiencies. Aventis submission includes evaluation of Study 3014 safety data with the results from the Kirkman-Campbell site excluded. Assessment shows that exclusion of Kirkman-Campbell data does not affect the study conclusions.
August 29, 2003	Dr. Kirkman-Campbell is indicted on fraud and false statements charges in Study 3014.
October 17, 2003	Aventis submits amendment to NDA, including its final response to FDA questions on Study 3014.
October 23, 2003	Dr. Kirkman-Campbell pleads guilty. (On March 24, 2004, Dr. Kirkman-Campbell is sentenced to 57 months imprisonment and ordered to pay $925,000 in restitution to Aventis. The Court finds that Kirkman-Campbell used "sophisticated means" to commit fraud in her conduct of Study 3014.)
March 4, 2004	European Agency for the Evaluation of Medical Products (EMEA) concludes that exclusion of the Kirkman-Campbell data from Study 3014 does not affect the overall conclusions of the study.
April 1, 2004	FDA approves NDA for Ketek®.

Whistleblower Timeline

Ketek integrity issues/hepatotoxicity timeline

28 Feb 2000 — Original New Drug Application (NDA) 21-144 submitted for Ketek (telithromycin) by Aventis. Review assigned to Division of Anti-Infective Drug Products (DAIDP). Review of the telithromycin safety database of 3,265 patients in Phase 3 trials reveals one patient who developed such severe hepatitis that a liver biopsy was required for management – a remarkable event in an antibiotic trial with a safety database of this size. Review of the biopsy at Armed Forces Institute of Pathology (AFIP) shows evidence of severe drug-induced liver damage; the liver damage is noted by one of the safety reviewers to be similar to that caused by trovafloxacin, an antibiotic linked to fatal liver injury. The incidence rate of Ketek-associated hepatotoxicity is 0.03% (1/3265) in the safety database; one of the safety reviewers notes that a fatal serious adverse event (SAE) rate of 0.001% would result in 80 – 100 deaths annually in the U.S., given the extent of antibiotic prescribing in this country. Hepatic safety review reports other evidence of liver toxicity in NDA. Other potential toxicities include cardiac, visual, and drug interaction toxicities. Overall and hepatic clinical safety reviews recommend against approval.

26 Apr 2001 — Anti-Infective Advisory Committee (AIDAC) meeting. Liver damage due to telithromycin shown to be similar to that caused by Trovan, based on discussion by head of hepatic pathology at AFIP. Based on toxicity data, AIDAC recommends large safety study, and recommends against use in young children; states that antibiotics are probably not needed in chronic bronchitis.

1 June 2001 — Approvable (AE) letter requests large safety study and additional efficacy data. Non-approval (NA) letter issued for streptococcal tonsillopharyngitis (strep throat), based on a review showing that telithromycin was not equivalent to penicillin, the gold standard for treatment of this disease

19 Oct 2001 — Aventis initiates Study 3014 (also designated TREAT), a large usual care open-label, active-controlled safety study conducted at 1872 sites; ~12000 patients receive Ketek and ~12,000 receive a comparator, Augmentin. The study is intended to be conducted under Good Clinical Practices (GCPs); study monitoring is performed by a contract research organization (CRO), PPD.

6 Nov 2001 — Aventis TREAT team minutes note that monitoring will probably be limited to high enrolling sites and sites with SAEs

9 Nov 2001 — Dr. Anne Kirkman-Campbell (site 1129, Gadsden, AL) enrolls her first patient in TREAT.

4 Dec 2001 — Initial monitoring visit by PPD finds no problems at Kirkman-Campbell's site.

6 Dec 2001 — Study newsletter congratulates Kirkman-Campbell for enrolling 94 patients.

17 Jan 2002 — PPD e-mails Aventis that Kirkman-Campbell is enrolling ~30 patients/day.

22 Jan 2002 — Aventis TREAT team minutes note site 1129 (Dr. Anne Kirkman-Campbell) as source of concern.

Annotated Ketek Timelines

29 Jan 2002	Kirkman-Campbell enrolls her 407th and final patient in TREAT. Dr. Kirkman-Campbell has ostensibly enrolled over 1% of the adult population of Gadsden in TREAT.
25 Feb 2002	Initial consultation by Aventis with internal statistician re: Kirkman-Campbell.
26 Feb 2002	New high enrolling site (William Terpstra, site #1622, Noblesville, IN) identified as source of concern. Continuing to enroll patients after being told to stop. Issues include: alterations of informed consent forms, multiple GCP violations, lack of awareness of GCP guidelines. Site ends up enrolling >160 subjects.
27 Feb 2002	PPD staff send Aventis e-mail detailing specific concerns about Kirkman-Campbell. Specifically: • Patients enrolled who did not appear to have an appropriate infection • Extremely rapid enrollment of patients, including enrollment at times when clinic was closed • Suspicious lab values • Limited documentation
5 Mar 2002	TREAT team decides to compare variability of Kirkman-Campbell's lab results with 2nd and 3rd highest enrolling sites (both of these sites will turn out later to have serious GCP issues; see entries for 4 Dec 2002 and 23 Dec 2002). No other steps documented. New site identified with possible forged patient signatures.
15 Mar 2002	PPD e-mail to Aventis notes lack of co-operation by Kirkman-Campbell with monitoring.
18 Mar 2002	Statistical analysis by Aventis shows no differences among top 3 enrolling sites; decision made that no action necessary.
19 Mar 2002	PPD e-mails reveal disagreement with Aventis over issue of forged signatures.
24 May 2002	PPD monitor notifies Aventis of another suspicious high-enrolling site (Vincent Sghiatti, site #0469, Los Angeles, CA); problems included no drug accountablility log, low reporting of adverse events, lack of PI signature on any informed consent forms.
5 Jun 2002	Aventis sends brief e-mail to PPD monitor about Sghiatti site, thanking her for a telephone conversation "confirming that no doubt exists regarding the reliability of the data collected from this site, and no misconduct could be suspected." No specifics given in e-mail about how potential GCP issues were resolved; no confirmatory e-mail from PPD documenting her agreement with Aventis's conclusions.
19 Jun 2002	E-mails reveal wide-spread problems with discrepancies in information from investigators.
25 Jun 2002	E-mails reveal two additional investigators not co-operating with monitoring visits. Aventis meeting minutes of 22 Jan 2002 indicate that FDA was to be

	notified; however, FDA project manager (Judit Milstein) did not recall being notified of these investigators.
24 Jul 2002	Resubmission of NDA with data from Study 3014 and additional efficacy data. Title page of Study 3014 report explicitly states that GCPs were followed; no mention of Kirkman-Campbell or other problematic Study 3014 investigators in study report.
4 Aug 2002	FDA reviewers note low reporting rate for adverse events (AEs) in study 3014.
9 Sep 2002	Decision made to inspect highest enrolling site in Study 3014 (Kirkman-Campbell). Formal consult sent to Division of Scientific Investigations (DSI) on 11 Sep 2002.
13 Sep 2002	Review of random sample of case report forms (CRFs) from Study 3014 shows multiple inconsistencies.
1 Nov 2002	DAIDP notified that inspection of highest enroller (Kirkman-Campbell) revealed multiple serious GCP violations; 407 subjects enrolled in catchment of. Significant GCP violations; 483 issued; Office of Criminal Investigation (OCI) referral. OCI interview with CRO informant reveals that Aventis had been informed of "red" flags (enrollment of patients every few minutes, and at times clinic had been closed; lack of AEs reported for first 100 patients.
13 Nov 2002	DAIDP requests DSI inspection of second and third-largest enrollers (Lang and Salermo).
4 Dec 2002	DAIDP notified that third-largest enroller (Egisto Salerno, San Diego, CA) had been on probation at time of study, with license suspended on emergency basis shortly after study ended because of drug, weapons, and assault charges.
10 Dec 2002	DAIDP notified of additional suspicious site at which company allegedly knew of problems. The investigator in question enrolled 2.5% of the adult population in his town, as well as family members.
18 Dec 2002	Aventis requests a "high-level debriefing" with Dr. Mark Goldberger (Office of Drug Evaluation IV (ODE 4) director) and Dr. Janice Soreth (DAIDP director) alone, in connection with a face-to-face meeting scheduling for the next day.
19 Dec 2002	Face to face meeting between Aventis and FDA. Company admits that it knew of "problems" at Kirkman-Campbell sites, but claimed there "were no other Kirkman-Campbells in 3014. (The following day, an FDA reviewer notes that technically Aventis is right since there is no other investigator names Kirkman-Campbell in the study, and suggests that there are no reliable sites in the entire study.) No explanation given for retention of investigator in study or failure to inform FDA re: possible data integrity problems. 20 Dec 2002 Definition of hepatic side-effects in Study 3014 found to have been significantly changed without notice to FDA.
20 Dec 2002	Dr. Goldberger requests team to look into possibility of post-marketing data from Europe as way of demonstrating safety of Ketek. Results show that majority of

Annotated Ketek Timelines

	Ketek post-marketing data is from countries with poor pharmacovigilance systems.
23 Dec 2002	Serious GCP violations found at second-largest enrolling site (Lang). Reviewers note common features of suspicious sites, and note that Aventis must have been aware of issues at high enrolling sites.
24 Dec 2002	FDA reviewers note improbably high enrollment of patients relative to local population. Analyses of high enrollers in study 3014 shows that 19 sites enrolled $\geq$1% of adults in the catchment area
2 Jan 2003	Safety Team Leader (Dr. David Ross) e-mails Dr. Goldberger (cc to Dr. Soreth) asking to discuss presentation of data integrity issues to Anti-Infective Advisory Committee. Goldberger responds that presentation of these issues "would not be productive", and urges that we focus on best possible presentation of post-marketing data.
8 Jan 2003	AIDAC meeting. Study 3014 data presented to AIDAC; no mention of data integrity issues at decision of office and division management. Applicant presents post-marketing safety data not available to Agency. Statistician (Dr. Janet Elashoff) on AIDAC notes that the trials do not demonstrate efficacy for any indication. Committee votes to recommend approval.
17 Jan 2003	Dr. Goldberger instructs Dr. Soreth not to have any more conversations by herself with Aventis.
21 Jan 2003	Dr. Sandra Kweder (Deputy Director, Office of New Drugs) sends e-mail to DAIDP outlining need to emphasize data integrity issues to Aventis. Dr. John Jenkins (Director, OND), and Dr. Janet Woodcock (Director, CDER) aware of data integrity issues and agree.
21 Jan 2003	Dr. John Alexander's review of efficacy concludes that there is no basis for granting a claim of efficacy for Ketek against macrolide-resistant organisms. This conclusion is based on: 1) the lack of any precedent for approval of this claim; 2) the lack of evidence to support the clinical impact of macrolide resistance; 3) the in vitro data suggesting partial cross-resistance between macrolides and Ketek; and 4) the lack of a significant difference between clinical cure rates against macrolide-resistant organisms between Ketek and macrolides, suggesting that macrolide resistance has no clinical import and that Ketek's activity against these organisms does not represent a clinically meaningful benefit, especially in view of its possible toxicity.
24 Jan 2003	AE letter issued. Major deficiencies cited: Unreliability of study 3014 data; incomplete post-marketing data. Post-marketing and audit data requested.
10 Feb 2003	FDA reviewers note major discrepancies in reported AE rates in European post-marketing data submitted by Aventis. Safety team leader estimates that Ketek could potentially cause as many as 2000 liver-related deaths annually in US.

Annotated Ketek Timelines

19 Feb 2003	Internal regulatory briefing with OND management. Chair of meeting is Dr. John Jenkins, director of OND. Discussants agree that issues with Study 3014 need to be resolved prior to approval.
4 Mar 2003	DAIDP and DSI continue work on data integrity issues with Study 3014; PPD informant offers to provide list of problematic sites.
7 Mar 2003	Telecon between ODE 4/DAIDP and Aventis in which Aventis is informed that a decision on 3014 acceptability will be necessary before Ketek can be approved.
20 Mar 2003	Additional clinical sites identified for inspection. Inspection of PPD and Aventis records also planned.
22 Apr 2003	DSI receives records from Aventis; all audit records related to study 3014 requested. Sponsor supplies records with virtually all lines blacked out.
1 July 2003	Meeting between Dr. Janet Woodcock and Aventis senior management; details of meeting unavailable.
11 Aug 2003	Inspection requests issued for five more investigators (Khan, Terpstra, Harker, Knecht, Achreja). All five have significant GCP violations; OCI opens two additional investigations (Knecht and Achreja).
29 Aug 2003	Kirkman-Campbell indicted.
Sep 2003	Goldberger receives e-mail from Center Director alerting him that investigation of Ketek is likely to be "big"
16 Sep 2003	Medical team leader safety review for 2nd cycle entered into DFS. "Softening" of final paragraph "requested" by Dr. Soreth.
17 Oct 2003	2nd resubmission of NDA. Aventis is allowed by DAIDP to submit only a limited set of audit and correspondence records, rather than full set requested in AE letter of 24 Jan 2003. Agreement is based on e-mails sent 12 Aug and 14 Aug 2003; no record in DFS of e-mail senders or recipients.
23 Oct 2003	Meeting between FDA and Aventis, with 17 infectious disease consultants in attendance at Aventis's request to provide "expert statements." Consultants had been briefed on study 3014 by company but were not aware of data integrity issues.
23 Oct 2003	Kirkman-Campbell pleads guilty to one count of mail fraud
6 Nov 2003	Revised Ketek safety team leader review entered into DFS.
5 Feb 2004	Dr. Soreth insists that an unrelated supplement be approved over reviewer and team leader's objections; despite objections, reviewer is eventually pressured into changing review.

Annotated Ketek Timelines

8 Feb 2004	Dr. Ross sends e-mail to David Roeder (Associate Director for Regulatory Affairs for ODE 4) e-mail documenting pressure to change Ketek review and 2nd review. No reply received from Roeder or his supervisor, Dr. Goldberger.
11 Feb 2004	Ross sends e-mail to his team with cc to Roeder regarding CDER policy banning pressure to alter reviews. No response from Roeder or Goldberger.
16 Feb 2004	Division director signs off on team leader safety review for 2nd cycle
16 Mar 2004	Original Safety team leader review (from 16 Sep 2003) for 2nd cycle entered and signed into DFS by Dr. Ross; TL documents that original review was altered at Dr. Soreth's direction.
25 Mar 2004	DSI consult issued concluding that none of the data in 3014 is reliable.
1 Apr 2004	Ketek approved. Office/division director memorandum mentions that there was "systemic failure" of the monitoring system for Study 3014, but does not mention suspicious behavior by company, or analyze risk of hepatotoxicity relative to benefit. Reliability of post-marketing data not addressed. Issues raised in Dr. Alexander's efficacy review regarding lack of evidence for clinical significance of macrolide resistance not addressed. No review of correspondence between company and PPD, in either safety review or office/division director review. No check with OCI regarding ongoing investigation.
28 May 2004	ORA investigator for Kirkman-Campbell site expresses concern over approval of Ketek despite evidence for fraud.
2 Aug 2004	Ketek launched in U.S.
May 2005	3 cases of severe liver injury noted at NC medical center; one death and one OLT, with liver from transplanted patient. MedWatch form submitted by Aventis with relatively few details. Report from physician has complete details.
June 14 2005	Consult from CDER Office of Drug Safety notes death of 26 year old man in NC from acute liver failure after taking Ketek. No regulatory action or other follow-up taken.
15-16 Jan 2006	CDER management holds emergency management on MLK holiday weekend to discuss impending publication of hepatotoxicity cases in *Annals of Internal Medicine*
20 Jan 2006	Electronic publication of hepatotoxicity cases in *Annals of Internal Medicine*. New hepatotoxicity case reported by Aventis via Medwatch; company claims few details available. Agency responds with Public Health Advisory describing study 3014 as pre-marketing evidence of safety.
20 Jan 2006	Division director for Ketek (Dr. Soreth) requests analysis of Study 3014 using unvalidated data mining system, despite overwhelming evidence that study is unreliable.

Annotated Ketek Timelines

23 Jan 2006	Primary medical officer prepares presentation on Ketek showing that hepatotoxicity rate in US is ten-fold higher than in other countries. Pivotal final safety assessment was based entirely on foreign data. Reviewer states in e-mail that he is suspicious of accuracy of company's reporting, but division director (Dr. Soreth) has repeatedly rejected his concerns.
26 Jan 2006	*Annals of Internal Medicine* informs FDA that it will stop accepting advertisements for Ketek; Dr. Jenkins (OND director) terms this an "overreaction". Center director (Dr. Galson) concurs.
7 Feb 2006	FDA learns of new case of severe Ketek-associated hepatotoxicity;
17 Feb 2006	David Ross (now of the Office of Oncology Drug Products) and Rosemary Johann-Liang (Office of Drug Safety) meet with John Jenkins and Sandy Kweder (Director and Deputy Director of OND, respectively); tell them of serious data, application, and review integrity issues with Ketek; warn them that Agency will be "crucified" if it does not act on these issues and story becomes public. Call for global reassessment of Ketek integrity issues. Inform Jenkins and Kweder that visual toxicity, especially in young children, is a huge concern. Also inform Jenkins and Kweder of corrupt scientific culture in Office of Antimicrobial Products (formerly ODE 4) with pressure to change reviews in order to approve drugs. JJ and SK given Ketek timeline and DSI consult, along with detailed analysis and examples of unscientific practices in OAP. Kweder responds by thanking them, but asking under what circumstances they would be willing to be publicly identified as having raised concerns.
18 Feb 2006	Kweder e-mails Mark Goldberger suggesting meeting on Ketek, to include previous reviewers, but does not insist on this. Ross suggests additional reviewers to attend. March 1 meeting scheduled without Ross or prior review team. Goldberger replies that he doesn't understand purpose of meeting to discuss Study 3014.
23 Feb 2006	Kweder asks Ross to meet with Goldberger to discuss Ketek integrity issues. Goldberger is out of the office, and Ross meets with Goldberger's deputy, Ed Cox.
23 Feb 2006	Ross furnishes Jenkins and Kweder with additional documentation regarding reviewers being pressured to alter reviews. He does not receive any reply.
27 Feb 2006	Ross e-mails Jenkins and Kweder re: conversation with MG documenting failure to respond substantively to concerns over Ketek, and renewing call for reassessment of Ketek integrity issues. Names of reviewers who have been pressured by Dr. Soreth given to JJ and SK; no attempt made by them to interview them

Annotated Ketek Timelines

1 Mar 2006	Ketek safety review meeting; Ross and prior members not present.
2 Mar 2006	Aventis receives letter from FDA requesting full set of post-marketing reports on hepatic safety.
21 Mar 2006	Print version of Annals article. Editorial in same issue cites Study 3014 as evidence that Ketek is no more toxic to liver than other antibiotics. Dr. Kweder responds to reviewer complaints about this by stating that useful information was obtained from Study 3014; does not refer to DSI consult of 25 March 2004 that concluded that data from this study was completely unreliable.
7 May 2006	Jenkins sends e-mail to Ross telling him to "disengage" from review teams in DAIDP; if he talks to reviewers there about scientific issues, he should include OAP management
16 May 2006	FDA Office of Drug Safety (now Office of Surveillance and Epidemiology) issues final analysis of Ketek-related liver events; finds that Ketek has >10 times the reporting rate of comparable antibiotics
22 June 2006	Acting Commissioner Andrew von Eschenbach meets with current Ketek review team; warns reviewers not to tell anyone outside the Agency about Ketek, and states that anyone who disobeys will be "benched" or "traded" from the "team."
29 June 2006	Ketek labeling revised; no written review prepared by review division to explain why risk of Ketek is outweighed by benefit.

Visual issues timeline

20 May 2002	IND 64,843 submitted for pediatric formulation of Ketek.
21 Nov 2002	Review of initial Phase 3 safety data shows that Ketek causes visual disturbances at 14 times the rate of comparator antibiotics.
11 Mar 2003	Review of visual safety from study 3014 reveals that Ketek is 15 times more likely to cause transient visual loss due to blurring of vision. Overall review of safety shows evidence that drug interactions may dramatically increase risk of visual toxicity, and risk of an event is directly proportional to concentration of drug in tear fluid. Mechanism unknown. **Effect appears to be most pronounced in younger individuals.**
22 Oct 2003	Internal FDA ophthalmology consultant states that he does not know of any other drug product causing visual toxicities in the same manner as Ketek.
31 Mar 2004	Review of post-marketing events shows large numbers of reports of visual blurring, loss of accommodation. Duration of event may be prolonged (hours).
1 Apr 2004	Ketek approved; label warns of severe cases of visual disturbance.
8 June 2004	DAIDP agrees to trials of Ketek in children in tonsillopharyngitis, despite poor performance of the drug in adults for this infection. Agrees to trials of Ketek in children in otitis media, despite availability of multiple agents for this indication.
14 Feb 2005	DAIDP agrees to informed consent forms for pediatric trials stating that there is no evidence of long-term risk to children's vision, despite any long-term safety studies. Issue of inability to monitor visual toxicity in young children is not assessed.
26 Oct 2005	At FDA-Aventis telecon, Aventis indicates that 150 children have been enrolled in otitis media studies; rejects need to perform nested substudy to assess vision. Complains that wording of informed consent form is limiting enrollment
25 Feb 2006	Cooper informs Goldberger informed of concerns over visual toxicity in children and potential measures to improve safety monitoring in ongoing trials in children; Goldberger informed that trials in children are ongoing.
27 Mar 2006	FDA receives report of 15 month child treated under IND with Ketek developing "staring spells". No referral to ophthalmologist or neurologist. Sponsor downgrades report from serious to non-serious.

<u>Abbreviations</u>

AE	Approvable letter or adverse event
AFIP	Armed Forces Institute of Pathology
AIDAC	Anti-Infective Drugs Advisory Committee – gives advice on new antibiotic NDAs
CDER	Center for Drug Evaluation and Research
DAIDP	Division of Anti-Infective Drug Products – responsible for Ketek review
DSI	Division of Scientific Investigations – supervises clinical site audits for FDA
GCP	Good Clinical Practice – standard clinical trial methodology used to guard against fraud
NA	Non-approval letter
NDA	New Drug Application
OAP	Office of Antimicrobial Products – new name for ODE 4 as of Oct 2005
OCI	Office of Criminal Investigation
ODE 4	Office of Drug Evaluation 4 (ODE 4) – supervises DAIDP
ODS	Office of Drug Safety
OND	Office of New Drugs – supervises ODE 4
ORA	Office of Regulatory Affairs – conducts field inspections
SAE	Serious Adverse Event
TREAT	Acronym for Study 3014

FDA NEWS

THE FOOD AND DRUG ADMINISTRATION / AN AGENCY OF THE U.S. DEPARTMENT OF HEALTH AND HUMAN SERVICES

FOR IMMEDIATE RELEASE
February 12, 2007
P07-19
Media Inquiries: 301-827-6242
Pr ss Officer: Susan Cruzan
su an.cruzan@fda.hhs.gov
Consumer Inquiries: 888-INFO-FDA

FDA ANNOUNCES LABEL AND INDICATION CHANGES FOR THE ANTIBIOTIC KETEK

The Food and Drug Administration (FDA) today announced revisions to the labeling for the antibiotic Ketek (telithromycin) designed to improve the safe use of Ketek by patients. The changes include the removal of two of the three previously approved indications -- acute bacterial sinusitis and acute bacterial exacerbations of chronic bronchitis -- from the drug's label. The agency has determined that the balance of benefits and risks no longer support approval of the drug for these indications. Ketek will remain on the market for the treatment of community acquired pneumonia of mild to moderate severity (acquired outside of hospitals or long-term care facilities).

In addition, the agency has worked with the company, Sanofi Aventis, to update the product labeling with a "boxed warning," FDA's strongest form of warning. The warning states that Ketek is contraindicated (should not be used) in patients with myasthenia gravis, a disease that causes muscle weakness.

FDA also worked with the manufacturer to develop a Patient Medication Guide -- that informs patients about the risk of the drug and how to use it safely. The Medication Guide (an FDA-approved patient information sheet) will be provided to patients with each prescription.

"Today's action is the result of comprehensive scientific analysis and thoughtful public discussion of the data available for Ketek, and includes important changes in the labeling designed to improve the safe use of Ketek by patients and give healthcare providers the most up-to-date prescribing information," said Steven Galson, M.D., Director, Center for Drug Evaluation and Research.

Other labeling changes included in today's action are a strengthened warning section regarding specific drug-related adverse events including visual disturbances and loss of consciousness. Warnings for hepatic toxicity (rare but severe symptoms of liver disease) were strengthened in June 2006.

The joint advisory committee, which met on December 14 and 15, 2006, advised that the available data including data acquired since the initial approval of Ketek support a conclusion that the benefits of Ketek outweigh the risks in patients with community acquired pneumonia, but not for patients with acute bacterial sinusitis or acute bacterial exacerbation of chronic bronchitis. They also recommended a boxed warning as well as Medication Guide for the drug. The joint panel consisted of FDA's Anti-Infective Drugs and Drug Safety and Risk Management Advisory committees.

The antibiotic Ketek was originally approved in 2004 and is manufactured by Sanofi Aventis.

For additional information, visit: http://www.fda.gov/cder/drug/infopage/telithromycin/default.htm

####

ATTENTION TV BROADCASTERS: Please use open caption for the hearing impaired.

FDA On The Internet: www.fda.gov

THE WALL STREET JOURNAL. ONLINE

February 12, 2007

COMMENTARY

The Clinical Trial

By MARK THORNTON
February 12, 2007; Page A14

On March 1, a federal appeals court will hear oral arguments in the case of the Abigail Alliance organization's lawsuit to change systems at the Food and Drug Administration to allow terminally ill patients access to promising drugs that have successfully completed initial stages of human safety testing. Because of my former role in the oncology division at the FDA, and in my eight-year experience as a cancer patient advocate on behalf of my son, I may be able to shed some light on the regulatory policy, medical drug development and patient rights issues surrounding this landmark case.

Abigail Burroughs was a young lady who developed a rare form of cancer in her mouth. As she was dying, her father fought to gain access to a drug that could possibly help her, but was denied access because the drug had not yet been approved by the FDA. After Abigail died, her father formed the Abigail Alliance, an organization which subsequently sued the government to force change in the policies that require FDA control over which dying patient does and does not receive approval to receive a drug not yet on the market. In the first round in the courts, the FDA won, but on appeal, the Abigail Alliance won. March 1 is the rubber match of the lawsuit.

If the Abigail Alliance is successful, drug companies could seek early approval of a drug for patients who are terminally ill and who are ineligible for participation in human testing of drugs that occur prior to FDA approval. The only requirement would be that the drug must have surpassed the initial safety phase of human testing, called "Phase I clinical trials." Critics of that position claim that current regulations and processes fully meet the needs of such patients -- doctors merely need to ask the government, on behalf of their patients, for access to any unapproved drug they wish. Change of the status quo is therefore unnecessary.

If these critics could be a fly on the wall at the FDA after such a special request is made by a doctor, they might change their tune. I can attest to the burden the physician-sponsors of these requests have to go through with FDA reviewers as they run the gauntlet. Manufacturing, pharmacology, toxicology, pharmacokinetic, clinical and even statistical "issues" raised by FDA staff, aimed at the applying physician, can sometimes rival receipt of an audit from the IRS. Requests are on occasion withdrawn by exasperated doctors or refused by the FDA, leaving patients to fend for themselves.

Other critics of Abigail Alliance also claim that at the threshold for early approval for the terminally ill, i.e., post-Phase I testing, the safety of the drug is still very much a concern; many more years of snuggling with the data will still be necessary before the FDA will feel things are just right. The fact is that all drugs, no matter what stage of development, have the potential to evolve new safety concerns. Since a drug is safe enough for the hundreds of patients in the "Phase II" of human testing, how is it not safe enough for a patient whose only option is the terminal progression of his disease?

Critics of early access also present doomsday scenarios of the impact of success of the Abigail Alliance case on the medical drug development process called "Phase III clinical trials." Over the last 25 years the U.S. has evolved an enormous engine for testing new drugs on patients at hundreds of medical centers in the country. If you have a life-threatening disease like cancer, and you want to try a drug not yet on the market, you better belly-up to a clinical trial, or wait a few years (or six or seven) before your doctor can prescribe it. It is a bloated and slow engine, but it is the best process we have to try to show if a new drug works or not.

Some with a vested interest in maintaining the status quo, such as medical society groups, might feel threatened by a victory by the Abigail Alliance if the perception is that a patient will be able to easily opt out of clinical trials and just get the drug directly. How will we ever get new drugs properly tested if everyone is slipping past the engine? In my opinion this threat is non-existent. One criterion of the patients under consideration by the court is that they cannot even be eligible for a clinical trial. In addition, the FDA will still have enormous authority in deciding who is truly terminal, who is eligible for other clinical trials, and whether other treatment options exist.

And what about the rights of the dying patient in all this? In the case of those with cancer, the patient turns not to the FDA but to his oncologist for options. These physicians are among the most well-educated and well-intentioned individuals in our society. The oncologist already has much access to off-label use of approved medications for patients in a terminal setting. The system is well suited to adapting should an Abigail Alliance victory add additional options to the patients and physicians faced with advancing and otherwise untreatable cancer.

Patients have valid arguments in demanding greater access to promising agents under development. Public servants should respect citizens who advocate that they be allowed to have a say in methods of their treatment when terminally ill, and government officials should have very compelling reasons for denying such access. New drug development will not suffer if a small minority of patients fighting for their lives, with no other options and in concert with their physician, gain access to a potentially beneficial agent with an established basic safety profile.

Mr. Thornton was formerly a medical reviewer in the oncology division at the FDA and is currently a senior vice president for GenVec, Inc.

URL for this article:
http://online.wsj.com/article/SB117124379156005353.html

THE WALL STREET JOURNAL. ONLINE

May 1, 2006

PAGE ONE

Infected Data

Fraud, Errors Taint Key Study Of Widely Used Sanofi Drug

Despite Some Faked Results, FDA Approves Antibiotic; One Doctor's Cocaine Use

Company Defends Safety

By ANNA WILDE MATHEWS
May 1, 2006

On Feb. 3, 2005, a 26-year-old construction worker named Ramiro Obrajero Pulquero walked into the emergency room at Carolinas Medical Center in Charlotte, N.C. Yellow from jaundice, he was running a fever and vomiting blood. Doctors quickly diagnosed liver failure, but a battery of tests couldn't explain its cause. He died three days later.

After seeing an autopsy report, physician Kimberly Clay and her colleagues concluded the answer might lie in a prescription bottle that Mr. Obrajero's wife brought with her to the hospital. It had contained the antibiotic Ketek, which her husband had taken a few weeks earlier after getting a sore in his nose. "When everything came back negative, the only thing we had was the Ketek," said Dr. Clay. An account of the death appeared in the Annals of Internal Medicine online in January.

Mr. Obrajero's widow, Ana Patricia Juarez, returned with the couple's two small daughters to La Concepción, his native village in central Mexico. "He was a healthy man, strong, and then suddenly we were watching him slip away," she recalls in an interview. "But we never knew why or how it could happen."

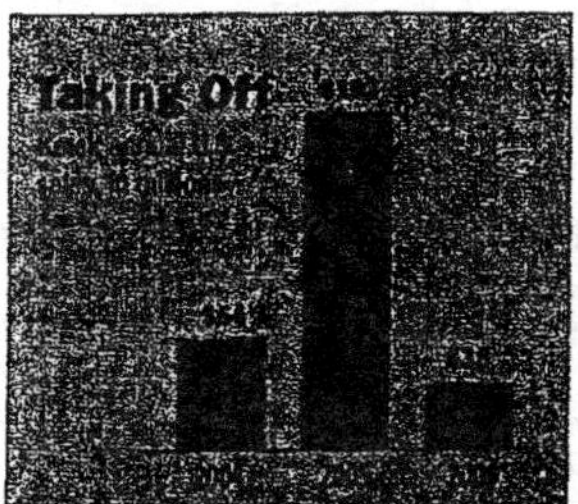

Ketek (pronounced KEY-tech) was approved by the Food and Drug Administration in April 2004. Its maker at the time was Aventis, a French-German company that after a merger is now called **Sanofi-Aventis** SA and based in Paris. Sanofi-Aventis, the world's third-largest drug company with 2005 revenue of $34 billion, says Ketek is an important weapon against respiratory infections. Last year the pills were prescribed 3.35 million times in the U.S. and brought in $193 million, according to IMS Health.

However, reports of severe liver damage among people taking Ketek have surfaced. An internal FDA analysis cited

10 reports of people suffering liver failure after taking Ketek, though it wasn't clear how many cases were caused by the drug. Agency officials say this is a preliminary estimate.

Now documents including internal Aventis emails reviewed by The Wall Street Journal are raising questions about a key clinical trial -- called study 3014 -- of more than 24,000 people that the company submitted to the FDA seeking approval for the drug.

The doctor who treated the most patients in the study, Maria "Anne" Kirkman Campbell, is in federal prison after pleading guilty to defrauding Aventis and others. An indictment says Dr. Campbell fabricated data she sent to the company. The documents show that Aventis was worried about Dr. Campbell early in study 3014 but didn't tell the FDA until the agency's own inspectors discovered the problem independently.

A doctor in California who treated the third-most patients in the study was on probation at the time with the state medical board for gross negligence and failure to keep adequate records. Shortly after his involvement in the study ended, police responding to a domestic-violence call found the doctor at home hiding a bag of cocaine in his underwear and holding a loaded semiautomatic handgun, according to a later complaint by the California medical board. The doctor lost his license.

The full extent of the study's problems has never been made public. Its results were cited last month in an article in the New England Journal of Medicine that suggested Ketek is as safe as other antibiotics. Five of the six authors of that article disclosed that they received consulting fees from Sanofi-Aventis, and the sixth was an Aventis employee at the time of the study.

Aventis originally undertook study 3014 in 2001 at the request of the FDA, which was worried about liver damage, blurry vision and other possible side effects from Ketek after reviewing the company's earlier trials. The agency said at the time that it couldn't approve Ketek without further research. It later concluded study 3014 was so rife with flaws that its data couldn't be relied upon.

An FDA official, Janice Soreth, says the agency nonetheless approved Ketek because of a key piece of information it didn't have in 2001: the drug's record in Europe and other countries. It was approved for use in Europe in July 2001. Dr. Soreth says Ketek was used about four million times overseas and reports of safety problems were minimal. The FDA typically prefers clinical trials to spontaneous reports of side effects partly because not all incidents get reported.

In a written statement to The Wall Street Journal, Sanofi-Aventis defends study 3014. "Although deviations were identified at several sites in the study, the data nevertheless provide important insight into the safety profile of Ketek," the statement says. Overall results from the study showed that Ketek was generally safe and didn't cause any cases of liver failure or death.

Sanofi-Aventis denies withholding any information that it was supposed to disclose to the FDA. It says it has reported "infrequent" liver events to the FDA but after a review the company "concluded that these events do not alter the overall benefit/risk profile of Ketek." The drug's label already mentions potential liver concerns, though not prominently.

Asked detailed questions about the emails and documents viewed by The Wall Street Journal, Sanofi-Aventis confirmed the gist of some but didn't comment on specifics.

The Senate Finance Committee is now examining issues raised by Ketek. "The Ketek allegations appear to be as serious as anything I've seen so far," said Sen. Charles Grassley, an Iowa Republican who is chairman of the Finance Committee, in a statement.

In the House, the offices of Democratic Reps. Edward Markey of Massachusetts and Henry Waxman of California are looking at the drug's history. Reps. Markey and Waxman also expressed their concerns in statements. Mr. Waxman said he is "deeply disturbed" by the approval of Ketek. He said Aventis "failed to disclose to FDA grave flaws in a key safety study."

Constant Tension

The Ketek case reflects the constant tension at the FDA between the push for new treatments and safety issues. As drug-resistant bacteria spread, the agency has faced pressure to approve new antibiotics. Even for antibiotics that raise safety issues, the chance that any individual will suffer serious damage is extremely low. The antibiotic Trovan was used by 2.5 million people as of 1999, and the FDA received 14 reports of liver failure. That was enough for the agency to severely restrict use of the drug.

John Jenkins, who heads the FDA's office of new drugs, says the agency and outside experts are assessing the recent reports of liver damage but the FDA still believes Ketek is "safe and effective when used according to the labeling." Dr. Jenkins says the rate of liver-related problems looks "not all that different than we would see for other antibiotics" for similar infections.

Aventis first sought permission to sell Ketek in the U.S. in March 2000. Fifteen months later the FDA refused to approve it. Eager to save a drug then seen as a potential big seller, Aventis hired a contractor called Pharmaceutical Product Development Inc., which specializes in coordinating clinical trials.

Starting in October 2001, the study enrolled patients with respiratory infections. They were given either Ketek or Augmentin, a widely used antibiotic. Aventis and its contractor, PPD, offered doctors $100 for each patient they signed up, another $150 when they submitted results and a final $150 after all questions were resolved, according to a contract with Dr. Campbell, the doctor who is now in prison. The contract became public during her court case.

Sanofi-Aventis says in its statement that it chose many primary-care doctors to conduct the study in order to mimic the real-world conditions in which Ketek would be used. It says most of the 1,824 doctors involved in the study had research experience.

Dr. Campbell oversaw a busy practice in Gadsden, Ala., that attracted patients by advertising weight-control treatments. By the middle of January 2002, she had signed up 287 patients and was receiving enough of the drugs to enroll 30 new people a day, according to emails sent by a PPD employee on Jan. 15 and 17.

The employee wrote that Nadine Grethe, an Aventis manager overseeing the study, had "put a cap" on shipments of the drugs to Dr. Campbell. Minutes from a study management meeting a week later showed that someone was a "little uncomfortable" with Dr. Campbell's site and the site required "additional monitoring." Ms. Grethe, who no longer works for Aventis, couldn't be reached for comment.

On Feb. 27, Ms. Grethe got an email from PPD warning that there were potential problems at the Campbell site including the lack of "proper diagnosis of an appropriate medical condition," medical charts described as "very limited," and laboratory test results that were "suspiciously similar" for multiple patients. PPD staffers also found that many patients signed on for the study during a lunch period when the office was supposed to be closed.

To check for possible fraud, Aventis directed a company statistician to analyze Dr. Campbell's lab information and other data, documents show and the company confirms. On March 14, 2002, the statistician wrote to Ms. Grethe and others that lab results for Dr. Campbell's site were "consistent" with those of two other top enrollers and a "systematic pattern is unlikely," apparently referring to a pattern indicating fraud. By then, however, Dr. Campbell was "refusing to address any issues via phone" or respond to faxes or FedEx deliveries, according to a March 15 email by a PPD staffer.

Sanofi-Aventis says in its statement to The Wall Street Journal that Dr. Campbell later did address questions raised by the monitoring, according to information the drug maker received from PPD. The company says it took several steps to deal with concerns about Dr. Campbell, including follow-up visits and training for her.

In a statement to The Wall Street Journal, PPD declined to discuss specifics but said it complied with FDA regulations and its contract with Aventis in monitoring the trial. It said it reported all issues including those involving Dr. Campbell to Aventis.

Red Flags

Emails from PPD staffers to Aventis officials indicate that PPD employees raised red flags about other doctors as well. A doctor in Indiana with more than 150 patients in the study had over 20 violations of the study instructions in an inspection, according to a PPD employee's email. The doctor, William Terpstra, says in an interview that there was no fraud but some "minor" violations of the instructions.

When Aventis turned in the results of study 3014 to the FDA on July 24, 2002, they included 407 patients from Dr. Campbell. At that point, Aventis "did not alert the Agency to any problems" with Dr. Campbell, according to a nine-page review of Ketek's history, safety and efficacy written later by an FDA official, David Ross. The review is posted on the agency's Web site.

The FDA's Rachel Behrman, deputy director in the office of medical policy, says in a statement that in general, if a drug company suspects fraud during a trial, "it is critical that...we be informed promptly, and we are considering new options to address this very issue." She says the FDA is planning a broad new effort to "modernize" how it monitors research.

An FDA inspector examined Dr. Campbell's office in the fall of 2002, selecting her simply because she had enrolled so many patients, according to Dr. Soreth, the director of the FDA division that oversees antibiotics. The inspector found serious problems. Some of Dr. Campbell's patients said they hadn't gotten any medication, even though records said they had, according to the review by the FDA's Dr. Ross. Others were allegedly being treated for weight loss and not respiratory infections, and some study patients were family members and friends of Dr. Campbell.

The FDA scrutinized the next-largest site, that of Carl Lange in Buffalo Grove, Ill., where 251 patients had been treated. That inspection, according to a public agency database of inspections, found Dr. Lange failed to follow the study plan and report adverse drug reactions. Dr. Lange says in an interview that he had never worked on a study before. He acknowledges he made some paperwork errors and didn't report an infection he thought was irrelevant, but he says "there was no question at all regarding the accuracy of the data."

The FDA also inspected the site of Egisto Salerno, a doctor in San Diego whose 214 patients made him the third-biggest enroller. Dr. Salerno's medical license was on probation during the study. The agency found deficiencies including use of white-out on some study records, according to the database and Dr. Ross's review.

In April 2002, police found Dr. Salerno with cocaine in his underwear and a loaded handgun, according to the state medical board's complaint that led to him surrendering his license. This happened seven weeks after Dr. Salerno saw his last patient in the study, according to Dr. Ross's review.

The complaint says Dr. Salerno was threatening to kill his wife and admitted using cocaine. Marijuana was also found in his home, it says. He pleaded guilty to a misdemeanor, which was expunged from his record after he did community service and completed drug counseling, says his lawyer, Gayle Askren. Dr. Salerno will soon receive his medical license back, says Mr. Askren.

Aventis told the FDA in December 2002 that it didn't know Dr. Salerno was on probation, according to minutes of the meeting.

As for Dr. Campbell, Sanofi-Aventis says in its statement that it had no "substantiated basis" to suspect fraud or serious problems with her work before the FDA's inspection of her site. As a result, the company says, "the conditions for reporting" Dr. Campbell as a potential problem to the FDA "were not met." Sanofi-Aventis says it was only after the government investigation that it discovered Dr. Campbell was fabricating data. The company notes it is named as a victim of her fraud by the court that ruled on her sentence.

The indictment against Dr. Campbell accuses her of cheating Aventis by sending the company false information through the mails. She pleaded guilty to one count of mail fraud in March 2004 and was sentenced to four years and nine months in federal prison. Through prison officials, Dr. Campbell declined requests for an interview.

When a committee of outside advisers to the FDA met early in 2003 to weigh a recommendation on Ketek, agency officials didn't mention the problems turned up by its inspections. The FDA's Dr. Soreth and Dr. Jenkins say revealing the suspicions might have biased the decision and impaired the investigation. The committee voted to recommend Ketek's approval. Two weeks later the FDA rejected the recommendation. It asked Aventis for more documents on study 3014 and potential side effects overseas.

Aventis complied. But the FDA ultimately decided the study was so flawed that the data couldn't be trusted. A March 25, 2004, FDA memorandum from the Division of Scientific Investigations says Aventis's monitoring program "uniformly failed to detect data integrity problems when they clearly existed." The report cited "noncompliance with FDA regulations and multiple instances of fraud" at four of the eight high-enrolling sites that inspectors visited. Dr. Campbell's site was one of the four.

One doctor who participated in the study, Jeffrey McLeod of Midlothian, Va., last year agreed with the FDA to stop doing research after an agency inspector accused him of backdating consent forms in study 3014 and failing to properly record which drugs his patients were taking. Dr. McLeod calls the accusations "nonsense" and says there was no fraud, although he acknowledges that perhaps "all the i's weren't dotted and the t's weren't crossed."

Sanofi-Aventis says that despite the FDA's criticism, the study still provided "useful information regarding adverse events" that was consistent with other data about Ketek's safety. It says PPD visited more than half of the study sites and took corrective action when problems were found.

Once the FDA found fault with study 3014, it still had to decide whether to approve Ketek. It had the same data Aventis had submitted back in 2000 -- which the agency had then found inadequate to demonstrate the drug's safety -- and overseas data on adverse reactions to the drug as well as some smaller new studies mostly on Ketek's efficacy against certain infections.

One document gives a hint of debate within the FDA about what to do. This is a version of Dr. Ross's review in which he calls approval of Ketek to treat sinusitis and bronchitis "doubtful," in part because of the drug's "risk profile." When he posted this version on an internal FDA document-sharing system, Dr. Ross appended a note saying his boss, Dr. Soreth, directed him to change that paragraph. The public version of the paragraph says neutrally that approval for those conditions "would depend" on further information.

Dr. Soreth denies ordering a change. "If he felt strongly, he was free to keep it," she says, adding that the review didn't reflect Aventis's final submission to the agency. In both versions, Dr. Ross's examination says Ketek could be approved for a third condition, pneumonia. Dr. Soreth says the Ketek application generated "discussion and the normal repartee about the merits of the data, no more and no less."

The FDA formally approved Ketek on April 1, 2004, for use in sinusitis, bronchitis and pneumonia acquired outside a hospital. Despite all the problems at the study-3014 sites, FDA officials say they believed the original Aventis data submitted in 2000, plus the data from the smaller studies and the drug's safety record overseas, justified approval.

Currently Sanofi-Aventis is studying the drug in children with ear infections and tonsillitis. The FDA rejected its application to sell the drug to adults with tonsillitis.

Meantime, study 3014 is still cited to back Ketek's safety. When the Annals of Internal Medicine published its article about potential Ketek liver damage, it also published an editorial that referred to study 3014 as a reassuring sign of the drug's safety.

The same day the Annals report came out online, the FDA said in a notice that based on data reviewed by the agency before approval, Ketek appeared no more dangerous to the liver than other antibiotics. The agency also cited study 3014. The FDA's Dr. Jenkins says he regrets that. "In retrospect, it probably would have been better not to reference it," he says.

In La Concepción, the revelation that Mr. Obrajero's death might have had a connection to a medicine he took has dredged up painful memories for his widow, Ms. Juarez. "After he died, I returned to Mexico and said to myself that I wouldn't leave again," she says. "The only reason I would ever go back to Charlotte is if I could find out what happened to my husband."

--John Lyons and Ricardo Millan in Mexico City and Henry van Wagenberg in Charlotte, N.C., contributed to this article.

THE ADEQUACY OF THE FDA TO ASSURE THE SAFETY OF THE NATION'S DRUG SUPPLY

THURSDAY, MARCH 22, 2007

HOUSE OF REPRESENTATIVES,
SUBCOMMITTEE ON OVERSIGHT AND INVESTIGATIONS,
COMMITTEE ON ENERGY AND COMMERCE,
Washington, DC.

The subcommittee met, pursuant to call, at 9:35 a.m., in room 2123 of the Rayburn House Office Building, Hon. Bart Stupak (chairman of the subcommittee) presiding.

Members present: Representatives DeGette, Waxman, Green, Schakowsky, Inslee, Dingell [ex officio], Markey, Whitfield, Walden, Ferguson, Murphy, Burgess, Barton [ex officio], and Blackburn.

Staff present: David Nelson, Joanne Royce, Kyle Chapman, Scott Schloegel, John Sopko, Alan Slobodin, Karen Christian, Krista Carpenter, John Halliwell, and Matt Johnson.

OPENING STATEMENT OF HON. BART STUPAK, A REPRESENTATIVE IN CONGRESS FROM THE STATE OF MICHIGAN

Mr. STUPAK. This hearing will come to order. Today, we have a hearing on the adequacy of the FDA efforts to assure the safety of the drug supply, part II. Each member will now be recognized for 5 minutes.

Today, the subcommittee continues its inquiry into the adequacy of the FDA's efforts to protect Americans from unsafe prescription drugs. The FDA has a long history of not adequately protecting the public from dangerous prescription drugs. The FDA has placed the approval on marking of drugs above its public safety mission. The Government Accounting Office and the Institute of Medicine, and members of the FDA old Drug Safety Advisory Committee have all released reports detailing the inadequacies of the FDA's drug approval process, post marketing surveillance, and inept leadership. Representatives from these organizations will present their testimony today, and we welcome their analyses.

This subcommittee has investigated three separate instances, the anti-depressant SSRI's, the anti-inflammatory medication Vioxx and Bextra, and the antibiotic Ketek, where senior officials in the FDA's Center for Drug Evaluation and Research, CDER, overruled competent, conscientious FDA medical officer's warnings that the drugs were not safe. The senior FDA officials who overruled the FDA medical officers performed no independent analysis of the data, nor did they solicit the opinion of unbiased, outside scientists. In fact, in the antidepressant and Ketek cases, FDA officials took deliberate steps to withhold critical information from the advisory committee on the most important facts regarding the issues under consideration.

In the Vioxx case, senior FDA officials refused to allow an FDA official to share his critical study with the FDA advisory committee. FDA officials responsible for protecting Americans overruled their own scientists and chose instead to listen to the self-interested pleadings of the drug companies.

In each case that this committee examined, the increased suicide risk in adolescents from antidepressant drugs, the unnecessary deaths from heart attack and stroke associated with Vioxx, and the liver deaths from the Ketek, the FDA has ultimately been forced to reverse its prior decisions regarding the efficacy of the drug. Amazingly, the FDA senior officials are still in a position of authority at the FDA and their actions have forced many well-respected and conscientious professionals within the FDA to leave their jobs. The American people cannot afford to have senior FDA officials overruling sound scientific analysis and approving dangerous drugs and forcing out professionals who exposed the problems within the FDA's approval and post marketing surveillance process.

On a positive note, our congressional investigations have resulted in strengthened warnings and provided more information to protect consumers. With the SSRI's, the FDA agreed to a black box warning and changed the labeling regarding efficacy in adolescents. With Bextra, the drug was pulled after our committee staff began an investigation. With Ketek, just days before our hearing the FDA announced a new black box warning and limited Ketek's approved use.

Following inquiries by our committee, the Office of Oncology Drug Products advocated for black box warning for the EPO drugs and convened an advisory committee to discuss the safety of EPO drugs. AmGen, Johnson and Johnson, and Roche worldwide sales are above $10 billion for these EPO anemia-fighting drugs, but in recent months, three off-label studies have been stopped because of serious adverse events such as blood clots, tumor growth, and death.

Another positive result of our bipartisan oversight investigation work was that in November 2004, the FDA requested the Institute of Medicine, IOM, to draft a detailed evaluation of the FDA's drug safety system. We will hear testimony today regarding the result of that IOM report and ways the FDA can improve its drug safety.

Today, we will also have an opportunity to hear from Dr. Andrew von Eschenbach, the Commissioner of the FDA. I look forward to the Commissioner's account of all his drug safety reforms to keep drugs like Ketek off the market. I also want to know what he will do to retain dedicated, competent medical officers who areleaving the FDA.

At our last FDA hearing, Doctors Ross and Powers were prime examples of scientists who became so disillusioned with the FDA's senior officials that they left the Agency. Our country needs to keep doctors and scientists within the FDA where their dedication is at the heart of drug safety.

As the full committee moves forward with the reauthorization of PDUFA, the Prescription Drug User Fee Act, and reviews the administration's draft, it is incumbent upon us to protect the American public and not help the pharmaceutical companies' profits. As this partnership between the FDA and the drug companies produced an Agency which views its clients as drug companies rather than the American public, I am curious to learn how Commissioner von Eschenbach's drug safety plan reverses the apparent partnership of automatic approval and encourages retaliation against those FDA employees who question the Agency.

I also want to hear what Dr. David Graham and other FDA employees think when they disagree with the efficacy and safety of the drugs. Will they be treated fairly? Will their voices be heard?

I also hope to hear the Commissioner say that instead of discouraging dissent, he will encourage dissenting views and the FDA's advisory committee will hear from every FDA employee, expert and consumer who may have concerns about the safety of a drug.

I also hope to hear that both the pre-approval and post marketing processes are going to become much, much more transparent so that data can be evaluated inside and outside the FDA. I hope to hear a commitment that advisory committees will consist of members that are free of conflicts of interest. The most trusted medical journals have no trouble finding qualified peer reviewers who have no financial ties to the medical issues they are reviewing. I cannot understand why the FDA cannot field advisory committee experts who do not have an interest in the drugs being approved.

I hope to see outside oversight of how the FDA treats its whistleblowers. Specifically, I want to see the abolition of the Office of Internal Affairs and termination of the Memorandum of Understanding that has stripped the Inspector General of the responsibility of ensuring integrity at the FDA. The Memorandum of Understanding is improper and has been systematically abused. FDA criminal investigators have been sent to harass and intimidate FDA scientists who have refused to compromise their scientific integrity. On the other hand, there have been no publicly disclosed investigations of senior FDA officials who violate whistleblower rights.

I want to hear that the FDA reviewers who uncover discrepancies, question data from drug companies or scientific misconduct at clinical sites will not be shunned. I hope that the Commissioner's statement that he will not tolerate public dissent from within the Agency has not discouraged whistleblowers from coming forward.

I want to hear that FDA supervisors will not abuse their authority by ordering safety reviews to be changed. Advisory committees will not be misled, and drug companies will not decide the content and placement of safety information on labels and that crucial safety data will not be ignored. I believe the FDA officials who abuse their authority by engaging in such activities can endanger the public health and must be removed from their supervisory capacity.

I wish to hear that the safety of the American public is paramount concern for the FDA when it comes to food, drugs, and medical devices.

More than just words, I wish the examples that the Commissioner of the FDA can renew the FDA's mission to protect the American people and not the pharmaceutical companies. Without meaningful actions, how can Congress be expected to hand the FDA another 5 years of unquestioned carte blanche under PDUFA?

With that, I will next recognize the ranking member of the subcommittee, my friend from Kentucky, Mr. Whitfield.

Mr. Whitfield, 5 minutes, please.

OPENING STATEMENT OF HON. ED WHITFIELD, A REPRESENTATIVE IN CONGRESS FROM THE COMMONWEALTH OF KENTUCKY

Mr. WHITFIELD. Thank you, Chairman Stupak, for convening this hearing. As you mentioned in your opening statement, today's hearing is this subcommittee's second hearing examining FDA's management of drug safety.

Recent reports by the Institute of Medicine and the Government Accountability Office and testimony at our first hearing make the case that the current system for monitoring drug safety needs improvement. I am delighted also that today Honorable von Eschenbach is with us. We appreciate your being here, Commissioner, and look forward to your testimony very much.

The FDA's responsibilities are great, and the American people want new drugs to be introduced into the marketplace to help fight deadly disease. Congress has asked FDA to promote public health by approving, when appropriate, applications for new drugs, drugs for which patients and physicians are often anxiously awaiting.

FDA has approved more drugs than ever before over the last 10 years, and while the numerical percentage of drugs withdrawn from the market has been stable over the years, the actual number of drugs withdrawn has gone up because there are more drugs on the market. Although this number is small compared to the total number of drugs approved, that number is still too great, as it represents patients whose health has suffered or who have even died because the drugs they were prescribed were not safe.

The Agency must balance promotion of public health with protection of public health by monitoring safety before and after a drug is approved. The FDA is asked to satisfy both these missions, which are often intentioned with each other under an ever-increasing workload.

We should also recognize that while we want FDA to act quickly, once it has strong scientific evidence of a safety problem there is also a risk of pulling a drug too early that may actually not have anything wrong with it. for example, several years ago it was mistakenly thought that Claritin caused sudden death like Seldane, but on further analysis it turned out not to be the case.

The Institute of Medicine and others have made a number of recommendations for improving safety, but in order for FDA to implement many of these proposals successfully, additional resources are needed. You can't do your job without necessary resources. With these resources, FDA would have the tools to spot potential safety problems much sooner, perhaps in a matter of months rather than years. According to Richard Platt of Harvard Medical School, if data from large health plans were pooled, more definitive evidence and potential safety risks, such as the cardiovascular events linked to Vioxx, could have been detected within just several months instead of nearly 3 years, enabling much faster action to address safety.

Today, as I said, we welcome Commissioner Andrew von Eschenbach who has been invited to discuss the FDA's drug safety initiatives, as well as issues related to the approval of Ketek. I would like to point out that this subcommittee's investigation of Ketek is at a preliminary stage. Dr. von Eschenbach's testimony in this regard is somewhat out of sequence. The standard practice is to have his testimony at the end of the investigation, and this subcommittee issued document requests to FDA 1 month ago, and FDA has produced some documents but is working to complete its production. We have not conducted interviews of the FDA staff involved with Ketek. And with respect to Ketek and specific factual matters, we are proceeding here today without the benefit of having a full record before us.

However, that is not the only focus of this hearing. I think it is also important to remember that many of the problems described in the IOM and GAO reports are not new and cannot be attributed only to certain individuals or personnel issues. Instead, these reports suggest that these problems are systemic and require comprehensive wide-ranging approach to solving them. There does seem to be particularly a problem with morale and some cultural problems within the FDA's Center for Drug Evaluation and Research, and I know that the Commissioner is focused on these morale problems, and it is something that he places priority in dealing with.

While he has been acting Commissioner, I guess, since September of 2005, he was confirmed by this Senate I guess about 3 months ago, and so we need to give him a chance to work with FDA employees, with experts, and with Congress to develop the Agency's response to drug safety concerns.

In addition to discussing the IOM proposals with Dr. von Eschenbach, I would also like to bring to his attention a letter that Ranking Member Barton and I sent to the Inspector General of the Department of Health and Human Services, requesting an updated evaluation of FDA's oversight of clinical investigators. Our request was spurred by FDA's delays in disqualifying scientists who have been convicted or found to be lying or cheating in studies used for FDA approval. For example, minority staff found that Dr. Ann Kirkman Campbell, a clinical investigator in the safety trials for Ketek who pleaded guilty in 2003 to misconduct related to her participation in the Ketek trial and has been in prison since 2004, has not yet been debarred by the FDA.

We look forward to the testimony of both panels of witnesses, and we know that they will offer valuable insight on this issue.

My time is expired, so thank you.

Mr. STUPAK. But we work in such a cooperative atmosphere, I was going to let you go a few more minutes.

With that, I recognize the gentleman from Michigan, the chairman of the full Energy and Commerce Committee, Mr. Dingell.

OPENING STATEMENT OF HON. JOHN D. DINGELL, A REPRESENTATIVE IN CONGRESS FROM THE STATE OF MICHIGAN

The CHAIRMAN. Thank you for holding this hearing. It is second in this committee's investigation of the handling of the food, drug, and safety issues by the Food and Drug Administration. I want to welcome Commissioner Dr. von Eschenbach to the committee, and I want to commend you for the vigor with which you are addressing the business of this subcommittee.

The Commissioner should know that the FDA's response to the committee's inquiries has been less than acceptable. Responses have been slow to our document requests regarding food safety, drug safety, and conflicts of interest. I would inform all, including the Food and Drug Administration, that this committee will see to it that our questions are answered properly and speedily.

The Commission appears here today was preceded a month ago by former FDA staff members who testified that they were forced to flee the FDA because they feared retaliation from their superiors. These are good doctors and good scientists that exposed bad decisions, decisions that appear to have needlessly cost American lives. This committee has a rather special interest in whistle-blowers and in their safety and comfort, and we will take whatever steps are necessary to assure that that intention by the committee is fully implemented by all who come before us.

Both private statements and public quotes attributed to the Commissioner indicate that he does not tolerate public dissent from FDA employees. Private protests, I would note, within the FDA do not appear to work either. For example, in the case of the drug Ketek, only after the Congress was informed by FDA former employees of the confused dictates of senior FDA officials did the Agency finally rectify its mistakes. We have heard testimony that the Commissioner told these same employees that anyone not willing to be a team player would be traded. That is unacceptable. Given that their protests went to congressional offices, including this committee, I must remind the commissioner and everybody else in the FDA, that threatening FDA employees with retaliation for talking to Congress is not only unacceptable, but it is illegal.

My concern is echoed in a letter dated March 9, 2007, by our former colleague and my good friend, Senator Chuck Grassley, to the Commissioner, and I believe that my committee colleagues should review that matter and that letter. I therefore ask that the letter be placed in the hearing record, Mr. Chairman.

Mr. STUPAK. Without objection.

The CHAIRMAN. Dr. von Eschenbach has been invited to tell us today why the Agency's new drug safety initiative will adequately express and address the cultural problems identified by a number of experts on FDA drug safety policies. That cultural problem comes down to what Senator Grassley calls having grown too cozy with industry, and preferring drug approvals over swift action when clear safety signals manifest potential post market problems.

At our last hearing, Dr. David Graham framed a question for today's hearing, and that is what in the FDA proposals would prevent another Vioxx? For example, what in the new FDA proposal would ensure that FDA reviewers would not negotiate for more than 14 months on label changes, even after receiving substantial evidence of serious cardiac side effects, as they apparently did with Vioxx? Will the new proposed Office of New Drugs act any differently upon the clear warnings regarding Vioxx from epidemiological work performed in the Office of Drug Safety? Under the new proposal, would the FDA medical officers in the anti-ineffective division been allowed to present their findings to the advisory committee? Under the new proposal, are the advisory committees more likely to hear about potential fraud or errors in political safety studies, or are they able to make an honest judgment as to whether or not these studies are sufficient to protect the public? Moreover, where in the new FDA proposal is there any provision to fully inform the public of the case risks and benefits prior to a drug's approval?

I, for one, do not see anything in the new FDA proposal that effectively responds to the many problems identified by this committee over the past few years. None of these reforms propose structural guarantees to stop the cultural bias that has skewed the Agency's judgment.

One of the concerns that I have that is very specific is how do these panels that would be set up or would continue to serve at the FDA do the job that they are supposed to do and to do so on the basis of an unbiased and independent group of members of those agencies? In the end, what the administration proposal really boils down to is a very simple word, "trust us". My old daddy taught me to trust everybody, but he also taught me to cut the cards.

We should then address this by understanding that it is easier to accept that "trust us" if the FDA and the Department of Health and Human Services were not resisting congressional oversight and threatening whistleblowers.

Regardless of the drug safety questions, those questions continue to be the central concern of this committee as reauthorization of the Prescription Drug User Fee Act, PDUFA, goes forward. I believe that all of us, including FDA, can trust this committee that with the strong support of my colleagues on both sides of the aisle, we will come up with changes to ensure against another Vioxx.

I want to thank you, Chairman Stupak and Ranking Member Whitfield, for holding this hearing. I believe that it is very valuable, and I look forward to the testimony of today's witnesses.

Mr. STUPAK. Thank you, Mr. Chairman. Next turn to the ranking member of the full committee, Mr. Barton from Texas.

Mr. Barton, sir.

OPENING STATEMENT OF HON. JOE BARTON, A REPRESENTATIVE IN CONGRESS FROM THE STATE OF TEXAS

Mr. BARTON. Thank you, Mr. Chairman and Ranking Member Whitfield for holding this second hearing on drug safety. I want to compliment all of the members that are here, especially on the Republican side. I think we have 100 percent attendance, so I want to compliment my minority members for all showing up and being ready to investigate this important issue.

As I said in my opening statement at the first hearing earlier this year, we on the Republican side support the important investigation of FDA's oversight of drug safety. In fact, as chairman of this committee in the last Congress, I requested a Government Accountability Office review of the FDA's organizational structure and decision-making processes for drug safety. The GAO issues its report last spring and it is going to present testimony on that report later today.

Recent drug safety incidents involving antidepressants and Vioxx have raised the public awareness about the monitoring and the safety of our drugs. In addition, there have been issues raised about an antibiotic called Ketek, which was the focus of the first hearing earlier this year. This subcommittee is currently investigating this matter with the GAO report followed by the Institute of Medicine's recommendations in 2006 to enhance post-market drug safety of the FDA, there is broad agreement that our current system for monitoring the safety of prescription drugs can definitely be improved.

This hearing can be, and I hope it will be, a constructive step in achieving improvement in drug safety monitoring. It is important to acknowledge and commend the FDA for making some progress in response to the IOM report. Much remains to be done, obviously, but the overwhelming need in responding to the IOM report is additional resources for the FDA. With more resources and more staff, more information and better quality data, the FDA can make better decisions and gain more staff consensus.

Of particular interest is what steps can be taken to improve the ability to identify most adverse events in a consistent and timely way. One possible solution would be to develop a true systemic approach to identifying safety signals in a broad part of the U.S. patient population by linking individual databases together, combined with electronic tracking of medication use and patient results. Recent analysis by Richard Platt of the Harvard Medical School shows that data from large health plans could be pooled to provide stronger evidence of potential safety problems in months rather than in years.

Finally, this subcommittee is examining the FDA's culture and morale, the concern over what effect, indirect or direct, this has on the FDA's ability to monitor drug safety. When the IOM issued its report in September 2006, one of the most important recommendations with regard to the FDA's culture and morale was to stabilize the leadership of the FDA. In particular, the report stated the absence of stable leadership at the Commissioner level has been a continuous problem for the FDA and its Center for Drugs. Thankfully, in December 2006, the Senate confirmed Dr. Andrew von Eschenbach, who is with us today, as the Commissioner of the FDA. FDA now has a newly confirmed Commissioner with full authority to lead. He happens to be somebody that I know personally, and I have full confidence he is going to do the very best that he can to lead the FDA.

I am glad that the subcommittee is giving Dr. von Eschenbach an opportunity to be heard today. He should be given an opportunity to actually lead, continue response to the IOM report, and a chance to work with the FDA employees, stakeholders, and the Congress to address drug safety concerns, to improve his Agency's morale.

It is understandable and legitimate to question Dr. von Eschenbach about the concerns raised by Senator Grassley and other witnesses from the first hearing about Ketek. That is what the oversight function of Congress is all about. I want to remind our members, though, that we are in an open investigation on Ketek. We are still gathering documents and we are still interviewing witnesses. With these circumstances, hopefully we will be careful not to make any premature judgments or allegations at this hearing. I believe that the members of this subcommittee on both sides of the aisle agree that we must move forward now, and we have to do our part to help the FDA address these problems. It is important, I think, that we do it in a way that is constructive.

I welcome Dr. von Eschenbach. I look forward to hearing his testimony. It is my hope that he is going to do everything possible to ensure that the FDA's processes with respect to drug safety are transparent, collaborative, and based on the best science available.

I am also looking forward to hearing our second panel of witnesses who are going to comment on improving the management and oversight of drug safety.

Finally, Mr. Chairman, I think as you understand, we have a telecommunication hearing that started about 30 minutes ago upstairs, so I am going to be scuttling back and forth like a little beetle, trying to listen down here and also participate up there.

With that, Mr. Stupak, I yield back the balance of my time.

Mr. STUPAK. I thank the ranking member and you are correct, I will be joining you upstairs here in a second as I am going to ask Ms. DeGette to take the Chair while I run up there and ask my questions, and I will be right back down.

Also, so the ranking member knows, we were able to work out, it looks like, our amendment for the 2:30 markup today. That is what we have been doing this morning, so things are progressing even though we look a little disorganized here this morning.

With that, I would recognize for 5 minutes Mr. Waxman from California for an opening, and then ask Ms. DeGette to take the chair, please.

OPENING STATEMENT OF HON. HENRY A. WAXMAN, A REPRESENTATIVE IN CONGRESS FROM THE STATE OF CALIFORNIA

Mr. WAXMAN. Thank you very much, Mr. Chairman. Dr. von Eschenbach, welcome to the committee. I am pleased that you are here.

I look at FDA, which was created a little over a century ago, as the premiere public health agency. Millions of Americans depend on it to protect us from unsafe foods, medicines, and medical devices, and it is held up throughout the whole world as the gold standard. It is an agency that deserves our support in every way.

Recently, there have been some very serious and concerning issues at FDA with respect to regulation of drug safety. A series of post-market safety problems in the past few years with Vioxx, Ketek has demonstrated beyond a shadow of a doubt that FDA's drug safety oversight is in serious need of repair. These examples make it abundantly clear that drug safety is at least as important after the drug has been approved as it is before, and the IOM has done an evaluation of this, and I am pleased that they are going to be here with us as well. They think it is seriously dysfunctional. Their report made one thing quite clear. FDA cannot protect Americans from unsafe drugs unless Congress provides more resources and more legal authorities.

Post-market drug safety oversight is currently grossly underfunded at FDA compared to drug approval side. This is in spite of the fact that there is now an increased risk of approving unsafe drugs, since PDUFA required that the timeline for drug approvals be accelerated.

In addition, the pharmaceutical industry has always fought giving FDA the modern enforcement powers it needs. I want to go through some of these enforcement powers that I believe FDA lacks and must have.

FDA lacks the authority to require post-market safety studies, even when they are necessary to determine a drug's risk. FDA lacks the authority to impose necessary restrictions on the distribution of drugs shown to have risks. FDA lacks the authority to place controls on the huge advertising campaigns at the launch of new drugs which cause excessive use of drugs before their safety profile is clear. FDA lacks the authority to demand labeling changes after approval. Their authority under the current system is so weak, it guarantees that drug companies will be able to delay and water down needed warnings on drugs. The case of Vioxx is a tragic illustration of this. FDA was forced to endure 14 months of haggling with the company before we finally saw a black box warning about the serious cardiac risks associated with the drug.

I think we simply have to fix these problems. We need strong leadership at the FDA to make the necessary changes, and I am eager to hear from Dr. von Eschenbach today about the steps he intends to take to address the very serious concerns raised in the IOM report.

Congress has to do its part. I have my own ideas about some steps we can take, and I introduced a bill this week to address many of these problems. We here in Congress owe it to the FDA to make certain that it has the basic tools and authorities it needs to fulfill its core mission, to protect the public health. We also need to do what it takes to get FDA adequate funding to fulfill this mission. To do our job right, however, we need full and complete information from the FDA.

For the last century, FDA has protected the health of the American people. It is now clear that a course correction is necessary to enable the Agency to continue its historic mission.

I applaud the chairman for calling this hearing, and I am looking forward to the testimony.

Thank you.

Ms. DEGETTE [presiding]. The Chair now recognizes the gentleman from Oregon, Mr. Walden, for 5 minutes.

OPENING STATEMENT OF HON. GREG WALDEN, A REPRESENTATIVE IN CONGRESS FROM THE STATE OF OREGON

Mr. WALDEN. Thank you, Madam Chairman. I will keep my remarks very brief.

I think Mr. von Eschenbach has heard from the committee already our concerns to make sure the American drug supply is safe and that when people go to the drugstore and get something that doctors prescribe, they know that they are going to get better and not worse.

And so, we look forward to the continuing effort to make sure this system works and works effectively, and we look forward to your testimony. Obviously, we will have some questions, so thank you for being here.

I yield back.

Ms. DEGETTE. The Chair recognizes herself for 5 minutes.

OPENING STATEMENT OF HON. DIANA DEGETTE, A REPRESENTATIVE IN CONGRESS FROM THE STATE OF COLORADO

As the full committee prepares to reauthorize PDUFA, I am confident that this series of hearings will be very informative to that process. Given the importance of PDUFA to ensuring that new drugs approved for the market are safe for patients, we need to make sure that the FDA has the systems in place to do the job effectively. As others have said today, we not want to find ourselves with another Vioxx-type situation that we could have prevented.

I would like to say that my questions for the panelists today focus on how to improve our drug safety systems to further improve protections for patients, but unfortunately I have set my bar a lot lower. My goal today is to have a system that avoids scenarios like Vioxx, Ketek, and SSRIs. At the very least, I hope our witnesses can show us how we can prevent those types of tragedies from occurring with some other kind of drug.

To that end, I have several issues today regarding drug safety at the FDA that I hope we can examine. First and foremost, I am interested to know how the FDA has made systemic changes to drug safety within the Agency to prevent large scale drug safety problems. In my mind, any one of these events should have spurred the FDA into corrective action, let alone, all three of these events together. I would hope that the FDA has not just tinkered around the margins this time, but has made a careful examination about what went wrong and has a large scale comprehensive plan for corrective action.

In light of our impending deliberations on PDUFA reauthorization, I am also interested to hear from the witnesses about how we might better address the issue of conflicts of interest, both real and imagined. Clearly, the current system makes it fairly easy for a collaborative, some would say cozy, relationship between the FDA and drug companies. While I certainly support the work done by pharmaceutical companies to develop the treatments and cures we have come to expect, we must maintain FDA's autonomy and its true role as a regulator. The FDA should not have to negotiate the black box warning label of a drug with the manufacturer. Once the FDA makes the decision after consultation, the decision should be in the hands of the FDA.

As I mentioned, there are a number of real problems with the system by which the FDA manages drug safety. At the same time, there is a feeling of mistrust by the public about the work performed at FDA that further exacerbates the problem. Instead of feeling that all drugs are safe and effective, people are now questioning the drugs that they take. Frankly, if we are going to maintain the health of the citizens of this country, then they need to feel confident that the treatments prescribed are safe. Furthermore, we need to prove to the public that clinical trials are safe.

I know that we can make the changes to the FDA that will improve drug safety. I can only hope that those changes will be made with the full cooperation of all stakeholders to enable true consensus on the approach. The American public deserves nothing less.

And so I yield back the balance of my time, and now recognize Mrs. Blackburn for 5 minutes.

OPENING STATEMENT OF HON. MARSHA BLACKBURN, A REPRESENTATIVE IN CONGRESS FROM THE STATE OF TENNESSEE

Mrs. BLACKBURN. Thank you, Madame Chairman. I want to welcome all of our witnesses today, and make note that Dr. Woosley is someone that I had the opportunity to work with when he was at our fine Vanderbilt University Medical Center as a researcher in the mid-1980's and I was the chairman of the board for the American Lung Association in Tennessee. We welcome you and look forward to hearing from you. Commissioner, we welcome you and look forward to hearing from you.

Very briefly, because I like to spend my time in questions, and I just want to highlight with you all that we all recognize that the public has an insatiable appetite for new therapies and new drugs, and they are quite frustrated with what they perceive to be a very slow process of commercialization and moving these drugs and therapies to the marketplace once they know that something is in to research or in to development.

We also realize, sir, that there is a responsibility that rests with the FDA to make certain that these reach the marketplace safely and in a timely manner. We will focus on that through our questions and our comments to you, on behalf of our constituents.

I look forward to both a conversation and a dialog, if you will, as we move forward on this, on how we go about it with fairness to everyone that is involved in this process: to you, to your employees, to our constituents who are the consumers and do have the desire for new things that will increase their quality of life.

I do want to highlight with you that any time we have constituents who hear about commissions or advisory committees, I think that is a sensitive area with many now. They feel as if that is a way that someone can toss aside a question or a concern that you can say well, we are going to study it. Studying never brings resolution to a problem. It is a form of procrastination, and unfortunately in the Government arena, many times when they hear "we are going to delegate this to a committee or a commission" they know that an answer will never be reached.

So we look forward to visiting with you, and we thank you very much for your time. I yield back.

Ms. DEGETTE. Chair now recognizes the gentle lady from Illinois, Ms. Schakowsky, for 5 minutes.

OPENING STATEMENT OF HON. JAN SCHAKOWSKY, A REPRESENTATIVE IN CONGRESS FROM THE STATE OF ILLINOIS

Ms. SCHAKOWSKY. Thank you, Madame Chairman.

We have heard a great deal about problems at the FDA, and I am glad that today we will hear from Dr. von Eschenbach about his proposals for solutions.

The time for action is long overdue. Two years ago, the National Center for Health Statistics told us "The Nation's medicine cabinets are more crowded than ever with almost half of all people taking at least one prescription medicine, and one in six taking three or more medications." Yet, in 2 years, little has been done to reduce the risk Americans face when they take their daily medications. You can't watch television or pick up a newspaper or magazine without being bombarded by direct to consumer advertising. Americans believe that when they go to their medicine cabinet or pharmacy to purchase FDA-approved drugs, they are getting medication that is safe and efficacious.

Unfortunately, as this subcommittee has documented, too often their trust is misplaced. We need to do better.

I was pleased that yesterday the FDA took steps to limit conflicts of interest involving advisory committee members, although I am interested in learning more specifics about the rules. This is just one of many problems that past witnesses and today's second panel have raised.

There are two issues that are of particular concerns to me.

First, I am deeply troubled by the atmosphere of secrecy and the harsh treatment of whistleblowers that seems to pervade the FDA, and in fact, most of the Bush administration. The members of this committee, healthcare professionals, and the public have a right to know about safety information. None of us is well-served when FDA experts feel unable or even threatened if they reveal serious and potentially deadly concerns.

Second, I believe that we must act to ensure that the policies and practices of the FDA reflect the needs of the public and not the drug companies. The imposition of user fees should not allow drug companies to dictate how those user fees are used. I hope that when we reauthorize the Prescription Drug User Fee Act, we make that clear. We should allocate funding and set post-marketing drug safety surveillance standards in order to protect consumers, not based on negotiations with the industry being regulated. In the meantime, however, we need assurances from the FDA that they are doing everything they can to prevent the drug companies from dictating safety reviews at the public's expense.

Thank you, Madame Chairman. I yield back.

Ms. DEGETTE. Chair now recognizes the gentleman from Texas, Mr. Burgess, for 5 minutes.

OPENING STATEMENT OF HON. MICHAEL C. BURGESS, A REPRESENTATIVE IN CONGRESS FROM THE STATE OF TEXAS

Mr. BURGESS. Thank you, Madame Chairwoman and Ranking Member Whitfield. I appreciate part two of this hearing. Part one, which was held last month, was very disturbing on several levels. The witnesses who testified told numerous troubling stories about what they observed during the approval process of the drug Ketek. While I was concerned about their personal accounts in their testimony, I was also very concerned that only one side of the story was told that day.

During the hearing, I called on the leadership of this committee to swiftly invite the FDA, the manufacturer of Ketek, Sanofi Aventis, to our committee so that they can address the serious allegations against them and tell their side of the story.

So thank you, Madame Chairwoman. I do wish the FDA had been invited to last month's hearing, but I do thank you for calling this hearing today and for inviting Commissioner Andrew von Eschenbach.

Dr. von Eschenbach, welcome. As the newly confirmed top administrator for the FDA, you have found yourself smack in the middle of some significant controversies. Some will be within your control, some are beyond your control. Last year when you were still director of the National Cancer Institute, you were kind enough to meet with me out at the NIH, and I thank you for your time then, and thank you for your time today, as well.

As director, as I recall, you proved yourself to the entire medical community to be, in fact a visionary leader. It was through that vision and that leadership that you were able to not only articulate, but to provide a roadmap of making cancer a manageable chronic disease in 10 years time, by the year 2015. You brought together researchers, clinicians, and politicians, and verbalized how we can accomplish that worthwhile goal.

Commissioner, while you are immensely qualified to lead the FDA, in my opinion, your leadership credentials are indeed impeccable, that is not to say that there are not problems, serious problems within the FDA. I feel that right now, this Agency needs leadership and you are, indeed, a proven leader for that job and indeed, I believe you to be the type of change agent needed to strengthen the drug safety system.

One of the most crucial aspects of all organizations is stable and steady leadership, but unfortunately that essential component has been absent at the FDA for far too long. Not a reflection of the FDA, but instead, a reflection on the Senate confirmation process. The political battles that have brewed over the years during this process have been a detriment to the Agency that is charged with America's health and safety. For the good of the American public, for the good of the FDA, the Senate must act in a more expeditious manner with regard to future confirmations. It is the only way we can assure a continuous form of leadership.

Madame Chairwoman, I believe this committee must continue our oversight regarding important public health issues. As a physician, I take this role extremely seriously and you have my commitment to work with you and Chairman Stupak and the entire committee on the vigilant pursuit of truth to our Nation's healthcare matters. As members of Congress, this is one of the most important roles that we will ever have, and I look forward to hearing from our witnesses today.

I yield back.

Ms. DEGETTE. The gentleman yields back.

The Chair now recognizes the gentleman from New Jersey, Mr. Ferguson, for 5 minutes.

OPENING STATEMENT OF HON. MIKE FERGUSON, A REPRESENTATIVE IN CONGRESS FROM THE STATE OF NEW JERSEY

Mr. FERGUSON. I am kind of in no man's land here between microphones.

Thank you, Madame Chair. Thank you for calling this hearing. Dr. von Eschenbach, welcome. We are glad you are here. We appreciate your service at the FDA and in your previous positions.

I want to address an issue, first, that you and I have been working on together with others since last summer, the enforcement of regulations concerning the distribution of FDA written medication guides, med guides to people who are receiving prescriptions. I think we can all agree that medication guides are an invaluable tool to inform people about the drugs they are taking. They are written in plain English, sometimes in a question and answer format, and they go a long way toward educating patients and parents of patients of potential concerns that can result when taking certain drugs, particularly in the cases that we have seen in children taking antidepressants.

I have been concerned that patients are not receiving the medication guides in every instance that they ought to be, and after examining medication guides and the supply chain for med guides, I and our staff found that there are gaps in the enforcement of med guide regulations. Drug manufacturers and pharmacist organizations and the individual State Boards of Pharmacy needs to be better informed and better instructed about what their duties are to ensure the proper distribution of medication guides.

After contacting a number of these different stakeholders, the New Jersey State Board of Pharmacy agreed to include the enforcement of medication guides as one of the protocols that they would investigate as one of their routine pharmacy inspections. Dr. von Eschenbach, I appreciate your willingness to work with me on this issue, and I welcome your thoughts today and in the future about what more the FDA could perhaps to do to help ensure that medication guide regulations are being enforced. You and your staff have been very, very helpful and forthright and cooperative as we have conducted this investigation in our office, and I am pleased. I do have your most recent letter from your office indicating some of the things that you are doing and will be doing in the future to help, in particular, with this issue, and in particular, if you could perhaps share with us today what the FDA may be able to do in terms of contacting State Boards of Pharmacy to inform them about medication guide protocols and what you might be able to do to enforce those protocols.

I have a couple of other topics I would like to get into during questions, but I just wanted to raise that during my statement here. I certainly appreciate your service and the work that you are trying to do. We have so many important issues that we are dealing with and that you are dealing with at FDA, and we look forward to continuing to work with you on these many important issues.

Thank you, and I yield back.

Ms. DEGETTE. Chair now recognizes the gentleman from Pennsylvania, Mr. Murphy, for 5 minutes.

OPENING STATEMENT OF HON. TIM MURPHY, A REPRESENTATIVE IN CONGRESS FROM THE COMMONWEALTH OF PENNSYLVANIA

Mr. MURPHY. Thank you, Madame Chair, and I want to thank everyone who is going to testify today.

Many of the issues about why we are here have already been raised from the standpoint of how we are concerned about drug safety, but we are also concerned about getting drugs into the hands of doctors and patients in a timely manner. I would like to demonstrate the importance of this with two calls I received just this week on Monday. One was a call from a friend of mine, we will call him "Joe", who a couple of months ago had approached me, saying that he had just come back from the doctor and was informed that because of the kind of aggressive cancer he had developed in several internal organs that he really only had a couple of months left to live. He was told to go home and put his affairs in order.

Joe doesn't operate that way. He has a business and he was not about to let his employees, all those lose their livelihood. He was going to do what he could to live for their sake. We made a number of calls and eventually got him involved in a trial program for a cancer drug. He began this medication, and a couple of weeks later called me to say that he had some blood tests, and there was no signs at all in his blood tests that he had cancer. They increased the dosage then of this experimental medication, and on Monday morning he called me and said I just got back from a CT scan, and the doctor called and said all my tumors are necrotizing. They are disappearing. Pretty incredible news from a man who was told he was dying.

Sadly, a friend of mine named Jackie, who had similar sort of aggressive cancer in the internal organs, I also had a call on Monday that she had died. A woman who had given her life helping so many causes, a young lady 41 years of age, gave much of her life to programs such as Habitat for Humanity, a loss for all of us to have someone like that gone.

Putting these two stories together tells me some of the things that the FDA has got to help us with to make sure that young women like Jackie do not go away too soon, and that standard therapies for cancer are seen as something of the past, and yes, indeed, we can treat this more as a chronic or acute illness in the future, and we can give moms like her hope that they will live to see their children grow up and help others.

We are excited about the things that happened to Joe, but still, all of this is experimental and we recognize part of the burden the FDA has to have is how you can bring medications to the market quick enough to save lives, but understand the safety and the risks all along. It is not an enviable position. I tell these stories to help us all understand, and the Nation understand that we are dealing with lives here. That anytime we have safety issues where someone has breached the scientific ethics and has withheld information or put information that is distorted, we are all deeply concerned about that, and we want to make sure that doesn't happen.

We also want to make sure that medications that are out there that show some promise, that show some possibilities, that they get in the hands of physicians and patients as soon as we can. We want to make sure that other lives are saved and others are not lost, and that none of this gets caught up in a bureaucracy and a whirlwind of paperwork that doesn't help anybody.

I hope that what we can find out from these hearings today and from future work with the FDA is that I believe the employees of the FDA have to be committed—and I believe they are. In their hearts, they want to make sure they are saving lives and they are doing it the right way. And I am sure that all of you that are testifying today will have that in your hearts as well. You want to make sure that we don't have other losses like Jackie out there.

Let us all make sure that what comes out of this hearing is ways we can do this better, ways we can save more lives, and ways that we can make more patients available to see their children grow up tomorrow.

I yield back.

Mr. STUPAK. That concludes all the opening statements.

Dr. von Eschenbach, we are ready for your testimony, but before you do that, we have a policy of this subcommittee to take all testimony under oath. Please be advised that you have the right under the rules of the House to be advised by counsel during your testimony. Do you wish to be represented by counsel at this time? Will you please rise, then?

[Witness sworn]

Mr. STUPAK. Thank you, Doctor. Consider yourself sworn in, and we will now hear from you for your opening statement, please.

TESTIMONY OF ANDREW C. VON ESCHENBACH, M.D., COMMISSIONER, U.S. FOOD AND DRUG ADMINISTRATION

Dr. VON ESCHENBACH. Thank you very much, Chairman Stupak, Mr. Whitfield, and other members of the committee.

This is my first opportunity to appear before the subcommittee as Commissioner of the FDA, and not only am I looking forward to adequately responding to your questions, but also to share my vision and commitment to ensure that the FDA continues its record of excellence as a regulatory agency dedicated to protecting and promoting the health of all Americans.

My formal written testimony provides details about the FDA's commitment to drug safety. My brief oral remarks this morning I hope will describe the kind of well-managed, efficient, and effective organization that I am committed to leading.

Let me first say a word about the personal commitment to that kind of effective leadership I hope to bring to the FDA. Before I became director of the National Cancer Institute in 2002, I served in various leadership positions for almost 26 years, caring for patients at the M.D. Anderson Cancer Center in Houston. While there, I strove to foster a multidisciplinary and integrated approach to addressing the complex problem of cancer, in order to bring the finest coordinated care to save the lives of cancer patients. From the patient's perspective, excellence depends not only on demanding the best from individuals, surgeons, radiation therapists, or oncologists or researchers, but also demanding effectiveness in combining and integrating these skills.

I believe the same approach is required at the FDA. As we manage the complexities of modern science and technology in an effort to bring lifesaving products to patients, and assessing the risk and benefit of drug, biologics, and medical devices, we must have the analysis of various individual skills, but they must also be integrated and coordinated.

At the FDA, we excel as individuals but patients and public will benefit best and most when we work together. To adjust the balance between understanding the benefits and risks of a new drug, we are integrating the work of our Office of Surveillance and Etiology, addressing drug safety with the work of the Office of New Drugs. We are doing this for one reason: it better serves patients and the public.

Throughout my career, Mr. Chairman, it has been my commitment, my passion, if you will, to offer leadership that fosters such an effective, efficient multidisciplinary and integrated organization.

With regard to the culture of such organization, let me assure you that I am committed to leading an FDA characterized by a culture that has commitment to excellence, based on and lead by science, and governed by a transparent and disciplined regulatory framework. FDA must always remain an organization dedicated to excellence, and that makes it a learning organization. We learn from experiences and we will change.

For example, one of the lessons we have learned in the pharmaceutical area of late is the need to address in detail drug safety issues throughout the entire life cycle of products, not just data coming in at the outset from clinical trials, but also data derived when the drug is used in large populations in a complex real world environment after approval. This has led to a number of changes that will improve our post-market surveillance and vigilance.

The FDA that I lead will be a science-based and a science-led regulatory agency as it has been in the past and must be in the future. New scientific discoveries are generating what might be now termed an emerging science of safety. Today, understanding of disease and its origin at the molecular level, as well as the patient, provides us with new methods and technologies for detecting molecular signals of both effectiveness and adverse events. These and many other scientific initiatives to be included in our effort are articulated in our recent report, The Future of Drug Safety. We are, as we speak, adopting 41 new measures to improve the safety of medical products as a major step, but not the only step, in an ongoing process of continuous improvement.

The FDA must also have a robust and disciplined regulatory framework. Our analytical and decision-making processes must be based on discipline and rigor. We must apply methods of scientific analysis with consistency, uniformity, and integrity. Our decision processes must be transparent and also open to scrutiny.

During my career, I have learned that the best decisions are those that are informed by diverse points of view and vigorous academic debate. At the FDA, I will continue to foster a climate of mutual respect that promotes dialog and informed decisions, because I know these robust exchanges will produce better public health decisions for American patients.

But even the best decisions, Mr. Chairman, can never declare any drug perfectly effective or perfectly safe. These decisions ensure the American people that in FDA's expert judgment, the expected benefits of the drug outweigh its potential risks for the intended use in a given population. The FDA's effort in the past has made it the world's gold standard as a regulatory agency, and I am determined that it remain so. There will be no other priority or agenda for the FDA than protecting and promoting the public health.

I look forward to working with you and the subcommittee as we pursue our shared goal of a strong and effective FDA.

Thank you, Mr. Chairman.

[The prepared statement of Dr. von Eschenbach appears at the conclusion of the hearing.]

Mr. STUPAK. Thank you.

Before we begin with questions of Dr. von Eschenbach, I want to take care of one housekeeping issue, and actually compliment Department of Health and Human Services. I would like to advise my colleagues as a result of our hearing last week into the current healthcare situation in New Orleans, Secretary Leavitt sent through Ranking Member Whitfield and me a letter expressing his willingness to work with local officials on a much smaller regional approach to address the health concerns in New Orleans. In addition, Secretary Leavitt also agreed to address the GME, Graduate Medical Education payments. This is a significant accomplishment for our oversight and investigations efforts, and I want to thank the Secretary as well as Ranking Member Whitfield, members of our subcommittee, and their staffs for their continued interest to improve the healthcare situation in New Orleans. We are looking for another hearing date in the near future to go down there and continue to push healthcare to a state of acceptability here in this country for the folks of New Orleans and the Gulf region.

So I want to thank the Secretary for his help and cooperation. Mr. Waxman.

Mr. WAXMAN. Thank you, Mr. Chairman.

Dr. von Eschenbach, I want to ask you about this post-market study commitment, also known as the phase 4 studies. I think we all agree that when a drug first goes on the market, we don't know all the information about that drug. It is not tested on hundreds of thousands of people. There is a small sample. We can't test drugs on tens of thousands. Very rare side effects often cannot be detected in this small number of subjects.

FDA often approves a drug on the explicit promise that the manufacturer is going to conduct post-market studies after the approval, and these studies are critical. They provide vitally important information about a drug that can't be learned pre-approval. In fact, these studies are so important, they are imposed as a condition for approval of the drug in about half of all new drugs, but by many accounts, a startling number of pharmaceutical companies are failing to uphold their part of the bargain that they need to do to make these studies and to complete them.

FDA is required to submit to Congress an annual report on how many of these post-marketing studies are completed, and according to your most recent report in 2006, there were over 1,200 open or ongoing commitments to conduct post-marketing studies, but manufacturers ended up completing or terminating only 11 percent of these studies. That means 71 percent have not even been started.

I would like to know your views on this. It seems to me that it shouldn't be acceptable that 71 percent of the studies are being delayed or pending. I want to hear what you think of the situation. What is the problem there?

Dr. VON ESCHENBACH. Thank you very much, Mr. Waxman.

I concur that this a process that definitely needs improvement, and I believe that the approach that I want to take is a process improvement approach from the perspective that, first of all, we need to be able to engage in a much more appropriate way in the kind of studies that should be conducted in the post-market setting. One of the initiatives that we are launching to provide the opportunity for much earlier consultation discussion and decision-making process about the assessment of the drug to define and determine both the need for a post-market study, as well as what the content of that post-market study should include.

By doing that in a much more strategic and much more effective way earlier on in the process, I think we, first of all, will have much better studies, studies that will be not launched sort of after the fact, but will be integral to the entire process of our entire life cycle management.

Mr. WAXMAN. That sounds good, but I am just concerned about what your Inspector General said. He looked at these post-market commitments last year and he found that in 1 year, about one-third of the reports were missing or incomplete. So for one-third of the studies that the companies promised to conduct, FDA was left in the dark about whether or not they were actually being done. So even if you consult with them earlier, we are not guaranteed they are going to do the work.

They also found that even when these required reports were provided to FDA, the information contained in them was so lacking that it wasn't possible to even assess compliance.

Have you done anything to respond to the OIG's concern that even when complete, the information contained in these reports is inadequate?

Dr. VON ESCHENBACH. Well, in addition to making sure that we don't have inadequate responses, by virtue of the fact the studies were not well developed and well designed and therefore, did not get implemented, we also need to be much more rigorous about that process itself. I believe we now have tools that will enable us to have much better oversight because of the ability to move to the post-market surveillance programs that are going to be based on larger databases, much more effective information technology tools, and we will be able to provide much more rigorous oversight of these trials——

Mr. WAXMAN. But do you have tools to make sure the companies do what they promise? Do you have the authority to require a company to look at their own drug when important safety things emerge after approval, or do you have to engage in discussions with the companies and hope that they will agree to be doing these studies that they promised they would do before the approval?

Dr. VON ESCHENBACH. Well, the development of the studies can be a condition in the process as part of the approval process. I think the important issue is to first make certain that we are creating a pathway and a post-market study scenario that is both effective, efficient, and rational to get better outcomes and better results.

In addition to that, we are engaged in informing legislation that is addressing the larger issue that you raised with regard to authorities. But my purpose and focus in addition to that and providing that technical assistance to considered legislation is to look at the process itself and make that better as well as oversight and authority.

Mr. WAXMAN. Well, your assumption is that the process is the problem, and I am submitting to you that ultimately, you don't have the tools. As I understand it, the only thing you can do is to take a drug off the market for failure to submit these studies. That is a pretty harsh sanction. Dr. Jenkins, who you know from the Director of the Office of New Drugs, said that pulling the drugs from the market for failing to complete a post-approval study is just not an attractive option.

Has FDA ever taken a drug off the market for failure to complete a post-approval study?

Dr. VON ESCHENBACH. Not that I am aware of, sir, but I would look at the record for that and provide further information for the record for you.

Mr. WAXMAN. Sir, do you agree with the OIG that you lack the ability to enforce compliance?

Dr. VON ESCHENBACH. Well, I believe the opportunity to enforce compliance is ultimately there. The effective way of achieving compliance I believe is to get much better studies in the first place, target them much more appropriately, monitor them——

Mr. WAXMAN. In the first place meaning before approval?

Dr. VON ESCHENBACH. As part of the process of approval, yes, sir, and the development of the studies themselves.

Mr. WAXMAN. Well, you are under pressure because of PDUFA and the user fees by the manufacturers to push for faster approval of the drugs, not to slow down and require that more studies be done that might give us signals for post-market problems that otherwise wouldn't be anticipated.

Dr. VON ESCHENBACH. Well, in PDUFA part of that process will provide resources, FTEs, talented individuals who are skilled in these areas to be engaged in the process earlier on so that I think the resources will match the need, and we will get the desired outcome that you are anticipating and wanting.

Mr. WAXMAN. I just want to leave this area by commenting that I don't think you have sufficient authority, but I also don't think you have sufficient resources, and I want to work to make sure that you have the ability to do that, because if you have to prioritize with inadequate resources, I am afraid that very important functions get cut.

I want to ask you about drug advertising because I think it plays a profound role in drug safety. When drug companies are permitted to oversell new products whose risks are not yet well established, the risks to the American public are substantially increased. The

Vioxx case was an example of that. And I want to ask you about the pattern at FDA that is so troubling.

In 2002, I issued a report that found that enforcement actions for false and misleading advertising dropped dramatically during the Bush administration. GAO later largely agreed with these findings. In 2004, I updated this report and found that enforcement actions against false and misleading drug acts continued to decline. The number of enforcement letters sent by the Bush administration in 2003 was 75 percent below the average for the last years of the Clinton administration. When enforcement actions did occur, they were mild mere slaps on the wrist and most of those were notice of violations letters that required no corrective action from the companies, rather than more severe warning letters. Even repeat offenders faced no increased actions or sanctions.

FDA has the authority to issue injunctions and fines to manufacturers, but none of these were issued in the timeframe of the report. I am concerned about the ability of your Agency to oversee these ads. At the time of my report, your Agency received over 3,200 promotional pieces every month. That is over 36,000 ads each year. How many staff are available to review 3,200 advertisements each month, do you know?

Dr. VON ESCHENBACH. As you point out, sir, the need to increase our resources to be able to address this is, in fact, part of our budget process for the current budget being considered, as well as included in the reauthorization of PDUFA, so that we will direct more resources to be able to more effectively monitor and act upon direct to consumer advertising, particularly from the point of view that is being presented in visual media television ads.

Mr. WAXMAN. I know you need the resources, but I understand the Bush administration decided it was essential, as they claimed, to first review all the enforcement letters that went to the companies, and then they said they want to just focus on the worst violations and take strong action to follow up.

Can you tell us in the last 5 years how many court actions the FDA brought against companies that have had repeated violations?

Dr. VON ESCHENBACH. No, sir, I will respond to the record for you on that one when I get the exact data. I don't have that.

Mr. WAXMAN. I would like to get it. I think it will show very little action. This is all before you got there. We want to work with you to change the situation. I think it has been troubling.

Dr. VON ESCHENBACH. Thank you, sir.

Mr. WAXMAN. Thank you very much, Mr. Chairman.

Mr. STUPAK. Thank you.

Mr. Whitfield for 10 minutes for questions.

Mr. WHITFIELD. Thank you, Mr. Chairman.

Mr. von Eschenbach, to follow up on a comment by Mr. Waxman of California, in regard to these post-marketing studies, he is making the point that the Agency needs additional enforcement authority, and the way to get that is through legislation. I am really not familiar with these post-marketing studies, but could you explain the process that companies go through in conducting these post-marketing studies, just in a brief way?

Dr. VON ESCHENBACH. Well, this is a very important area and opportunity, I believe, Mr. Whitfield, where we now have tools that were literally not available to us even 5, 10 years ago. We are now able to look at large populations, be able to acquire and analyze, if you will, data mine the actual experience of that drug being used in that real world environment. Often, diverse populations that were not included in the original trials and clinical trials, often populations, as has been pointed out by others, that are taking other medication. So that opens up for us an entirely different database with which we can learn about the drug both from the point of view of unexpected, unpredicted adverse outcomes, but also importantly, unpredicted and unexpected efficacy or benefit that could give even further insight into the drug development process.

So this is an extremely important part of a discovery, development, delivery continuum, and it is essentially, in short phrase, being able to gather data from large diverse populations about the actual experience of the drug.

Mr. WHITFIELD. And what can you as an Agency do if a drug company does not complete a post-market study? What options do you have?

Dr. VON ESCHENBACH. Well, as the ultimate option as part of a commitment, our ultimate option is to withdraw, but——

Mr. WHITFIELD. Other than withdrawal.

Dr. VON ESCHENBACH. Working directly with making that data and that information known about lack of compliance and publicizing that, so that there is a significant awareness in the medical community of the fact that there is a lack of compliance to that commitment.

Mr. WHITFIELD. I would think that publicizing would be an important tool to have, and how often does the FDA really publicize the fact that a post-marketing study has not been completed or not——

Dr. VON ESCHENBACH. Well, data is provided, obviously, to Congress in the form of an ongoing report, but I think it is true and important to point out that as we direct any kind of action, there is both the goodwill of the sponsor, there is also the publicity that is associated with lack of compliance, and then ultimately, a regulatory authority.

Mr. WHITFIELD. Right. Mr. Stupak mentioned, I believe, in his opening statement that Dr. David Ross, who is a former FDA employee, testified before this committee about a meeting on Ketek in late June 2006 with the Center Director, Dr. Stephen Galson, and that you were invited to attend that meeting. I think Mr. Ross talked about that you compared the FDA to a football team, and having worked for a Fortune 500 company myself before being in Congress, I do know the importance of team building and people having that relationship. I think that is very important, certainly, in a Federal Agency as well.

But Dr. Ross evidently came away with the impression that an effort was being made to silence dissent on concerns of particular drugs and a frugal process. You were at that meeting, and I would just like you to respond to that. I am assuming that you certainly would not discourage dissent at the Agency.

Dr. VON ESCHENBACH. Thank you, Mr. Whitfield.

First of all, let me emphatically express to you, to the chairman, and to all members of the committee that I am adamantly in support of and committed to the perfection of legal rights for every single employee within the FDA or any organization that I am associated with. That will be unwavering on my part.

I deeply regret if there was a misunderstanding on the part of Dr. Ross in terms of my comments. I would hope to have had the opportunity for him to raise that, his misperception with me directly so I could have corrected it. but in terms of the question you posed, it reflects the perspective that I shared earlier about my approach to the need for the FDA to be a science-based and science-led academic-like organization that I wish to provide an environment, if you will, a locker room, an environment in which people with diverse points of view, completely different perspectives on an issue or problem can come together with mutual respect and vigorously, even aggressively, debate and discuss those issues, and do that in the comfort of that being respected and supported and even encouraged—even, quite candidly, from my standpoint, expected. That was the intent of my remarks was to create the awareness among everyone that I really fully wanted to support diverse opinion and vigorous discussion and debate.

I think the issue that is important to point out is that that is where that kind of process can go on and be very constructive to informed decision-making. When people don't choose to participate in that and aren't willing to be a part of that, and then simply express opinions independent of that, I don't think that is helpful to the process.

Mr. WHITFIELD. I am not sure you were at the FDA at this time, but officials in the Office of Drug Safety at FDA evidently on the issue of serotonin reuptake inhibitors had prevented a scientist from presenting to an advisory committee his findings that the SSRIs posed a significant risk of increased suicidal tendencies in a teenager.

Now, I am assuming that there would be—is there ever a time when it is just not appropriate for a scientist to go before an advisory committee to express his concerns? I am not a scientist but I am assuming that it is non-scientific data that it would not be suitable. Am I wrong or not?

Dr. VON ESCHENBACH. Well, in general, Mr. Whitfield, as one approaches an advisory committee, I think there is a very significant commitment to presenting all the data that is appropriate for that particular decision-making process. It may be that if all of that data is not available at the time, it would be perhaps not helpful to just present one part of it. You would want to wait until you got the other parts of the data from other sources, perhaps, or other studies, and then present it all as a package so the advisory committee could see it all. That may be one reason why you ask someone to withhold presenting their data at a particular meeting, but not to suppress data or not to prevent it from being presented or surfaced, but to do it in the context of a full portfolio of information.

Mr. WHITFIELD. Because you have to have transparency, that is where you come up with your best product, when everyone has an opportunity for input and to express their opinions, and then the committee makes their decision based on that.

Dr. VON ESCHENBACH. Absolutely, and I am adamantly committed to creating a culture, if you will, an environment at FDA that both encourages and expects everyone to have an opportunity to express their perspective and their point of view about a particular issue.

Mr. WHITFIELD. Weren't you the chief operations officer at M.D. Anderson at one time?

Dr. VON ESCHENBACH. Executive vice president and chief academic officer.

Mr. WHITFIELD. Yes. So you always have these scientific medical debates going on.

How do you deal with situations where maybe it is a disgruntled employee, sometimes maybe it is an employee who has a legitimate scientific dispute, when they go out to the news media outside the spectrum of the organization, how do you as a chief executive officer deal with that and balance that?

Dr. VON ESCHENBACH. I think it is very important, in addition to creating the environment and the opportunities and the appropriate forums for the kind of discussion debate, to also have pathways and mechanisms where people who have issues, either about the process itself or have issues about the conclusion that may have been drawn, that there are alternative pathways for them to be able to bring their individual point of view. That can be done through a grievance process, that can be done through an appeal to a superior, it can be done in a variety of different mechanisms.

One of the things that we need to always be sure of is that we are providing multiple pathways where people feel that they can have their perspective or point of view both heard and appreciated and valued.

Mr. WHITFIELD. Thank you.

Mr. STUPAK. Thank the gentleman.

I recognize the chairman of the full committee from Michigan, Mr. Dingell, for 10 minutes for questioning, please.

The CHAIRMAN. Mr. Chairman, thank you for your courtesy, and again, thank you for this hearing.

Commissioner, these questions will almost all be answerable by yes or no. First of all, Senator Grassley sent you a letter dated March 9, 2007, requesting that you clarify your position on the rights of the FDA employees to talk to the Congress. Yes or no?

Dr. VON ESCHENBACH. I fully support their opportunity to——

The CHAIRMAN. No, but he sent you that letter? Is that right, he sent that letter?

Dr. VON ESCHENBACH. My recollection is that is correct, sir, but I would——

The CHAIRMAN. Commissioner, the Lloyd LeFaud Act passed in 1912 protects Federal employees who blow the whistle to Members of Congress. It states as follows,

> The right of persons employed in the civil service of the United States, either individually or collectively, to petition the Congress or any member thereof, or to furnish information to either House of Congress or any committee or Member thereof, shall not be denied or interfered with.

Are you aware of this provision of law?

Dr. VON ESCHENBACH. Yes, I am, sir.

The CHAIRMAN. Now, Commissioner, do you understand that FDA employees then are free to share information with the Congress without notifying their supervisors or the Office of Legislative Affairs?

Dr. VON ESCHENBACH. Yes, sir.

The CHAIRMAN. Now, Senator Grassley suggested that you notify all FDA employees that they are free to talk to Congress, and that you do not intend to interfere with their rights to share information with this Congress. Have you done that?

Dr. VON ESCHENBACH. Yes, Mr. Chairman. November 30, I issued to all FDA employees as Acting Commissioner a three-page memorandum that specifically addresses, I think, the concern and issue that you are raising. I didn't do it in response to Senator Grassley's letter, I had done this as a matter of policy back in November 2006.

The CHAIRMAN. Now, Commissioner, I assume then you understand that neither you nor any other manager at FDA or any other Government agency may interfere or retaliate against an FDA employee or an employee of any other agency who shares information with the Congress. Is that so?

Dr. VON ESCHENBACH. Yes, sir.

The CHAIRMAN. Now, are you aware that the Office of Internal Affairs has been used to attempt to identify and threat whistleblowers?

Dr. VON ESCHENBACH. No, sir.

The CHAIRMAN. Are you aware of any instance when the Office of Internal Affairs has investigated allegations of unlawful harassment of whistleblowers?

Dr. VON ESCHENBACH. No, sir, not to that specific.

The CHAIRMAN. Now, Commissioner, this committee has made document requests involving Ketek, the closing of FDA labs, and conflicts of interest in FDA contracting. The responses to these requests have either been late, incomplete, or redacted, or all three. Do you recognize this committee has a right to full, complete, timely answers to the questions regarding those or any other subject?

Dr. VON ESCHENBACH. Yes, sir, I am committed to providing the information that is appropriate in response to those inquiries, and doing it in a timely fashion.

The CHAIRMAN. Now, Commissioner, have any of the problems with regard to the response to these requests come because of intervention by lawyers or other HHS employees?

Dr. VON ESCHENBACH. Only to the issue of the appropriateness of the information being provided.

The CHAIRMAN. Only to the what?

Dr. VON ESCHENBACH. Appropriateness of the information being provided with regard to, for example, redacting confidential proprietary information, or access to a line investigator who was in the midst of an investigation. That kind of guidance has been provided.

The CHAIRMAN. What steps will you then take to assure that investigations by this committee are not delayed or slow-rolled or misled by incomplete or redacted document production?

Dr. VON ESCHENBACH. My commitment to fully cooperate with the committee and any of those investigations and to continue to live up to that assurance by providing appropriate information upon request, and providing in the appropriate way.

The CHAIRMAN. Now, Commissioner, Senator Grassley has introduced a bill to improve drug safety by establishing the independence and the authority of a post-market safety office. Do you agree with that proposal?

Dr. VON ESCHENBACH. No, sir, I do not.

The CHAIRMAN. You do not. Why?

Dr. VON ESCHENBACH. I believe that we have and are entering into an entirely new era of science and technology in which integration and coordination is far more an effective way of being able to accomplish the goal of assuring effectiveness and safety of the application of these drugs in the market, and doing that in silos that tend to then be separate and apart and do not then benefit from the opportunities to, first of all, integrate the science of safety and effectiveness, and also to be able to integrate the tools of our being able to understand and analyze the real world experience of these drugs.

The CHAIRMAN. Thank you, Commissioner.

Mr. Chairman, this will surprise everybody. I yield back the balance of my time.

Mr. STUPAK. You are correct. We are stunned.

Mr. Barton for 10 minutes of questions, please.

Mr. BARTON. Thank you, Mr. Chairman. I needed that extra three minutes and 50 seconds to get ready. I am somewhat at a loss here, but I will try to make up for it.

Dr. von Eschenbach, you were very active down in Houston at the M.D. Anderson Cancer Center. I think that is where I first met you. How many people were under your direct supervision, ultimately, in your leadership position down there?

Dr. VON ESCHENBACH. As far as faculty itself, independent of fellows and residents and interns, but as far as faculty of physicians, scientists, clinicians, over 1,000.

Mr. BARTON. I don't want you to pat yourself on the back, but my recollection is that your position down there, you were universally recognized as one of the more outstanding cancer center directors in the country. You had a positive reputation.

Dr. VON ESCHENBACH. Thank you, sir.

Mr. BARTON. You would agree to that.

Dr. VON ESCHENBACH. My mother certainly does. Yes, sir.

Mr. BARTON. You weren't unhappy in Houston; you were not into self-promotion to come to Washington to—you would have been happy to stay down there and do great things at M.D. Anderson?

Dr. VON ESCHENBACH. Yes, sir.

Mr. BARTON. The President, basically, recruited you to come to Washington and ultimately because of the prior Commissioner's problems, to some extent you were the white knight asked to go in and—I won't say save the FDA, but reestablish morale and credibility to the FDA. I am not trying to make you pat yourself on the back, but there was quite a bit of hope when you were nominated to be Commissioner at the FDA, that you could reestablish the credibility of the Agency. Is that a fair statement?

Dr. VON ESCHENBACH. I think the best way, perhaps, I can express it is I did come to the FDA in response to a crisis not by my own choosing or by my own intent or aspiration. That is correct.

Mr. BARTON. Now, we have an ongoing investigation that the minority supports the majority looking into some of these allegations of the whistleblower, Dr. Ross, with response to the drug Ketek and whether it should be on the market or not on the market and under what conditions, and we fully support. I don't want there to be any misunderstanding. We fully support the document requests, we fully support trying to get to the bottom of it, but we want to do it in an open, transparent, constructive way. We do have this investigation, we are supportive, so I don't want to preclude any of that.

But I do want to ask a few questions, since Senator Grassley testified, and I think it is fair that when we have you here under oath that we can go into that a little bit.

This meeting where you made the comments about trying to be a team player, whatever it was, that was not a meeting that you called, is that correct?

Dr. VON ESCHENBACH. That is correct, sir.

Mr. BARTON. You were invited by the Senate Director?

Dr. VON ESCHENBACH. Yes, sir.

Mr. BARTON. OK. And Dr. Ross was at that meeting, is that correct?

Dr. VON ESCHENBACH. Apparently he was.

Mr. BARTON. How many people were in the meeting?

Dr. VON ESCHENBACH. The room was full and I would estimate probably 30.

Mr. BARTON. Thirty or 40 people.

Dr. VON ESCHENBACH. Forty, something like that.

Mr. BARTON. And at some point in time, the Senate Director turned to you and asked if you wanted to make any remarks, and you kind of felt compelled at that time, were you the Commissioner or were you Acting?

Dr. VON ESCHENBACH. Acting.

Mr. BARTON. Acting. You felt compelled to participate. What was your frame of mind when you made those remarks? Were you in an intimidating frame of mind, were you in a healing frame of mind, were you in a I would rather be anywhere but here frame of mind? What was your frame of mind?

Dr. VON ESCHENBACH. Well, as you point out, Mr. Barton, I came to the FDA in the sense of in response to a crisis. I became very acutely aware of the duress that the Agency had found itself in for a variety of reasons. The stresses and the strains of the enormous amount of responsibility that that Agency bears, the increasing complexity of the products that it is being asked to regulate, both in scale and scope, et cetera, et cetera. And what I found my most important responsibility was was to begin to talk to the people of FDA and bring them together, create an enhanced environment of morale, and begin to bring us together to look more positively at the future as to how we were going to be able to together address the challenges, to address the issues, and to continue to improve. There was an agency that was beginning to celebrate its 100th anniversary of being the world's gold standard, and I wanted us to look forward to the next century, the 21st century, and be the FDA of the 21st century.

Mr. BARTON. So you were really there to listen, to participate if asked, but you weren't there, in your mind, to try to single out individuals and intimidate them to keep their mouths shut?

Dr. VON ESCHENBACH. Absolutely not, just the opposite. I was there to reinforce the model that I learned at M.D. Anderson where it was so important to not have people working in isolation and silos, surgeons here and medical oncologists there, but a woman with breast cancer needed all of us coming together, working for her behalf. I believe that is the way that the FDA can best become the FDA of the 21st century is coming together as an organization, working together. And that is what I was there to indicate to them was my vision of leadership and what I was hoping to promote.

Mr. BARTON. At the time of this meeting, had you met Dr. Ross?

Dr. VON ESCHENBACH. I can't recall ever meeting Dr. Ross.

Mr. BARTON. To this day you have not met him?

Dr. VON ESCHENBACH. No, sir, not that I can recall. He might have introduced himself to me at some point, but not——

Mr. BARTON. Based on what you know of Dr. Ross, do you have a high opinion of him, a positive, professional opinion? I understand he is no longer at the Agency and I think he has moved to the VA, so——

Dr. VON ESCHENBACH. My understanding of his credentials and background, I have a high opinion of him, but I don't know him personally.

Mr. BARTON. And I would assume you support the investigation to try to—if there are things that we can do to make sure that the FDA is run in an up-front, transparent fashion, you would be supportive of that?

Dr. VON ESCHENBACH. Absolutely, absolutely. I welcome the opportunities for oversight. That is the only way we continuously improve is to be thoughtful and even self-critical of that process. I never did an operation in my entire life, no matter how well it turned out for that particular patient, my response and duty to the patient was to follow, how could I do it even better? So no matter how well we perform at FDA, I will constantly be asking how can we do it even better, and I will seek input and insights from a whole host of sources, both inside and outside the Agency, to address that question, how can we be even better.

Mr. BARTON. Well, we have had ongoing issues with the FDA, really, I would say for the last 20 years. We had issues with Dr. Kessler when he was chairman of the FDA. Congresswoman Eshoo and I introduced an FDA reform bill that is now law. It is so important that we operate—and the FDA is one of the most important Federal agencies, because we are the gold standard for drug approval and safety issues for our drugs, medical devices for our country and the world, and so this subcommittee has a long bipartisan history of paying very close attention to your Agency and very close attention to the way it reviews these drugs and medical devices. And in order to have the best, you have to have the ability within the Agency to dissent on some of these literally life and death issues, and from all I know, Dr. Ross was doing exactly what he felt he should do, acting in a very positive, professional fashion. Some of these are tough judgment calls. All I ask that you do in your position of leadership at the FDA is insist that we have these high standards and that we have a mechanism within the FDA. There can be dissent, there can be debate, that people are not punished for speaking out on policy grounds, and that we have a method of reconciliation in the FDA to resolve these issues in a fair fashion. Do you agree with that?

Dr. VON ESCHENBACH. Yes, sir, I do.

Mr. BARTON. Madame Chairwoman, I yield back.

Ms. DEGETTE. [Presiding] Thank you very much.

Commissioner, the first thing I want to ask you. You had mentioned to the chairman, Mr. Dingell, that there was a memo that you sent to the staff that Senator Grassley requested. I am wondering if you could provide the committee with a copy of that memo?

Dr. VON ESCHENBACH. Madame Chair, just so I think I clarify my response, I sent a memo to the staff on November 30, and I will be happy to submit it for the record. I don't believe the timing of this memo was in response to Senator Grassley's letter. It was independent.

Ms. DEGETTE. OK. If you could provide us with a copy, that would be great.

Dr. VON ESCHENBACH. Yes.

Ms. DEGETTE. Commissioner, I know you will agree with me that FDA credibility is its most important asset, and there is a lot of concern that the pharmaceutical user fees that are contained in PDUFA which support FDA operations have contributed to a significant loss of public trust in the FDA. So my first question is, how can restore the public faith in the FDA when so much of the funding from PDUFA funds the speed of drug approvable, and arguably, sometimes at the expense of drug safety?

Dr. VON ESCHENBACH. Well, Madame Chair, I think there are a number of points I would like to make in response to the question, because there is not one thing but many things that I think we need to do to assure the confidence of the American people that we are, in fact, serving them and no one else.

First of all, it is the issue of openness and transparency in the decision-making process, regardless of where the sources of resources or funds are coming from to provide that infrastructure of the decision-making process is open and transparent.

Ms. DEGETTE. And I agree with you on that. Are there ways we can improve the transparency, because that is one of the critiques of the approval process.

Dr. VON ESCHENBACH. Yes, ma'am. I believe that there are a number of ways we can improve process as it relates to our decision-making and our communication of that decision-making. I also believe that there are opportunities that, for example, making certain that those fees are compartmentalized, used only for the purposes for which they were applied. Investigators do not have any direct knowledge of where their support is coming from with regard to their own professional functions, which is another important component. We want to separate this idea that people are motivated by a source of their resources. They work for the FDA.

Ms. DEGETTE. Right. What else?

Dr. VON ESCHENBACH. In addition to processes that are continuously improved, I think one of the important parts of PDUFA IV negotiations is, in fact, that many of these funds will now be used to specifically address the safety dimension and component of drug approval, not just decisions about efficacy or streamlining the approval process.

Ms. DEGETTE. Have you put these improvements in place or are you working on that?

Dr. VON ESCHENBACH. Some of the improvements as outlined in our report following the IOM study that we commissioned, some of them are in place. Some of them we are actively engaging in as we speak, and some of them will be implemented as we get further resources in the budgetary cycle.

But I want to just emphasize, Madame Chair, that even those 41 initiatives that are currently as a part of that report is a major step, but not the only step, and I am committed to even further efforts to continue to improve this process.

Ms. DEGETTE. Do you think that all of these efforts that you have undertaken will take the inherent conflict of interest out of PDUFA? We have had witnesses come in to talk to us, and they just flatly said no matter what you try for transparency and the compartmentalization of the fees and so on, you still have an inherent conflict of interest.

Dr. VON ESCHENBACH. Well, I view the issue of the user fees to be a service to the American people, not a service to the FDA or to the industry, even though there is a way of creating this process so that it benefits all three. It is so that drugs can be more efficiently approved and understood with regard to their expected benefit and their expected risk. And the sooner we bring them to the American people with the better information to define their use and be able to continue to monitor their use even after we approve them, I think really then serves the American people best.

Ms. DEGETTE. Yes. How are you going to monitor all of those things, because you know, we agree that it is important to bring drugs quickly to market, but we also think that it needs to be, obviously, safe and so how do you monitor that?

Dr. VON ESCHENBACH. Well, that is the opportunity to take advantage of what is emerging with regard to science and regard to technology. Literally we now have information technology tools and data mining tools that are being used in other industries like banking, for example, or even your supermarket, knowing about the purchases of the food that you are making. Those kind of information technology tools can be applied now to databases where we have large populations of patients, for example, our agreement with the Veterans Administration, our agreements that are emerging with the Center for Medicare and Medicaid Services, and even large healthcare systems like United Health, as they go to electronic medical records, we can begin to really engage in a much more profound post-marketing opportunity of pharmacal vigilance that I think will give us——

Ms. DEGETTE. And you think that data mining will be sufficient post-market? I think it will be a tool, but will it be enough of a tool?

Dr. VON ESCHENBACH. Well, I think it is a major step. Other steps that we can continue to define, as I said, I see this as a process of continuous improvement. As other opportunities present themselves, I look forward to engaging in those.

Ms. DEGETTE. The IOM report, and also four former FDA commissioners, said last month that the Nation would be better served if rather than funding PDUFA the way we do, Congress just directly appropriated the money that the FDA needs to review these drugs and get them to market. What do you think about that?

Dr. VON ESCHENBACH. Well, as I indicated, we are attempting to build a resource base that presents both to the American people and to the Congress options as to how we can fund that. PDUFA happens to be one of the options that has been in place. I think it is an option that has served us well. It needs to be constantly continuously monitored, as you indicate, but it is an important part of the resource base.

Ms. DEGETTE. But my question to you is, we are funding PDUFA right now through these fees, and so the question I am asking you—and I know that is the way we are doing it, but the question is would it be better as the IOM and the FDA Commissioners said, to just eliminate that portion which creates a conflict of interest and go to direct congressional appropriations?

Dr. VON ESCHENBACH. Well, I think that the issue there is it puts an even further burden on the American taxpayer, and when there is an opportunity for others to contribute or participate in the support of this process, I think it is appropriate as long as it is done in an appropriate way.

Ms. DEGETTE. So you think that we can take the inherent conflicts of interest out sufficiently through the ways that you talked about to continue this funding?

Dr. VON ESCHENBACH. I think we can be vigilant and vigorous in that process, and at the same time, have the industry contribute a share of the burden of being able to get these drugs to patients in a much more efficient and effective way.

Ms. DEGETTE. What percentage of the CDER staff would you estimate are focused on review and approval of new drugs? Do you have a sense?

Dr. VON ESCHENBACH. I cannot give you an exact percentage of that. I would be happy to respond to that for the record of an exact number.

Ms. DEGETTE. What about how much of their resources are focused on the post-market safety of drugs?

Dr. VON ESCHENBACH. Well, up to the present time, there has not been a significant investment in post-market. It has been evolving and I intend to accelerate it.

Ms. DEGETTE. In fact, we have had an estimate that Dr. Graham estimated that 90 percent of the staff are focused on review and approval of new drugs, and just a small 10 percent or so are post-market safety review. Would you generally agree with that?

Dr. VON ESCHENBACH. I would generally accept a number. I would have to look back to give you my own precise number, but the fact of the matter is, I think we are changing that. I know we are changing that. We are integrating the Office of Surveillance and Epidemiology much more effectively and efficiently into the new drug application process, and my idea of——

Ms. DEGETTE. What is your timeframe for doing that?

Dr. VON ESCHENBACH. We are doing it as we speak.

Ms. DEGETTE. So if we had you come back here in 3 months, you could talk to us about the improvements that you have made?

Dr. VON ESCHENBACH. Yes.

Ms. DEGETTE. Does the FDA have the funds to do the data mining that you say you are going to do?

Dr. VON ESCHENBACH. Well, we look forward to the appropriations—that request is before Congress now to provide these additional funds.

Ms. DEGETTE. So you don't have the funds right now, you are going to need an additional appropriation?

Dr. VON ESCHENBACH. We have requests for additional appropriations, both in PDUFA IV, as well as in our appropriations.

Ms. DEGETTE. And if that request does not come through, is it your testimony that you won't have the funds to do it?

Dr. VON ESCHENBACH. There will not be adequate funds to do all the things that we have to do. We may make decisions with regard to the use of our funds to apply them to this as a priority, as opposed to something else within the Agency, but we would have to find the funds somewhere else.

Ms. DEGETTE. Thank you.

Chair recognizes Mr. Burgess for 10 minutes.

Mr. BURGESS. The last remaining member of the committee. Thank you for the recognition. Again, thank you, Dr. von Eschenbach, for being here. We appreciate you taking time out of your schedule to be with us.

Let me just ask a question that is a little bit off the point. I know when I was in clinical medicine, I resented the fact that FDA took so darn long to approve anything. Europe could have drugs decades before we could. And then we hear from the committee this morning that maybe the FDA moves too fast on approving some products. And then in a few weeks, we are going to be talking either in this committee or the health subcommittee about the concept of generics for biologics, big large biologic molecules that some people believe that the Federal Government can save billions of dollars if we move to a generic process for that.

So do you see a problem with our consistency?

Dr. VON ESCHENBACH. Well, I think, Dr. Burgess, we are moving very much into an era where I don't believe that the idea of moving the approval process through more efficiently and more effectively necessarily means that it is therefore allowing more dangers on drugs to be applied to patients. I think the science is allowing us to both understand adverse outcomes, as well as effectiveness, in a much more profound way than we did before. As we move that process more efficiently and more effectively, I think we are bringing both safe and effective drugs to patients.

Mr. BURGESS. Are we making unreasonable requests on the FDA, asking you to approve the safety of generic biologics since these are different from, say, a statin or an antibiotic? These are much more complex molecules.

Dr. VON ESCHENBACH. Well, that speaks exactly to the point of science having to be the basis upon which those decisions are made. As it relates to follow on proteins, as many have appreciated, the complexity that is involved in complex proteins is orders of magnitude different than what we experience in small molecules that are drugs. And therefore, the science that is required for us to be able to approve an abbreviated application for a follow on protein is radically different and much more complicated, much more sophisticated, and some of it is not even developed. So we have to take an appropriate approach to the particular issue.

Mr. BURGESS. Let me ask you a couple of questions dealing with the questions that Chairman Dingell was asking you about Senator Grassley's letter. My understanding is a lot of that came out of a newspaper article that was written after you addressed a group called the Center for Public Medicine and Interest, and the Newark Star Ledger reported that you would not tolerate whistleblowers who go outside the Agency. Do you think that article accurately reflected your remarks that day?

Dr. VON ESCHENBACH. No, sir, it does not, and interestingly, for purposes of recording my speech for the Web site, that presentation and that question and answer period afterwards actually was taped, which there is a transcript, and my remarks were not in any way, shape, or form addressing the issue of whistleblowers. I never used the word. They were simply talking about a culture in which you have vigorous academic debate and how constructive that can be when people participate within that construct and within that opportunity, rather than choose not to.

Mr. BURGESS. Have you taken steps to address that?

Dr. VON ESCHENBACH. Well, with all the other important things to address, I didn't chose to respond. I think there has been a second article written by that same newspaper, and there is a letter to the editor that is now being prepared, since it has occurred the second time in terms of a misquote of what my comments were. So I hadn't before, but we are in the process of doing it now.

Mr. BURGESS. Then I guess just for the edification of the committee, can you tell us your position on whistleblowers?

Dr. VON ESCHENBACH. I fully support the legal rights of every single individual at the FDA to exercise their response—whistleblower, in that context, yes, sir.

Mr. BURGESS. Going back to some stuff that Ranking Member Barton was asking earlier, I believe Mr. Barton and Mr. Whitfield have sent a letter to the HHS Inspector General requesting an evaluation about the delays in FDA's disciplinary actions against clinical investigators who have been convicted or found to have engaged in misconduct during a clinical trial regulated by the FDA. Do you have concerns over delays in the FDA disqualifying individuals convicted or found to be falsifying data submitted to the FDA?

Dr. VON ESCHENBACH. Well, I respect the fact that there is a legal process, and that legal process has its own inherent pathway, if you will, that is beyond any control that we have. Having said that, I believe that the FDA must be rigorous and must be efficient and take rapid steps when those kind of actions need to be employed.

So I can't control how long a legal process may take, but I certainly expect the Agency to act promptly in initiating any kind of process, once it has been recognized that there is an issue.

Mr. BURGESS. Currently, there is a Memorandum of Understanding reached between the Inspector General of HHS and the FDA, going back to 1994 and the HHS Inspector General seated its authority to investigate the FDA matters—seated that authority to the FDA. Assuming that the Inspector General of HHS receives additional resources and wants to resume its investigative authority over the FDA, would the FDA be open to working with the Inspector General of HHS and letting the IG's Office resume direct responsibility over FDA employee misconduct cases and thus render unnecessary the FDA Office of Internal Affairs?

Dr. VON ESCHENBACH. Yes, sir, I would be open to any discussions about how we can improve the process. I think that we have always welcomed the Inspector General's participation in any investigation, any process. There is value to having the Office of Criminal Investigation within the FDA as at least a part of that process because it provides the opportunity to have individuals who are really extremely knowledgeable and skilled about the unique particulars of the business of the FDA in terms of the complexity of drug reviews and manufacturing, et cetera, so that as we engage in investigations, they really are both content experts and imbedded in the knowledge base by being part of the FDA.

Now, they may not need to be the sole participant, but I think to totally completely dismiss that element in favor of something else might lose things that you want to retain while you're trying to address another issue. So I am open to discussions. I look forward to continuing to improve that process, as I will any others, but I would just mention that I think there is an important role for the internal process within FDA.

Mr. BURGESS. Thank you. You have a lot of written testimony about the drug Ketek, which came to be available after I had left the practice of clinical medicine, so I have had no experience with that antibiotic. Do you think it is a worthwhile addition to our antibiotic——

Dr. VON ESCHENBACH. Yes, sir, I do, because as you know as a physician, we have constantly struggled with continuing to find and develop new antibiotics that would overcome resistance that generally can occur with organisms that adapt and with serious infection, the need for newer, more effective antibiotics is a constant ongoing process, and any addition to that can be a very valuable contribution to public health.

Mr. BURGESS. The FDA has been criticized for going forward with its advisory committee meeting even though the individuals connected to the large-scale clinical trials were still under criminal investigation and scientific misconduct investigations. In a briefing with the staff, Dr. Jenkins, the head of the Office of New Drugs, stated the same factual pattern, if it presented itself to the FDA in the future, he was of the view that the FDA would postpone the hearing and get the results of the investigations first. Do you think that is worthwhile position to take?

Dr. VON ESCHENBACH. Yes, sir. This occurred prior to my arrival at the FDA, but as I have looked at this process and have been briefed on it, I believe that they made the best decision they could at the time, given the information that they had. But again, this concept and commitment to process improvement and continuous improvement, as we look back upon that in terms of lesson learned, I agree that it would—going forward, not bringing that advisory committee together until the issue of the data had been resolved would have been a more preferable and ideal way to approach it, and the way we should approach it in the future.

Mr. BURGESS. And just for purposes of clarification for the committee and the record, many of those events took place prior to the time you were appointed Acting FDA Administrator, is that correct?

Dr. VON ESCHENBACH. That is correct, sir.

Mr. BURGESS. In the very brief time I have left, let me just ask you a quick question about post-marketing surveillance process, post-marketing safety process. In a perfect world, what would be your vision of the correct type of post-marketing surveillance that the FDA should undertake?

Dr. VON ESCHENBACH. I believe we have the opportunity with electronic databases to be able to access the real world experience of the drug in the context of not just the drug itself, but the unique characteristics of the person taking that drug, because that will vary widely as we all appreciate, based on a whole host of factors, gender and on and on. And in addition, the interaction of that drug with other substances that that patient may be taking, because we are seeing an era in medicine of patients taking multiple medications simultaneously.

So with those kinds of opportunities to see that drug in that context, I think that will provide enormous insight and information to us in terms of not just how to manage that drug, but how to continue to improve the process of discovery and development on the front end with the next generation of drugs in that class or of that variety.

Mr. BURGESS. Or for that individual, given their individual genetics?

Dr. VON ESCHENBACH. And by being able to, for example, identify populations, we will have tools in terms of genetic or genomics to stratify. We are seeing that even now for an old drug like lophine, a blood thinner, where we now can begin to stratify and understand patients based on their genetic makeup in terms of what the right dose could be.

Mr. BURGESS. We are going to restrict your access to genetic data this afternoon, so hurry up and gather that.

I yield back, Mr. Chairman.

Mr. STUPAK. Well, you are well over, so nothing to yield.

For 10 minutes, Mr. Inslee. We are going to try to get Mr. Inslee in before votes. We have 10 minutes and 30 seconds, so Mr. Inslee for 10 minutes.

Mr. INSLEE. Thank you.

Commissioner, in regard to Ketek, there has been some discussion about use of non-inferiority trials as opposed to a test with placebos, and as I understand it, there was a recommendation to go to a placebo test rather than just a non-inferiority test. That makes some sense to me, given the nature of some of the problems we have encountered. Could you tell us if you have any plans to review that?

Dr. VON ESCHENBACH. Well, this is an important part of an ongoing effort to look at the entire clinical trial's construct, Mr. Inslee. We are evolving in science and we are evolving in our utilization of clinical trials. New statistical models like basian statistics that will enable us to use adaptive trial designs are now emerging so the old traditional models that we used in the past are evolving. The movement within, particularly, the reference you are making to non-inferiority studies is a part of that ongoing process of learning as far as how we can apply the right kind of trial design to the right question.

Mr. INSLEE. So I am not sure what the answer is.

Dr. VON ESCHENBACH. The answer is we are evolving based on our learning and understanding of the utilization of trials as new models become available to us, and recently, the Center has issued and is in the process of issuing guidance to where and when non-inferiority trials are appropriate and where other trial designs are preferable.

Mr. INSLEE. I want to ask you about disclosure, the summary basis of approval documents. There has been a recommendation that they essentially be available publicly except for genuine trade secrets, and that, as I understand, that issue is still stalled. Is there any progress in that front?

Dr. VON ESCHENBACH. I will respond to the record with regard to the specific details of the issue and the trajectory, but overall, I am continuously committed to providing information and data to be open and transparent in the processes, while we, at the same time, respect and protect, for example, confidential information, proprietary rights, the other kind of issues that frame our ability to legally disseminate information.

Mr. INSLEE. So I will ask you just a little more pointed question. Would you support amending the current FDA regulations to require public disclosure of those except for genuine trade secrets?

Dr. VON ESCHENBACH. I have to be certain that there weren't other issues besides genuine trade secrets that might impact upon that, but I am committed to looking to provide as much disclosure as is legally and appropriately possible.

Mr. INSLEE. But legally is what you decide, so you decide what is legal. And I hope you will consider that public confidence in this system is very, very important.

Dr. VON ESCHENBACH. I understand.

Mr. INSLEE. We have had real concerns about that. I understand the nature of propriety and information. I come from a biotech community. We understand intellectual property. It is very, very important. But I think that those two things should be reconcilable to maintain and build public confidence and still protect that property. I believe that can be done. I would encourage you to look at a way to accomplish that.

Dr. VON ESCHENBACH. And I am committed to continuing to work through those kinds of processes to move us to a better place. I give you that commitment to work with you and others who have a vested interest in this.

Mr. INSLEE. Thank you. I yield back.

Mr. STUPAK. We have about 6 minutes left in this vote, so we will take recess until 12:15 and we will be back.

Commissioner von Eschenbach, that three-page memo of November 26, do you have copies made on whistleblowers that you said you sent to all your employees?

Dr. VON ESCHENBACH. I have to——

Mr. STUPAK. We will have one of our staff people get it from you and make it be available for everybody. I will ask questions when we get back, and whoever else arrives, and we will be finished.

Thank you. See you at about 12:15.

[Recess.]

Mr. STUPAK. Mr. Commissioner, thank you again for appearing here.

Go to tab three of your book there. Do you have a book there with documents in from the committee? Go to tab No. 3 if you would, please. In there is the March 9, 2007 letter from Senator Grassley to you concerning treatment of individuals who may not agree, and in particular talking about the whistleblower issues.

In the first paragraph it says "Careful congressional oversight of the FDA is especially important to ensure the FDA upholds its responsibilities to the public safety by properly regulating the Nation's drug supply. Proper role of an agency leader is to cooperate with legitimate congressional oversight activities, not to impede congressional inquiries, or conceal information from Congress." Do you agree with that statement?

Dr. VON ESCHENBACH. I am sorry, sir. I was just trying to find it.

Mr. STUPAK. Paragraph one, middle of the page, starts "Careful congressional oversight".

Dr. VON ESCHENBACH. As I indicated, Mr. Chairman, previously——

Mr. STUPAK. Do you agree with this statement?

Dr. VON ESCHENBACH. I agree that individuals at FDA should appropriately cooperate and participate with Congress.

Mr. STUPAK. Very good.

Mr. Burgess and Mr. Whitfield both asked you about a 2006 conversation with Dr. Ross about an analogy to a football team and having to be on part of that team, and you indicated that you saw this as being constructive to have adversity on the team and in no way did you indicate that you have to be on the team—you can't be off the team. Is that right?

Dr. VON ESCHENBACH. As I indicated, I was discussing my perspective on being able to create an environment to have the opportunity for vigorous, aggressive scientific discussion and debate, and participating in that is constructive. Not participating in that does not contribute to the well-being of the institution.

Mr. STUPAK. So they have got to be on the same page as the rest of the team or they are not contributing to the institution?

Dr. VON ESCHENBACH. No, sir. What I am intending to say, and hopefully continue to always express clearly, is it is not a matter of being on the same page, it is a matter of bringing your point of view, your opinion, your diverse perspective to the process of deliberation and discussion.

Mr. STUPAK. Are you going to allow scientists and doctors within your Agency to bring their diverse view to advisory committees and things like that if it is not with what the supervisor at the FDA feel it should be?

Dr. VON ESCHENBACH. Yes, sir. We need to provide information to advisory committees and do that in a proper and appropriate way.

Mr. STUPAK. If that was November, then the second paragraph of that letter says "I was extremely troubled by the statements that the Star Ledger reported you made on February 21 at a conference sponsored by the Center for Medicine and the Public Interest. Star Ledger reported that you expressed your unwillingness to tolerate whistleblowers who go outside the Agency because they disagree with the final outcome." You are further quoted as saying "The people have to understand to go outside that process is not constructive, it is actually destructive." Did you make that statement?

Dr. VON ESCHENBACH. That statement does not apply in any way, shape, or form to whistleblowing——

Mr. STUPAK. Did you make the statement, sir?

Dr. VON ESCHENBACH. I did not make a statement about whistleblowers, Mr. Chairman.

Mr. STUPAK. I am not saying anything about whistleblowers. The quote is "The people have to understand to go outside the process is not constructive, it is actually destructive." Did you make that statement?

Dr. VON ESCHENBACH. I made that statement with regard to the process of deliberative discussion, scientific debate——

Mr. STUPAK. Well, what is the difference of, let us say, Dr. Ross who wishes—or Dr. Graham, who wishes to testify at an advisory panel that may not be in keeping with the position of the FDA. Are you going to allow them to do that?

Dr. VON ESCHENBACH. As I indicated before, the appropriate way and the appropriate fashion of bringing all the data and all the points——

Mr. STUPAK. No, what I asked is if Dr. Graham wants to go before an advisory panel, let us say on Accutane, one he has been really involved with and one he has been denied to present testimony. Are you going to continue to deny Dr. Graham the right to testify at advisory panels on, let us say, Accutane?

Dr. VON ESCHENBACH. I would not deny to Dr. Ross, Dr. Graham, or any other individual within the FDA the right to express their professional opinion and point of view about an issue.

Mr. STUPAK. OK. You indicated that there was a tape of your statements, and did that include the questions and answers at this conference on February 21?

Dr. VON ESCHENBACH. Yes, it did, sir.

Mr. STUPAK. OK. Will you provide that tape to the committee?

Dr. VON ESCHENBACH. I would be happy to do that, sir.

Mr. STUPAK. Great. Would you go to tab No. 4 please, in that same big book? It is called "Open Letter to Members of Congress" dated March 14, 2007. Sixth paragraph, right on the bottom of the page. It says "With expiration of PDUFA this year, the FDA and PHARMA have negotiated terms for a 5-year reauthorization. This negotiation completed behind doors had only limited input from the public. Unfortunately, the proposal crafted by the FDA and PHARMA does not come close to addressing the problems identified by IOM." Has that agreement been published at all?

Dr. VON ESCHENBACH. The agreement was published in the Federal Register and has been subject to open public discussion and debate during——

Mr. STUPAK. After it was published, not before, right?

Dr. VON ESCHENBACH. The negotiation resulted in a proposal——

Mr. STUPAK. And that was open to public discussion, and now is being presented to Congress.——

Mr. STUPAK. And that was just FDA and PHARMA?

There has been no public discussion, not until after it was published, right?

Dr. VON ESCHENBACH. It was published in the Federal Registry, it was——

Mr. STUPAK. After the publication, it is now——

Dr. VON ESCHENBACH. Further modification before the proposal was——

Mr. STUPAK. How does one discuss it publicly if it is already published, it is already agreed upon? How do we have input into the process?

Dr. VON ESCHENBACH. The proposal was agreed upon. The proposal was still subject to modifications and based on input from a variety of sources through both public commentary to the Agency prior to its coming to Congress as a final proposal.

Mr. STUPAK. Will you provide us the documents of those who have had input into this process, the closed door process, and the rest will be provided to this committee when asked?

Dr. VON ESCHENBACH. Provide the information regarding the process that——

Mr. STUPAK. No, no, the information that went into the negotiations from the closed door meeting that you had with PHARMA. Are you willing to submit those documents to us so we can see them, see who had input in the FDA and PHARMA?

Dr. VON ESCHENBACH. The discussions that went on between FDA and PHARMA were done with negotiating teams that were made up of content experts on the part of the FDA to work through the package.

Mr. STUPAK. Sure. And that was done behind closed doors, and we want to see what input drug companies had in that process, so will you make those documents available to us?

Dr. VON ESCHENBACH. They were part of the discussion in the process.

Mr. STUPAK. I know they were.

Dr. VON ESCHENBACH. The documents that are available, I would be happy to look at that and provide the appropriate documents to you in that regard.

Mr. STUPAK. Not appropriate, all documents we asked for. There is no proprietary interest in those negotiations.

Dr. VON ESCHENBACH. Mr. Chairman, at this point in time, I cannot certify or testify to all the content of whatever materials are available. I would have to go back, look at that, gather that together, and be responsive to you.

Mr. STUPAK. Sure. Let me go to page 9 of your statement. You didn't mention much about Ketek, but let me ask you. Page nine of your statement you allege that "Based on the information available, the concerns [data, integrity issues] study 3014 apply to only one site out of more than 1,800." In fact, every site that the FDA investigators looked at had serious problems. Look at tab 20 and you will find a series of e-mails relating to the integrity—the data integrity at the largest sites in study 3014, including an e-mail dated December 10, 2003, where the lead investigator says it looks like the new drug application, NDA, will have to be put on hold.' Were you shown the e-mail traffic between the review division and the field inspection force relating to this study when you prepared your testimony?

Dr. VON ESCHENBACH. No, sir, I was not aware of e-mails as I prepared for this testimony.

Mr. STUPAK. Then who prepared your testimony, someone else in your office, or did you prepare it?

Dr. VON ESCHENBACH. I prepared it along with my staff, and based on briefings and information that had been provided to me over a series of meetings with the people who were involved and engaged in this process.

Mr. STUPAK. Were the individuals that presented the Ketek case to you aware that you would be testifying under oath and have written statement would be sworn testimony?

Dr. VON ESCHENBACH. I would assume they were.

Mr. STUPAK. OK. Then let me ask you this. Also on pages nine and 10 of your testimony, you state "After considering the fact that the investigation results were preliminary and we have not received formal recommendations about how to take the results into account in review of the application, and the fact that only in very rare cases do inspection results from individual sites lead to the exclusion of an entire large clinical trial, FDA decided to hold the advisory committee meeting as planned. In fact, in an e-mail dated January 2, 2003, the office director writes David Ross stating that it would not be 'productive' to present the data integrity concerns to the advisory committee." So do you believe it is appropriate to withhold from an advisory committee a study when the integrity of that study is the principle study of the drug in question?

Dr. VON ESCHENBACH. When there is an issue about a particular part or piece of the study that has been withheld in previous circumstances and situations, when it is apparent——

Mr. STUPAK. This is part parcel. I think that was very clear, wasn't it, in that e-mail? Do you have the e-mail right there? I think we provided it there in tab 20, there are number of e-mails. It is really the second to last page of tab 20 there, all those e-mails, if you look at the second to last page. It says "E-mail of January 2 from Mark Goldberger to Mr. Ross. In general, I don't believe spending time on these issues, part parcel to these issues to the AC will be productive. I do feel that having the company make the best possible presentation of their PM data, focusing on information from countries where we have confidence in the reporting would be useful." So it sounds like you are not trying to discourage Study 3014 from being presented.

Dr. VON ESCHENBACH. First of all, Mr. Chairman, in preparation of my testimony, I do not recall ever seeing this particular e-mail or others that you may be alluding to. I prepared my testimony based on the principles and fundamentals of oversight of studies and their presentation to committees, and it has been the policy, as I have come to understand at the FDA, that certain parts of the study would be excluded——

Mr. STUPAK. This is your testimony. You bring up all these issues. Your statements and your testimony on Ketek do not correspond to the e-mails that are right there in front of you. That is why I asked you who prepared the testimony. Because what you said in your testimony, which is under oath, is contradicted by tab 20 and the e-mails contained therein.

So either you are not being forthright with us, when I believe you are, but whoever is doing your work is trying to lead this committee down the wrong path. We know these issues, we are on top of these issues, so when you come and give us testimony that isn't accurate, we are going to call you on it.

Dr. VON ESCHENBACH. I fully appreciate and understand that, Mr. Chairman. What I was hoping to communicate to you was the fact that as I have viewed and understood this matter, the decision to remove a part of the study or not present a particular part or element of the study has been done prior to this case——

Mr. STUPAK. But you didn't remove it. 3014 was presented, it was relied upon by FDA and by the advisory committee and the FDA—even on your Web site you relied upon Study 3014. To approve Ketek, that is contrary to what you say in your testimony.

Dr. VON ESCHENBACH. No, sir. May I clarify what I was intending to say? 3014 was not used as part of the decision to approve Ketek.

Mr. STUPAK. That is not what your Web site says.

Dr. VON ESCHENBACH. The Web site was incorrect, sir, and it should not have been presenting that information. The decision to approve Ketek was made after 3014 had been removed entirely from the analysis. The decision when 3014 was presented to the advisory committee was not to approve Ketek, even though the advisory committee recommended doing so. That decision to approve Ketek came after 3014 had been removed.

Mr. STUPAK. Well, that is what you continue to claim. In fact, on page 11 you say "Study 3014 was dropped for consideration, making the decision whether to approve Ketek."

Dr. VON ESCHENBACH. To approve Ketek, yes.

Mr. STUPAK. That is false. See the March 21, 2006 e-mail from Queter. "In addition, the FDA cites 3014 as part of evidence it had before Ketek's approval of the drug safety." Again, look at your Web site. Also "Prior to approval, FDA looked extensively at the potential for hepatitic toxicity in patients treated with Ketek. The data examined included a 25,000 patient study." If it wasn't used for approval, why was it cited on your Web site and why it in the 2006 e-mail, March 26, saying we used it as the evidence to approve Ketek?

Dr. VON ESCHENBACH. Mr. Chairman, it should not have been presented on the Web site. That was an error.

Mr. STUPAK. Nor in your testimony.

Dr. VON ESCHENBACH. My testimony, sir, it was never intended to indicate Ketek was used to approve—3014 was used to approve Ketek. My testimony was to indicate the approval decision was made after 3014 had been removed from the analysis.

Mr. STUPAK. Well, we hope to hear from the manufacturer of Ketek, once they ever get the information, so we can go through it, and we will have you come back up and explain it then with them in the room. Maybe we can sort this thing out. I would strongly advise you to correct your Web site, if it is wrong. And your testimony be reviewed before you come so it is accurate.

Mrs. Blackburn for questions, 10 minutes.

Mrs. BLACKBURN. Thank you, sir, I appreciate that, and thank you for your endurance and your patience this morning. We appreciate that.

First, I have got two or three different questions, and then hopefully I can yield back, Mr. Chairman, so that we can move on with the other witnesses and the rest of the hearing.

I want to go to page four of your testimony, and you talk a little bit about the IOM and their recommendations, and as I mentioned in my opening statement, they do recommend the establishment of an advisory committee. So many times now, our constituents, they know that these are not going to get us where we want to go. They have grown weary of seeing advisory committees and commissions and things of that nature, and view it as a procrastination mechanism. I know that you have mentioned that you can do this administratively and work with an advisory committee administratively.

So I would like for you to do a couple of things very quickly, so that we can move forward. Lay out how you feel like you can go about administratively instituting some reform on these IOM recommendations, and then also what we repeatedly hear from individuals that deal with the FDA process is their frustration with the bureaucracy and the desire to see some efficiency there. So if you can do this administratively, how can you do this and not increase the bureaucracy over there? Not increase the number of people, not increase the paperwork load on individuals who are trying to go through your process.

Dr. VON ESCHENBACH. I am going to be happy to provide much detail in that regard for the record, but let me just quickly address the issue from what I believe I can do administratively from the Office of the Commissioner leading this Agency.

I address this from the point of view of talent, tools, and structure. We can continue to increase and provide expertise that will look at the safety issues specifically and integrate them and coordinate them much better into the approval process. We will have better tools, both scientific tools to our critical path initiative with which to make those decisions, as well as information technology tools, as I have indicated before, in post-market surveillance. Even structural changes that we are making by much greater integration between the Office of Surveillance and Epidemiology and the Office of New Drugs, simple facts of how they are now engaging in meetings on a much more regular and frequent basis, how they are dialoging and communicating by virtue of the fact that we have colocated them in our facilities at White Elk as they have been constructed.

So very briefly and quickly, I see this as a multi-step, multiphase way of bringing this organization into a much, much better integrated coordinated and efficient in functioning organization that will make these decisions, enhance our decision-making about safety and effectiveness, and do that without creating more bureaucracy.

Mrs. BLACKBURN. You mentioned the critical path initiative as a structural tool, and I would like to hear from you a little bit about the value of the public private partnerships that are over there, if you think there is a value, and what that is bringing to the table as far as the critical path initiative goes, and also the value of having some outside consultants with a different set of eyes that are looking to the problems and the workload, the paper load, the documentation load that is a part of that process, a frustrating part of the process.

Dr. VON ESCHENBACH. I think one of the important areas of public private partnership and collaboration is the fact that industry and academia both have an enormous amount of data and information and insight into molecular mechanisms associated with these drugs and to their unique impact on various organs, both beneficial and perhaps adverse, and having FDA be able to access and participate and acquire and analyze that data further informs our regulatory decision-making.

Mrs. BLACKBURN. Does the same thing apply to international data? Do you use it in the same way in your communications?

Dr. VON ESCHENBACH. Well, all of the data that is available for an application is required to be presented to the FDA, and that includes international data, which is always looked at, and then weighed and valued in terms of the impact that it can have on our approval process.

Mrs. BLACKBURN. One other question on your guidance on communication of drug safety. As you laid out that guidance, quickly, what did you use to formulate those guidelines and then on the workload, how much of that was done internally and how much did you outsource?

Dr. VON ESCHENBACH. I would respond to the details of that with regard to the record in giving you accurate information about outsourcing and how that was developed and defined, and I will be happy to provide that for you.

Mrs. BLACKBURN. That would be wonderful.

I yield back, Mr. Chairman.

Mr. STUPAK. Thank the gentle lady for yielding back.

Mr. Green from Texas for 10 minutes.

Mr. GREEN. Thank you, Mr. Chairman.

Mr. Chairman, I apologize and Dr. von Eschenbach, this has been one of those mornings where I have three committee meetings and the problem is I am on the Ethics Committee, and that is like serving on the jury that they don't do it unless you are there, too. I am glad to be through with that for at least a little while.

Mr. Chairman, I would like to have my full statement placed into the record.

Mr. STUPAK. Without objection.

Mr. GREEN. One, I want to welcome Dr. von Eschenbach, because having known you for many years before and your career at M.D. Anderson and University of Texas there both as a physician and researcher and a cancer survivor, and I sometimes wonder why you left the National Cancer Institute and came to the FDA, and sometimes under questioning from my colleagues, you might wish you were back there.

Some of the questions I have, and because I am also on the health subcommittee, and so this fits right in with some of my concerns is that the culture of the FDA, and I know you rejected the

IOM recommendation to appoint an external advisory board to develop a strategy to change the organizational culture, and you set off to hiring an external management consultant. Was the external management consultant something that you personally felt, or is that something that came from somewhere else?

Dr. VON ESCHENBACH. The consultant was engaged by the Center itself. They had been actively involved in internal assessment and brought in the opportunity of an external consultant to help them address issues of culture. I in particular feel that this is my responsibility to be actively engaged in that process and to provide leadership and direction for that process as well. I am continuing to do that.

Mr. GREEN. How was the consultant selected?

Dr. VON ESCHENBACH. I cannot tell you the specific criteria that the Center used in selecting the consultant——

Mr. GREEN. When you say Center, I apologize——

Dr. VON ESCHENBACH. Center for Drug Evaluation; CDAR.

Mr. GREEN. Do you have any idea on how long this review will take?

Dr. VON ESCHENBACH. I believe they have a preliminary report thus far. I have seen some of that information regarding some of the principles of enhancing interaction, communication within the organization, within the Center. I don't know if they have the final report at this point, but I have seen some preliminary findings.

Mr. GREEN. Will that final report be made public?

Dr. VON ESCHENBACH. I would be happy to provide that to any appropriate source that would be interested in it.

Mr. GREEN. Mr. Chairman, I would hope our Oversight and Investigation Subcommittee, and frankly, the Health Subcommittee, because since we have direct oversight on FDA, but I would like to see—because it is structural reforms that may need statutory consideration. Our committee needs to look at that.

Will you post commitment to the zero tolerance retaliation for FDA employees, you speak candidly with these consultants?

Dr. VON ESCHENBACH. Well, I am certainly, as I stated before, completely dedicated and committed to preserving and protecting the legal rights of every member of the FDA.

Mr. GREEN. And I know that without a permanent advisory board as recommended by the IOM is the director—will you assure that the recommendations from the consultant will be enforced?

Dr. VON ESCHENBACH. Well, I look forward to it in a couple of ways, Mr. Green.

One is to directly address issues that may be particular to that Center, as well as really addressing this issue more broadly across the entire Agency. I have engaged within the Office of the Commissioner changes that will specifically address our ability as an Agency to continue to enhance the environment that I have spoken to earlier in my testimony. Changes I made with regard to deputy commissioners, bringing in a deputy commissioner and chief operating officer to specifically address our management functions and make them much more efficient and effective, including our communication tools. But also, particularly creating the deputy commissioner and chief medical officer position that Dr. Woodcock will now occupy that will specifically focus on our issues of us being a science-based and science-led regulatory agency.

Mr. GREEN. That brings up my next question. The FDA response to the Institute of Medicine report puts a great deal of weight on the science of safety to address the problems of FDA drug safety programs. But a recurrent criticism is that politics is put ahead of science, and why will the science of safety fair any better with new initiatives than it did with the science of Vioxx or Ketek or some of the other things that we have heard about? Do you feel comfortable that we are actually going to see that culture change?

Dr. VON ESCHENBACH. I am very confident that the FDA will continue to be a science-based Agency, and I want it very much to also be science-led. The nuance there is that we are integrating these tools that are enhancing our opportunity to make better informed decisions, both about safety and efficacy of these drugs, and the processes by which we do that will be both disciplined and rigorous and precise, and I believe that will enhance our performance, rather than slow it down.

Mr. GREEN. Thank you.

Mr. Chairman, I know that in substantive work it is other subcommittee, but I will just say this in addition to my statement that will go in the record.

Some of us who voted for PDUFA never intended for that to be the ultimate decision-making on someone paying a fee ahead of time, and that is what worries me and that is what some of the interest is, and so both from our report from this committee and hopefully our Subcommittee on Health will be able to deal with the issue.

Thank you.

Mr. STUPAK. Thank you, Mr. Green. We are going to hold just a minute for Mr. Markey, who is on his way down. He is chairing a hearing upstairs, the one I have been bouncing back and forth on.

While we wait a minute, any questions from Mr. Whitfield?

Mr. WHITFIELD. No, sir.

Mr. STUPAK. Let me ask a question, if I may. I don't want to waste this valuable time, since we have got the Commissioner here.

Mr. Waxman indicated that there are about 1,200 studies pending, or about 1,200 post-market studies that should be done that have been promised to be done that are not being done, and 71 percent have not even started. Who determines of these 1,200 which ones are going to have priority to get done to urge the drug companies to do them? Do you have some kind of priority list, or do you just sit back and wait until drug companies submit them?

Dr. VON ESCHENBACH. Well, it is one of the important issues that needs to be addressed and will be addressed, Mr. Chairman, in terms of our prioritization of our resources and using these post-market studies in a way that they are designed extremely well——

Mr. STUPAK. Well, wouldn't the drug companies do the studies, not you?

Dr. VON ESCHENBACH. The drug companies carry out the studies, but they carry them out at our direction.

Mr. STUPAK. So it depends on the severity of the issue, or how do you prioritize them?

Dr. VON ESCHENBACH. They should be designed and developed in ways that answer questions——

Mr. STUPAK. Correct. How do you prioritize those, those are life-saving drugs, or how do you do it?

Dr. VON ESCHENBACH. Some of those may have questions having to do with adverse outcomes that might be expected. Some of them may have to do with our ability to learn and how to better utilize that drug, dosages, for example, or a particular population.

Mr. STUPAK. Let us take Accutane, a controversial drug. They have been talking about dosage studies for a long time, and Roche has been asked to do it. As far as I know, it has never been done. Why don't you do that one? It is sort of a controversial drug. We have birth defects, we have suicides related to it. Why hasn't a dosage study ever been done? There is a question that the dosage is maybe 200 percent greater than what it should be.

So why hasn't a study been done on that? I think we have been waiting for if one has been done, correct me, but I don't think one has been done, and I think it has been about 8 years now, 9 years maybe?

Dr. VON ESCHENBACH. Accutane has been available as a very important part of the armamentarium to treat nodular acne, and there is a very rigid and very stringent process called I Pledge to manage the utilization——

Mr. STUPAK. No, I am talking about dosage.

Dr. VON ESCHENBACH. I am not aware of a need for a specific dosage study.

Mr. STUPAK. I sent you a report back on, I think it was like November 2006, very lengthy, about 23 pages, laid it all out for you, the things that had to be done, and I got this letter back saying yes, we continue to monitor it. But I asked specifically about the dosage study, why wasn't anything done on that?

Dr. VON ESCHENBACH. I would be happy to look into that again, Mr. Stupak, and give you that specific response with regard to dosage itself.

Mr. STUPAK. Yes, just when are you going to do this dosage study?

Dr. VON ESCHENBACH. I am not sure that a dosage study is necessarily required, but I would be happy to——

Mr. STUPAK. It was recommended about 8 years ago or 9 years ago. Take a look at it.

Mr. Markey is here. Mr. Markey for 10 minutes, please.

Mr. MARKEY. I thank you very much, Mr. Chairman, for your graciousness.

Dr. von Eschenbach, on the first day of this series of hearings on FDA issues, several former and current FDA employees testified about the truly frightening problems at FDA, including a culture of scientific censorship and intimidation, a lack of transparency in the review process, the inaction of FDA management in response to serious drug risks, and a lack of scientific freedom and the inability of FDA reviewers to have their concerns heard by senior management FDA advisory committees and the public.

It was clear from the whistleblower's testimony that the FDA is an Agency that needs to be changed, in the best interest of the public. I would say that I was disturbed by your responses to Chairman Stupak regarding your testimony and the apparent contradictions between your testimony on Study 3014 and the internal FDA e-mails. It is clear that we are not getting an accurate and complete picture of what went on at the FDA during the lead up to the Ketek approval.

It is this kind of lack of transparency and openness about serious issues at the FDA that has made this Congress and the public very concerned about the FDA's ability to communicate effectively to the public and to be a true watchdog for public health.

My first question, Dr. von Eschenbach, is I would like to ask you about the FDA's policy of providing complete information to advisory committees. In response to Mr. Stupak's excellent questions about allowing FDA employees to present to advisory committees, you testified that you believe that employees should be able to present to advisory committees even if their managers do not want them to. Just to clarify, do you believe that any FDA employee working on a matter related to an issue before an advisory committee should be allowed an opportunity to make a presentation to the committee?

Dr. VON ESCHENBACH. Mr. Markey, if I can clarify. I believe that employees of the FDA that have material contributions to make should have opportunities to present that. Presenting to an advisory committee is something that would include, if and when it was appropriate. There may be reasons why it might not be appropriate to present, for example, only one portion of the data, when other portions or other perspectives were not available. That may need to be withheld from that particular meeting until those other parts and pieces are assembled.

So there may be reasons to not be allowed to present at that specific meeting, but that is not to say that that is equivalent to suppressing important, valid information that has to bear on the decision. I will not tolerate that.

Mr. MARKEY. Would you support the provision in my bill H.R. 1165, the Safe Drug Act, which would clarify that any FDA employee working on a matter related to an issue before an advisory committee should be allowed an opportunity to make a presentation to the committee?

Dr. VON ESCHENBACH. I think they should be allowed opportunities to have their position and point of view made and included in the process, the deliberative process. How that comes about, whether it is by direct presentation to the advisory committee, whether it is a submission of a report, or whether it is including their particular point of view in an overall analysis is something that I think needs to be determined on a case-by-case basis.

Mr. MARKEY. I believe that the provision in my legislation to ensure that advisory committees have access to complete information is necessary because of not only what we saw with Ketek, but also because in 2004, this committee conducted an investigation that found that the FDA had prevented a scientist from presenting data to an advisory committee that SSRIs increased the risk of suicidality in adolescents. I am worried that the FDA has a pattern of restricting information presented to advisory committees, and believe that Congress needs to act to clarify the scientific censorship because I don't think that that is acceptable.

So in my opinion, the purpose of an advisory committee is to examine all the available scientific data, to make a recommendation to the FDA. If the FDA puts its thumb on the scale and only presents part of the story, then the public will not get the benefit of having the best scientific minds examine all of the information and give unbiased recommendations regarding the best course of action at the FDA.

I have a second question for you.

At our last hearing, former FDA employee Dr. David Ross testified that Ketek happened because there were no penalties for FDA managers who engaged in suppression of reviewers and dissemination of false information. Do you believe that it is acceptable for managers to ask their subordinates to exclude or alter scientific information for non-scientific reasons?

Dr. VON ESCHENBACH. I believe it is never permissible for anyone to ask or influence someone else to change their scientific data or their scientific opinion.

Mr. MARKEY. Well, according to a 2006 survey conducted by the Union of Concerned Scientists, of the 997 FDA scientists who responded to the survey, nearly one-fifth, 18.4 percent said that they have been asked for non-scientific reasons to inappropriately exclude or alter technical information or their conclusions in an FDA scientific document. Do you agree with that conclusion reached by the Union of Concerned Scientists in their survey? Are you aware of a culture of suppression at the FDA?

Dr. VON ESCHENBACH. I am aware of the fact that there are times in the development of any particular body of information that there is an opportunity for drafts of that information to be changed, modified, or altered, depending upon input that comes from a variety of sources. That is a different issue than asking someone to change or alter scientific data or alter their particular conclusions. They have the opportunity to present that, to stand behind that. Others who disagree with that can provide alternative rebuttal if they have a different point of view. That is different than preparing a report that requires distillation of information from a variety of sources.

Mr. MARKEY. Well, would you agree that it is important to have penalties in place for FDA employees who do seek to censor or suppress scientific information for non-scientific reasons?

Dr. VON ESCHENBACH. When someone acts inappropriately and illegally to suppress that type of information as you are describing it, that is clearly in violation of what would be considered law, then that should have penalties associated with it, and those penalties can include disciplinary action of that individual, including severance of their relationship with the FDA.

Mr. MARKEY. Would you also agree that if an FDA employee reports through the appropriate channels that censorship or suppression of scientific information has occurred at FDA, then that person should be protected under the whistleblower laws?

Dr. VON ESCHENBACH. I believe all legal rights having to do with whistleblowers should be protected. I believe that when someone issues a complaint or a concern or registers an issue, that needs to be investigated, evaluated, the certainty of that needs to be determined, and then actions need to be taken. I believe that is an important part of managing and meeting this kind of a complex scientific-based organization.

Mr. MARKEY. So do you believe that we should ensure that reporting of scientific censorship is covered under the Whistleblower Protection Law?

Dr. VON ESCHENBACH. I believe that the legal rights of people need to be protected.

Mr. MARKEY. So if we made that more clear, that those whistleblowers——

Dr. VON ESCHENBACH. If Congress passed a particular law with particular language, I would always be committed to enforcing that law. That is correct.

Mr. MARKEY. So I thank you, Doctor, very much, and I do believe it is important for Congress to act in order to give the FDA employees a scientific bill of rights so that there is no misunderstanding that the fact is that full scientific discussions must be at the center of all FDA decisions. The Safe Drug Act that I have introduced is designed to do just that, and I look forward to continuing to work with you, Doctor, and members of the committee towards the goal of giving these protections to the workers at your Agency.

I thank you for your testimony here today.

Thank you, Mr. Chairman, again, for your more than generous tolerance of my tardy arrival. Thank you.

Mr. STUPAK. And you put up with me all morning running back and forth, so that is the least I can do. Thank you.

Thank you, Mr. Commissioner, and we look forward to working with you on this reauthorization of PDUFA, pediatric exclusivity, and some other pieces of legislation.

There will probably be written questions and follow-ups to you, and we look forward to documents we requested from you. Thank you for being here today.

Dr. VON ESCHENBACH. Thank you, Mr. Chairman and Mr. Whitfield, and other members of the committee for your consideration this morning.

Mr. STUPAK. We will immediately go into our second panel. They have us under a timeframe again today, and at 2:30 we have a full committee markup, so they want the full committee room. So we will try to move along with panel 2 here. I would ask panel two members to come up. Bruce Psaty, a doctor, professor of medicine, Epidemiology and Health Services at the University of Washington, School of Public Health and Community Medicine.

Next we have Marsha Crosse, Director of Public Health and Military Healthcare Issues, U.S. Government Accountability Office.

We have Dr. Curt Furberg, professor of Public Health Services, Division of Public Health Services, Wake Forest University School of Medicine. And we have Dr. Raymond Woosley, president and CEO of Critical Path Institute.

As you know, it is the practice of this committee to take all testimony under oath. I would ask each witness to stand and raise their right hand, please.

[Witnesses sworn]

Mr. STUPAK. Let the record reflect all witnesses answered affirmatively as to the oath.

We will start with Dr. Psaty.

TESTIMONY OF BRUCE M. PSATY, M.D. PROFESSOR, MEDICINE AND EPIDEMIOLOGY, UNIVERSITY OF WASHINGTON

Dr. PSATY. Mr. Chairman and members of the committee, my name is Bruce Psaty, a professor of medicine and epidemiology at the University of Washington. I served on the IOM Drug Safety Committee.

The IOM safety review was undertaken at the request of the FDA after the withdrawal of Vioxx had raised questions about the integrity of the U.S. drug safety system, and this testimony reflects my views as a public health scientist.

According to one former FDA Commissioner, the only novel IOM recommendation was the proposed 6-year term for future Commissioners. All the other recommendations had been made in one form or another in a dozen previous reports, yet in the FDA response to the IOM report, all actions are listed as recently initiated, new, or planned in PDUFA IV. What happened to the scores of previous recommendations? Whether this time the FDA responses will eventually improve drug safety remains to be seen.

The FDA, which has many outstanding scientists, has a difficult job. The interests of the pharmaceutical industry and risks and benefits are not symmetrical. There is little short-term economic interest in safety, and some sponsors lack imagination when it comes to the design of safety studies, hence the need for a strong, science-based regulation to protect the health of the public.

The current business model pre-market evaluation drug approval and marketing, which is mirrored at the FDA, is the primary structural flaw that allowed the Vioxx drug disaster. The current drug safety system, in which approval largely signals the end of evaluation, could hardly be weaker. The FDA centerpiece, the Adverse Event Reporting System, creates a case series, the weakest form of epidemiologic evidence.

Other major drug safety efforts are the post-marketing study commitments, and as some of the questions have pointed out today, 71 percent, 899 remain still pending. The completion rate has dropped from 62 percent in the 1970's down to 24 percent in recent years.

To improve the system, the IOM Committee recommended a life cycle approach to drug evaluation, an ongoing, systematic effort to identify safety signals, translate them into high quality studies, evaluate both health benefits and health risks, and integrate the information into risk-benefit analyses and communicate that information to patients and physicians.

FDA needs additional resources. While some FDA responses to the IOM report were excellent, or were limited by inadequate resources, others seemed to embrace the culture, vision, and values of the status quo at the Agency. For all new molecular entities, the IOM recommended a reevaluation of post-approval data by the FDA, an idea that will merely be pilot tested. Leaving the review of new safety data in the hands of industry may, on occasion, be a hazard to the health of the public. The IOM recommended public release of the FDA's risk-benefit analysis after the completion of post-marketing studies. FDA plans to do so only on a case-by-case basis.

Transparency is, however, essential. Although the Agency usually needs to make one decision, physicians and patients deserve to hear not one constrained voice, but the range and the quality of the evidence that underlie a regulatory decision, and scientific disagreements should be incorporated into that information that is released. It should not be a matter of legality and whistleblowers. We need to know what the scientific disagreements are. They will be good predictors of drug safety problems. Otherwise, the FDA fails in its mission to serve as a trusted intermediary of complex information.

The IOM recommended joint authority for the Office of New Drugs and the Office of Surveillance and Epidemiology. The FDA plans a few pilot projects. This response, which fails to acknowledge even a future commitment to the spirit of joint authority does not signal a major cultural change at the FDA. The IOM recommendations to involve advisory committees in the review of all new molecular entities was largely ignored. The failure to recognize the importance of independent review provided by advisory committees is not in the spirit of broad cultural change.

These responses, taken together, do not represent “fundamental changes that will entail a cultural shift within the FDA.” A fundamental change would involve actively embracing an ongoing lifestyle evaluation that includes both transparency and independent review. Cultural changes need to come first. They need to come from the top, and include leadership that relies on science in its decision-making process, leadership that values and harnesses scientific disagreement to improve the drug approval process, and leadership that is at once courageous under outside pressure and passionate about the health of the public.

Thank you.

[The prepared statement of Dr. Psaty follows appears at the conclusion of the hearing.]

Mr. STUPAK. Thank you. Dr. Furberg, please, for 5 minutes. Thank you, sir.

TESTIMONY OF CURT D. FURBERG, M.D., PROFESSOR, PUBLIC HEALTH SCIENCES, WAKE FOREST UNIVERSITY SCHOOL OF MEDICINE

Dr. FURBERG. Mr. Chairman and members of the committee, I am Curt Furberg. I am professor of Public Health Sciences at Wake Forest University School of Medicine, with expertise in drug evaluation and safety. I also serve as a member of the FDA Drug Safety and Risk Management Advisory Committee. This testimony reflects my personal views.

I am a firm believer in law and order. Congress has a very critical role in developing and passing laws to protect what is right and fair. Laws and regulation are effective, because violations have consequences. Our citizens cherish the notion that no one is above the law. Therefore, it troubles me that drug makers can violate FDA regulations, commitments, and public trust without apparent consequences.

Here are some examples. One company, testing its depressant in adolescents, reported and made public only three of its 13 trials. The other 10 did not support the company’s claim for efficacy and safety. Despite this suppression, the FDA has taken no action against the sponsor. Another company delayed for several years submitting unfavorable safety data from a trial of its COX–2 inhibitor in Alzheimer's disease. The FDA has taken no action. The third company submitted falsified data for an FDA hearing of its antibiotic, as discussed in the previous hearing on drug safety. Again, the FDA has taken no action against the company.

Thus, it appears to me that regulatory violations have no consequences in the United States.

The fourth company stalled negotiations for 14 months over label changes that would add an important black box warning to its COX–2 inhibitor. Decisions about label warnings should take only 1 to 2 weeks. This irresponsible delay had no consequences for the drug maker.

These cases illustrate the industry's malfeasance. They are alarming and have serious implications for public health. Tragically, they represent only a small fraction of the total problem.

These examples pale in comparison to the potential public health harm caused by industry's unmet commitments to conduct post-market safety trials. The approval of many new drugs is based on these commitments. As of last fall, there were 1,259 unmet commitments, with more than two-thirds not even initiated. What has the FDA done? Nothing.

In my view, it is critical for Congress to provide FDA with enforcement tools, give the FDA legal authority to change drug labels, and to withdraw unsafe drugs without negotiation, ensure, through Congressional oversight that the FDA utilizes this new authority appropriately and in a timely manner.

I was asked to comment on the FDA's responses to the IOM recommendations. Overall, I find them disappointing. Although many of the responses have merit, there are several shortcomings.

First, the Agency's apparent unwillingness to ask Congress for more authority to enforce drug safety regulations is troubling.

Second, FDA's plan lacks concrete and constructive steps to bring drug safety to parity with drug benefit in the evaluation process. After all, decisions about drug approval and later, use of a drug, are based on the balance between benefit and harm.

The Office of Surveillance and Epidemiology needs more experts in drug safety, public health, and surveillance. The Director of this Office should report directly to the Commissioner, and the Office should have its own external advisory committee.

Third, another concern not addressed is FDA's lack of transparency. Prescribers and the public are not given safety information known to FDA officials in a timely manner. The reasons for disapproving a drug, and the reasons for requesting post-marketing safety studies are kept secret.

Fourth, also missing in FDA's response is an evaluation plan. Progress towards improvement of the drug safety problems needs to be closely monitored and reported, and corrective actions being taken if goals are not met.

Finally, the measure of FDA's performance needs to be changed. It should not be based only on the number of drugs approved within a certain time period. Full credit should be given for disapproval of drugs for safety reasons. These were the problems highlighted in the recent article entitled "The FDA and Drug Safety: A Proposal for Sweeping Changes," which I would like to add to my testimony. This article was written by me and four other current and past members of the FDA Drug Safety and Risk Management Advisory Committee.

Thank you so much.

[The prepared statement of Dr. Furberg appears at the conclusion of the hearing.]

Mr. STUPAK. Thank you, Doctor. And that article, I think we all have it, and it will be made part of your opening statement. Thank you.

Dr. Marcia Crosse.

TESTIMONY OF MARCIA G. CROSSE, Ph.D, DIRECTOR, PUBLIC HEALTH AND MILITARY HEALTH CARE ISSUES, U.S. GOVERNMENT ACCOUNTABILITY OFFICE, ACCOMPANIED BY MARTIN T. GAHART, PH.D., ASSISTANT DIRECTOR

Dr. CROSSE. Mr. Chairman and members of the subcommittee, I am pleased to be here today as you examine FDA's process for decision-making regarding post-market drug safety.

My remarks today are based on GAO's March 2006 report on this topic, and on steps FDA has taken that respond to the recommendations we made in that report. Our work focused on two FDA Offices that are involved in post-market drug safety, the Office of New Drugs, OND, and the Office of Drug Safety, ODS, which has since been renamed the Office of Surveillance and Epidemiology. Consistent with our report, I am referring to this Office as ODS.

As we reported in March 2006, we found a failure to appropriately manage the post-market drug safety process. We found a lack of clarity about how decisions were made, and about organizational roles. There was insufficient oversight by management, and there were significant data constraints.

Importantly, there was a lack of criteria for determining what safety actions to take and when to take them, which contributed to disagreements over decisions about post-market safety.

Specifically, certain parts of ODS' role in the process were unclear, including ODS' participation in scientific advisory committee meetings that were organized by OND to discuss specific drugs. We found examples of the exclusion of ODS staff from making presentations at certain meetings.

For example, in the case of Arava, an arthritis drug with concerns about liver toxicity, ODS staff were not allowed to present their analysis of post-market safety at a meeting held to review Arava's safety risks and benefits. We also found that insufficient communication between ODS and OND was an ongoing concern, and hindered the decision-making process.

For example, ODS did not always know how or whether OND had responded to ODS' safety analyses and recommendations for safety actions. ODS management did not systematically track information about the recommendations its staff made, and OND's response. This limited the ability of management to ensure that safety concerns were resolved in a timely manner.

Moreover, FDA faced data constraints that contributed to the difficulty in making post-market safety decisions. In the absence of specific authority to require drug sponsors to conduct post-market studies, FDA has relied on drug sponsors voluntarily agreeing to conduct these studies, but studies have not consistently been completed.

FDA was also limited in the resources it had available to obtain data from outside sources. Annual funding for this program was less than $1 million a year for 2002 through 2005, and was $1.6 million in 2006, which allowed for four data contracts.

The problems we identified were not new. For example, FDA conducted a lessons learned review in 2000, of the withdrawal from the market of the nighttime heartburn drug Propulsid following safety concerns about serious heart arrhythmias. In its internal review, FDA identified the need for better communication between the organizational groups, and called for the development of a standard approach to post-market safety, including what types of evidence to use, when labeling changes or other safety actions are warranted, who should be involved in the process, and how to present the issues to advisory committees. Yet when we conducted our review more than 5 years later, FDA had not acted on its own recommendations.

Today, almost a year after our report was issued, FDA has begun to take steps that could address the goals of three of our four recommendations. First, we recommended that FDA systematically track post-market drug safety issues, and the Agency is in the process of implementing a tracking system.

Second, we recommended that FDA revise and implement its draft policy on the decision-making process for major post-market safety actions, and FDA has made revisions to, but not finalized, its draft policy. Third, we recommended that FDA clarify the safety staff's role in scientific advisory committees, and the Agency is developing, but has not finalized, guidance to clarify their role. And fourth, we recommended that FDA improve its process to resolve disagreements, but FDA has not taken actions in response to this recommendation.

In conclusion, while FDA has taken positive steps, its actions are not yet fully implemented, and it is too soon to evaluate their effectiveness in addressing these longstanding concerns.

Mr. Chairman, this concludes my prepared remarks. I would be happy to respond to questions you or other members of the subcommittee may have.

[The prepared statement of Dr. Crosse appears at the conclusion of the hearing.]

Mr. STUPAK. Thank you, Dr. Crosse. Dr. Woosley, please, for 5 minutes. Your opening statement, sir.

RAYMOND L. WOOSLEY, M.D., PRESIDENT AND CHIEF EXECUTIVE OFFICER, THE CRITICAL PATH INSTITUTE

Dr. WOOSLEY. Mr. Chairman, members, thank you for the opportunity to provide testimony to the subcommittee on this very important topic. As mentioned, I am Raymond Woosley. I am President of the Critical Path Institute, a publicly-funded nonprofit that is based in Tucson, Arizona and Rockville, Maryland.

I am a pharmacologist and a physician for the last 40 years. I have had a lot of experience with the study of medications, and often working very closely with the FDA and its scientists. I was at Georgetown for 13 years. I appear here today because I am very concerned about the future of the pharmaceutical industry, not an easy stand to take. But even more, I am concerned about the patients who need their medicines, and the new medicines.

This industry that everyone thinks is so successful and profitable is, in fact, threatened by the inefficiency, threatened by the resulting unacceptably high prices for its new products, and threatened by the unacceptably high rate of product failure during development and after development.

After millions are spent in the laboratory, 90 to 95 percent of drugs that enter clinical testing today fail to make it to the market. We can't survive with those statistics. The rare success that gets to the market requires an estimated investment of 15 years and $1.3 billion. Therefore, as you consider how to improve drug safety, which we must do, you must do, we must also maintain and create incentives for innovation.

I can't resist quoting a colleague and friend, Hugh Tilson, who said: "Without innovation, all we have are the products of yesterday." So innovation is important, and safety is even more important.

In the remaining few minutes, I would like to share with you some of the lessons I have learned about drug safety over the last 40 years. I am sure others have testified that the complete profile of a drug's risk or benefit can never be fully defined before a drug reaches the market.

Also, though, patterns of use can change on the market, in the marketplace, meaning that drugs must be carefully evaluated throughout their lifecycle, even decades after they have been on the market. That must be paid for, and it is not even covered in user fees today.

I have learned that surveillance signals that suggest harm are just that, signals. Before alarming patients with public, early disclosure of premature data, these signals need to be confirmed, and many will turn out to be false alarms, and I could cite you many of those. Also, I have learned that when a drug has to be removed from the market due to toxicity, it is not necessarily the result of mistakes made by anyone, including the developer or the FDA. Some new drugs will have adverse effects that could never have been anticipated. We must find those problems early, though.

Yet today, there are some important opportunities to do better. Some of those have been discussed. Prior to administering drugs in humans today, we rely on the same laboratory tests that we developed over 50 years ago. As part of the Critical Path initiative, the FDA has helped create pre-competitive collaborations with groups of companies that now share and validate their testing methods. This work will result in safer drugs entering human testing, and eventually reaching the market.

It will also identify biomarkers. These are the clinical tests that can predict which patients are at risk for harm before they receive the drugs. This is the essential first step before we get what we all have asked for, personalized medicine.

The FDA, though, needs more resources to fully participate in these collaborations, and to incorporate the results of that work into new standards for testing. Post-marketing safety assessment can also be greatly improved with a modest investment, in fact, by using the modern information technology that is already available. The U.S. does not have a system capable of rapid and accurate detection of adverse drug events. The AERS system is effective, but it is too slow.

For the last 19 drugs that were removed from the market, their average time on the market was 6.6 years. That is too long. We must do better. We have got the tools to detect those adverse events much more quickly.

For example, the ARC funded centers for education and research on therapeutics that was mentioned twice this morning, Rich Platt. Those centers have access to medical records from health plans that can readily be expanded to form a network of health plans that serve approximately 100 million people. A network such as this could readily serve as an early detection system.

Lastly, does the FDA need extensive reform? I don't think so. I think they need the resources, the permanent leadership, to do the job we are asking of them.

In closing, I remind all of us. For some time now, we scan the barcodes of everything in our grocery basket. We know how many suitcases were lost by every airline in the Nation each month. We can tell which cell tower picked up our friend's call, yet we don't have a safety system in place today. Clearly, we have the technology available today to establish a world-class safety surveillance system, and at the same time, maintain the path for safer, innovative new therapies to each patients.

Thank you, Mr. Chairman.

[The prepared statement of Dr. Woosley appears at the conclusion of the hearing.]

Mr. STUPAK. Thank you, Dr. Woosley.

Tab four in that big binder has the open letter to Chairman Kennedy, Chairman Dingell, and members of this committee.

You were talking about, and I quoted it earlier, at the bottom of the page, where it said the FDA and pharma have negotiated terms for a 5-year reauthorization. This negotiation, completed behind closed doors, had only limited input from the public. The proposal crafted by FDA and pharma does not come close to addressing the problems identified by the IOM.

Care to expand on that just a little bit more? You signed it, I believe.

Dr. PSATY. Yes, I did. I would be happy to comment.

Under PDUFA, the U.S. has become increasingly the country of first launch, the kind of testing ground for new drugs. For the first 10 years of PDUFA, the FDA was prohibited from using any of those fees for safety.

This occurred during Kessler's time, when he was Commissioner. He indicated that they wanted to use some of these fees for safety, but industry said no. So Congress enacted PDUFA legislation that really entrusted safety to the pharmaceutical industry, and did not adequately fund the FDA. So, this has been a problem that has existed for some time, and will take some time to fix.

In the implementation, and this is part of the issue that you are getting to, the appearance is that FDA has industry as its primary client.

There are negotiations that take place between the regulator and the regulated that exclude the Academy and patient groups, and just about everyone else, until things are published in the Federal Register. So, there have been problems with the implementation as well.

The IOM report expressed a preference for general appropriations and we did this largely because we think drug safety is a public good.

Mr. STUPAK. Dr. Furberg, would you care to comment on that at all?

Dr. FURBERG. I would like to add the safety aspect, the rush to meet deadlines and be paid. That is a price, and the price, according to new scientific evidence, is there is an increase in adverse effects, when those drugs are rushed through. And overall, since 1997, there is a two and a half fold increase in serious adverse events in the United States.

Mr. STUPAK. Should PDUFA and the scope of PDUFA be limited, then, to those drugs that we need for life-threatening illnesses like AIDS and cancers, that are almost incurable? Should we use that kind of a timeline in approving those types of drugs? That is how PDUFA sort of got, politically got its legs, because they were saying it was taking too long for AIDS drugs, if I remember correctly 15 years ago.

Dr. FURBERG. Yes, but there is another solution that is used in Europe, conditioned approval, which wouldn't slowed down introducing a drug on the market. You just put restrictions on the approval, so during the period of probation, basically, companies wouldn't have to provide the safety information that you don't have at the time of giving approval.

Mr. STUPAK. One of your testimonies had to do with, when you approve a drug, it is like a 2-year conditional approval, and then after 5 years, go back and look at all the adverse events that have been reported, and things like that. So, it is like a 2-year approval, which is on the package, to show that it is still in its, sort of like trial stage, and then go back after 5 years, and look at it. Is that what you are——

Dr. FURBERG. Yes. And that is done in several countries in Europe.

Mr. STUPAK. Doctor?

Dr. PSATY. Part of the problem is that the approval process almost ends the evaluation. Companies commit to these post-marketing studies and then don't do them, and the FDA doesn't have resources to do studies, and the AERS system is not adequate. What we need is a kind of lifecycle approach, where there is an ongoing evaluation, integration of that information, assessment of risk and benefit, so that the approval process doesn't signal the end of an evaluation.

Right now, companies put together teams to get these drugs approved. Once they are approved, they disband those teams, put them to other drugs, and create marketing teams. We need a system that evaluates drugs throughout their entire lifecycle.

Mr. STUPAK. What about off-label use? Do you believe the FDA currently, is currently structured—Dr. Crosse, you may want to hit this—off-label use, do they have a right to restrict off-label use?

Dr. CROSSE. Mr. Chairman, no. The FDA has the responsibility to approve the marketing of the drug for the labeled indications. The usage of the drug is then in the hands of the medical community, and oversight is by state medical boards, if there are, if there is a belief that a particular use has been inappropriate.

Mr. STUPAK. But do the state medical boards actually try them—for off-label use——

Dr. CROSSE. In instances where there are malpractice charges brought.

Mr. STUPAK. I see.

Dr. CROSSE. Or where there is a concern about a particularly unusual prescribing pattern. But in general, FDA has no responsibility or ability to contain——

Mr. STUPAK. Do you believe they should be given the ability to limit off-label use?

Dr. CROSSE. I don't think I am qualified to comment on that. I think the concern is whether FDA is monitoring the promotion of the off-label use of drugs.

Mr. STUPAK. OK.

Dr. CROSSE. And FDA does have the ability and the responsibility to oversee whether inappropriate marketing is being done by the pharmaceutical companies, but the practice of medicine, I think, particularly in the area of cancer, has often extended the use beyond the labeled indication, but there are certainly accounts out in the public about more unusual uses of a drug, and that is something, I think, that is part of policing within the medical community.

Mr. STUPAK. OK. Dr. Woosley, if I may. The article you co-authored, entitled "A New System for Moving Drugs to Market," contains your recommendation that newly approved drugs should be given a defined population under observed conditions only. Wouldn't this require an initial ban on most of the direct to consumer advertising, since a newly approved drug would be approved for a carefully defined population?

Dr. WOOSLEY. Well, I think the problem is that the direct to consumer advertising, as originally conceived, would not require that, but the way it is executed today, it should. The direct to consumer advertising was created so that patients who had an illness knew they could go to the doctor, but instead, the direct to consumer advertising has become hyping one drug against the other, and selling the drug, and trying in a 30 minutes sound bite to convey risk and benefit. That is a very dangerous situation, but I think the patients could be told, under the system I suggest, that if they have an illness and certain characteristics, they should see their doctor, but not try to sell the drug to them on the TV.

Mr. STUPAK. I asked the Commissioner this question. Let me ask this panel, and maybe you have some suggestions. As we have heard, there is over 1,200 studies or commitments to do studies, on post-marketing issues.

Is there a way, should they be prioritized on which ones the FDA should put pressure on these manufacturers to develop them, or do we just sit back and let the FDA, let the manufacturers bring forth their studies whenever they feel like getting them?

Dr. PSATY. I can comment briefly. There have been about 800 studies in this pending category for a long time. Some of them are old, and many of them were developed rapidly within a couple of weeks before the approval time. Many of them aren't well designed, and probably 20 percent don't deserve to even be done. I think the FDA needs to go through all of these studies, take a look at them, decide which ones need to be done, drop the rest, assign a start date to all of them. Many of them don't have a start date. They are going to remain pending in perpetuity here. And you will see them on this list year after year, so some need to be dropped, some need to be redesigned. They all need a start date, and the medical officers in the OIG report in March 2003, many of them were uncertain about what sort of post-marketing commitments to ask of companies.

And we need epidemiologists to help the medical officers think about the proper design, independent review would help. In the current system, in which there is a rush to create these studies right at the last minute, under the PDUFA guidelines, really contributes to the weakness of the U.S. drug safety system.

Mr. STUPAK. Doctor.

Dr. FURBERG. Yes, I would like to add that we also need a completion date, and hold the sponsors responsible for those, and if they don't produce the studies on time, there should be consequences. Staggered consequences, eventually with drug withdrawal, if these studies are not done.

Mr. STUPAK. Well, Doctor, you also brought up in your testimony, the average time to make label changes, and I mentioned pediatric exclusivity, I lost a battle 5 years ago, but I am ready to fight it again. Here is a chart here, this is based on 2001, pediatric exclusivity, where you get the patent for doing the study, but then if there is a label change that is required, on this one here, it could be as high as 18 months. The average was 14 months back then in 2001. I am sure it has only grown, so we do the study, we see for the adolescent community, you have to prescribe it, dosage, or it may be contraindicated use, but we don't know about that until months, on average, 14 months after you get your patent extension.

That is insane. There is no incentive, then, to do the study or to change the labeling. The extension should be given after the label change, after the study is completed, not before.

Dr. FURBERG. That is correct. Then you can add to that the delay in getting the new package inserts out to the customers.

Mr. STUPAK. Sure.

Dr. FURBERG. It could be up to a year before all packages have the new insert.

Mr. STUPAK. Let me ask you one more. Subpoena power. I have gone around and around with the FDA on subpoena power. I know in Accutane they are looking for an eye exam, the raw data, they have been waiting over 14 years for that. They still can't seem to get it. Every time I ask the FDA about it, they say oh, we don't need subpoena power. Without subpoena power, how do you compel, or how do you get the information you need, especially raw data? If they submit a study, you see maybe a flag goes up, you want to see the raw data, how do you obtain it if you don't have kind of subpoena power? I think the FDA is about the last regulatory body we have in the Federal Government that doesn't have subpoena power.

Dr. FURBERG. I agree with you. I think it is essential. If you are going to see any change in the problem with drug safety, we have to have consequences for the drug makers. And what is interesting in the meeting with the former Commissioners, they all admitted we have no enforcement power. The best we can do is to go public and embarrass a company. What kind of a system is that?

Mr. STUPAK. Well, I asked them the last time they tried that, and they said they have never done it. So, even your so-called bully pulpit, they are even afraid to use that.

Dr. FURBERG. Yes.

Mr. STUPAK. I could go on forever, but my time is up, so I am going to turn to my friend from Kentucky, Mr. Whitfield, for 10 minutes, please.

Mr. WHITFIELD. Thank you, Chairman Stupak, and thank you all for being so patient today. We welcome you, and appreciate your interest in this important issue.

Dr. Psaty, you are a member of the IOM, and I was curious, how, as a person selected to be a member of the IOM, are you appointed, or——

Dr. PSATY. I am actually not a member of the IOM. I was a member of the IOM Drug Safety Committee, and I can't really speak to the selection process, since I was on the other end. The members included a diverse group, who had expertise in epidemiology, pharmacology, law, regulation, organization, but I don't, I can't speak to how we were selected.

Mr. WHITFIELD. And how were you appointed to the committee that you are a part of?

Dr. PSATY. I was asked by the IOM if I would be interested. I was screened for conflicts of interest. Personally, I have worked on drug safety issues for many years. So, I suspect that is why I was asked.

Mr. WHITFIELD. And Dr. Furberg, now, you are a member of the FDA Advisory Committee on Drug Safety. How were you selected for that?

Dr. FURBERG. Again, it was an invitation that came from the FDA.

Mr. WHITFIELD. From the FDA.

Dr. FURBERG. I went through the same screening, and like Dr. Psaty, I have been in the field for many, many years.

Mr. WHITFIELD. Yes. I am assuming that all four of you would agree that when you are having an Agency like FDA, as complex as it is, and I don't know how many employees they have, 9,000 or 10,000, I guess, over 9,000 or 10,000, but it is my understanding they have only had a Commissioner, full-time confirmed Commissioner two out of the last 6 years, at the top spot. Does that concern any of you, or does that bother you?

Dr. FURBERG. It bothers me, and I think what bothers me is this is a little bit too much a political process.

Mr. WHITFIELD. Yes.

Dr. FURBERG. And that is what the Commissioner has pointed out, the four former Commissioners. It is too much politics going in, and we are getting away from science.

I wish we would appoint Commissioners based on credentials, scientific credentials, management skills, and so on, the way academic institutions do it.

Mr. WHITFIELD. Yes. Well, Dr. Woosley.

Dr. WOOSLEY. I would just add I agree completely, and it is not just at the Commissioner's level. They have had acting Directors for Center, all the way down the line, it is acting everybody, and the inability to make decisions, the inability to plan, the inability to make change, is crucial to that organization, and without the resources, and without somebody in power, it is not going to happen.

Mr. WHITFIELD. Yes. Dr. Psaty.

Dr. PSATY. The IOM Committee did recommend a 6-year term for the Commissioner. It is an effort to get someone in there to stabilize the process, and 6 years crosses a Presidential term.

Mr. WHITFIELD. Right.

Dr. PSATY. And the idea is to create stability at the top.

Mr. WHITFIELD. Some continuity.

Dr. PSATY. Yes.

Mr. WHITFIELD. Dr. Crosse.

Dr. CROSSE. Yes. We also found that there was significant turnover in the leadership of the Office of Drug Safety, and we believe that was a major contributor to some of the problems and some of the lack of followup on issues that were uncovered.

Mr. WHITFIELD. Yes.

Dr. CROSSE. Because there was frequent turnover of leadership in that Office.

Mr. WHITFIELD. And is that a political appointment?

Dr. CROSSE. That is not a political appointment.

Mr. WHITFIELD. It is not a political appointment. Yes.

Dr. WOOSLEY. Just to follow up on that. A lot of the criticisms have been because the Agency hasn't done this or hasn't done that. A lot of this comes down to just lack of simple infrastructure. They don't have, and they are starting to gather, a database of what the previous commitments are. They don't even know. How can they enforce it?

Mr. WHITFIELD. They don't know what the post-market commitments are?

Dr. WOOSLEY. They have no database of that. Two years ago, they had a three ring binder on the desk inside the Commissioner's office, where people handwrote when they received an NDA. Now, it is getting better, but it is unbelievable the restraints in resources that those people have to live through.

Mr. WHITFIELD. Yes. Well, to appoint for 6 years, is that something we would need to do legislation on?

Dr. PSATY. I believe that is true.

Mr. WHITFIELD. OK. Listening to your testimony, and talking about the integrity of the drug approval process, and the post-marketing process, it sounds so bad that it would almost lead one to believe that our drug approval system, as it currently exists, is presenting a major concern for safety of the American people. Would you agree with that statement, or is that not true?

Dr. PSATY. It is possible we actually in some cases don't know, because the questions don't get asked and answered. I have to say that the FDA does many good things, and the medical officers who review these drugs, who think about them, who work with the companies, and the pre-approval process is a good process, and it generally works well. I think they need to work on how they handle scientific disagreement. That needs to be incorporated into the information that is provided to the public. But in general, the FDA does a good job in the pre-approval process. Once a drug is approved, in the old days, we let the drugs come on the market in Europe, and let Europe detect the problems, and then, we didn't have to worry about them.

Mr. WHITFIELD. Right.

Dr. PSATY. And with the speedup of the drug approval system——

Mr. WHITFIELD. Is there anything wrong with that?

Dr. PSATY. Well, the issue is, that then Americans don't get drugs that we would benefit from.

Mr. WHITFIELD. Right.

Dr. PSATY. And that is the problem with that. But we need a correlative, strong drug safety system if we are going to move them in the U.S., if we are going to move them to market quickly.

Mr. WHITFIELD. Right. Dr. Furberg.

Dr. FURBERG. Well, thank you for asking that question. I am supportive of a strong pharmaceutical industry. They have changed the whole face of medicine over the past decades, improved survival, reduced complications, alleviated symptoms. That is wonderful, but it has come at a price, and I am not prepared to pay that price. I like the benefit side. Let us support that. But on the safety, the situation could be much improved, and that is why I am here, to argue for better ways of reducing the safety issues.

Mr. WHITFIELD. Dr. Crosse, do you have any comment?

Dr. CROSSE. I would agree that I believe the pre-approval process is very rigorous. I think that they work really hard to try to be sure that those decisions are correctly made. I think there are some fundamental problems in the kind of information that the Agency has had available, and in the support for pursuing that sort of information and figuring out how to best use it in assessing the problems that occur once a drug is on the market.

Mr. WHITFIELD. And Dr. Woosley.

Dr. WOOSLEY. I think we need to look at the full spectrum. Our Nation invests $90 billion in research and development every year, and we spend only $300 million to see if it was worth giving to the public, and I think that is the problem. We haven't invested in that final tip of the filter.

Mr. WHITFIELD. Are talking about the post-marketing aspect?

Dr. WOOSLEY. No, I am talking about the process of reviewing all that science. And because we have not invested well in that, because we only spend that much money at the FDA, what I am getting at is the incentives for new product development are drying up. The number of new products submitted to the FDA has fallen by 50 percent, even though we have increased our R&D by 250 percent.

Mr. WHITFIELD. Fallen by 50 percent?

Dr. WOOSLEY. Right. The number of new, innovative chemicals submitted to the FDA, not sitting there being reviewed, coming in the door, and that is in spite of more than doubling our investment.

Mr. WHITFIELD. Well, everyone has to be concerned about that, because we hear as laymen that more and more people are becoming, certain antibiotics are not having any impact on them, and so we need more R&D and more drugs coming to market, and then your comment that the average cost to take a drug to market is like $1.3 billion, and it takes 15 years. Is that a concern to you all, or does that bother you, or does that not bother you? Dr. Furberg.

Dr. FURBERG. Yes, it bothers me, and I think the solutions are on the industry side. They need to be more efficient, and really focus on innovations. Right now, much of what they are doing is driven by profit motives. They are developing me-too drugs, rather than focusing on the new ones. They should really be, they should be encouraged and rewarded if they bring new products to the——

Mr. WHITFIELD. How do you do that? How do you encourage and reward them for doing that?

Dr. FURBERG. Well, there are different suggestions. One is to extend the patent period for certain drugs.

Mr. WHITFIELD. Extend the patent period.

Dr. FURBERG. Yes.

Dr. WOOSLEY. And you could have the market exclusivity that they get today to be dependent upon innovation.

Mr. WHITFIELD. Yes.

Dr. WOOSLEY. I think there are many ways that we could create carrots. Honestly, I think we have got far too many hammers that are hitting our own thumb in many cases.

Mr. WHITFIELD. Yes. One other question, Dr. Psaty. You have made the comment that there is little economic, little short-term economic interest in safety.

Dr. PSATY. Yes, sir.

Mr. WHITFIELD. Now, are you referring to the drug companies?

Dr. PSATY. Yes, sir.

Mr. WHITFIELD. What about this issue of the lawsuits, the class action lawsuits, and things like that? I have never worked for a drug company, but I know some of these are pretty expensive, and I would think that that would be a motivating factor to be concerned about safety, but——

Dr. PSATY. There are large numbers of safety studied that are designed by companies, that can't answer useful questions, that will not answer useful questions, and if you don't have the answer to the question, then you don't have the information.

And industry does not pursue questions about safety with the same vigor, interest, and aggressiveness that they do questions about efficacy, and I think it is in their, as you point out really, in their long-term disinterest. Merck now faces billions of dollars in lawsuits but I think that that could have been prevented had patients known about the risk associated with Vioxx in a timely fashion, and had the company studied it and informed people. But instead, it was on the market for 6 years.

Mr. WHITFIELD. Thank you.

Mr. STUPAK. I understand Ms. Blackburn's coming, or Burgess, one of them. While we are waiting here, just a general question.

Has PDUFA helped our drug safety issue, or has that hurt it? In hindsight now, it has been over 10 years since we have had it here. Has PDUFA been a good bill for drug safety in this country, and the drug approval process?

Dr. FURBERG. Well, for the first two version of PDUFA, nothing could be spent on safety, so they had no impact whatsoever, and now, they are slowly moving up and allowing some of the funding to go towards safety, but even in the new, behind closed door development agreement between FDA and industry, the ratio is 13 to 1, so $13 slated for approval reviews and general expenses per $1 going to safety. So it is a total imbalance.

Mr. STUPAK. Do you have a comment?

Dr. WOOSLEY. I would say that PDUFA wiped out the backlog. Back when it was taking 40 months to review new drugs, it got, it is down now for important new drugs to be 6 or 8 months. So it worked in that sense. I agree there should have been money there for safety from day one. That needs to be made clear.

The other part of it is, and one of the advantages of almost being, and there are few advantages of almost being 65, is looking back, and I was very opposed to PDUFA entirely. I would say in a perfect world, we would have only money coming from the Government. But I thought about it and realized that the FDA approval process gives the company a better product, so yes, they should pay for that better product, and it is a gold stamp of approval that helps them market their drugs, and they should pay for that. But the public needs to maintain control, so if we have to have user fees, I think there is a rationale for it, but I think it has to be kept in balance. To have more than half of the money coming from user fees right now at the FDA is not a good balance.

Mr. STUPAK. Mr. Burgess for 10 minutes.

Mr. BURGESS. Thank you, Mr. Chairman. Dr. Woosley, I guess let us stay with you, if we could. When a drug is taken off the market, does that mean that someone at the FDA messed up, did something wrong?

Dr. WOOSLEY. No. I think one of the things that the public expects, that when a drug is approved, it is absolutely pure as the driven snow, and when something goes wrong, somebody should be blamed, but in fact, drugs are very, very potentially toxic agents. We are all very, very different people, and there will be examples where we could not have anticipated, no matter what we had done, the toxicity. Drugs being taken off the market is not a bad thing. Taken off the market too late is a bad thing. So, I think that is a very important thing. It is very difficult for people to understand, the public.

Mr. BURGESS. Pfizer Corporation just had a very famous, a few months ago, the drug that they had thought was going to be the next generation of LDL lowering medication, I don't remember the name of it now, but had to be withdrawn. In all likelihood, the scientists at Pfizer learned something along the way in that process. Would that not be a fair statement?

Dr. WOOSLEY. Yes, they did. They learned it too late, though. I think after $1 billion of investment, that is not a success.

Mr. BURGESS. But is there a likelihood that by changing the molecule, by changing something about the character of the medication, that they could come up with one that would ultimately be beneficial and not toxic?

Dr. WOOSLEY. Absolutely, and I think that is one of the things that we miss in post-market surveillance. We don't do a post-mortem, as you will understand, to find out what could we have done differently next time. We continue to make the same mistakes with drugs, unfortunately, so an investment into what went wrong, and I am sure Pfizer will do it for their product, but what about the other companies that won't learn from that process? I think we need an open, and when I wrote the paper that was cited earlier, we talked about the need for an NTSB. When planes go down, we need to look at the system. When drugs go down, we need to look at the whole process openly, and see are our standards right? Was there something wrong with the science, which has been the case, or is there something wrong with the regulation?

And that kind of independent overlook, I think is missing in all this. I would quickly say I am not calling for separating the decision-making on risk and benefit. I am saying something that is looking at not within the Agency, but from a societal point of view. In many cases, 60 percent of the drugs taken off the market were safe when used as directed, so as a former medical educator, am I to blame? Did I not teach doctors how to use those drugs?

So, again, I think when the problem occurs, we need to——

Mr. BURGESS. You are under oath. Let me instruct you to answer the question. Just kidding, Mr. Chairman. And you are quite right. I can think of Bendectin, some 15 years ago, removed from the market, and withdrawn voluntarily by the manufacturer, never actually withdrawn by the FDA. The Copper–7 IUD, famously went away because of liability, potential liability costs, not because of anything wrong with the product itself, and Vioxx, that we are all familiar with most recently.

Is there a risk of the FDA mistakenly concluding that a drug does have a safety problem when in fact none exists?

Dr. WOOSLEY. I think it is a great risk. There have been examples where they have spent an enormous amount of money and time to investigate signals, and then find out at the end that it didn't occur, and you and I are probably—we will remember the days when we used Reserpine for treating high blood pressure.

Mr. BURGESS. I am not that old.

Dr. WOOSLEY. Sorry. But there was a signal that it may cause breast cancer, and a lot of extra studies were done, and finally concluded that it didn't. There are many examples like that, that have to be looked at carefully.

Mr. BURGESS. Well, I do recall synthetic progestins were, at one time, thought to cause endocardial cushion defects in newborns, and now they are used for the early days, or perhaps to prevent a pregnancy, if clearly that would be a risk, if that had really been true.

What was the rate of withdrawal of drugs from the U.S. market before the user fee that you have been talking about, before PDUFA?

Dr. WOOSLEY. It was about 3.1 percent, as I recall. It was slightly higher after PDUFA, but not significantly different.

Mr. BURGESS. Has PDUFA, though, made an impact? Again, I reference my earlier question to Dr. von Eschenbach. When I was a clinician, we used to gripe about how long the FDA took to approve anything, and that the great doctors over in Europe could have drugs available to them 10 or 15 years before we got our hands on them. Has PDUFA been useful in speeding up that timeline?

Dr. WOOSLEY. It has. Now, significant new drugs are reviewed in 6 to 8 months. For AIDS drugs, it was only 3 to 4 months. In one case, it was 1½ months of review. So we can do better. AIDS drugs were developed in 3 to 4 years, not 12 years.

So, we can, and there were no shortcuts. No AIDS drug has ever been taken off the market. There has been no surprises with AIDS drugs. So, we can do it faster and safer when somebody puts a gun to us.

Mr. BURGESS. We don't need that mental age, but the avian flu might be a similar situation, should that come to be the problem that some people feel it might, where it will be necessary to develop a vaccine under a very, very short timeline.

Well, since I brought up Europe, in our first hearing, some witnesses raised concerns about the reliance on foreign post-marketing data. Do you think that there is a place for us to change here? Is there some other system that we should adopt?

Dr. WOOSLEY. I think we need our own system. We buy data now from the UK on how drug experiences occur post-market there, but we have different drugs on the market in this country. We have different uses and patterns in this country, so we need our own active surveillance system that responds very quickly. We should look at the data from the rest of the world, absolutely, but we should compare it to ours, not rely on it entirely.

Mr. BURGESS. But if there is a glaring example, such as Thalidomide, yes, sir, I am sorry. Someone was raising a finger there?

Dr. FURBERG. Yes. No, I being the European on the panel.

Mr. BURGESS. Please. We have got some other European questions here, too.

Dr. FURBERG. Thank you. No, I think we can, we should collaborate and work with Europe. Europe has made major strides. They introduced conditional approval for new drugs. They have a risk management program that is mandatory, and they have a very successful pharmacovigilance system in many countries. They pick up side effects long before we do, in a shorter time period.

So, we can learn a lot from collaborating with those. Thank you.

Mr. BURGESS. Thank you. Director Woosley, just one, and I think you, in fact, tried to answer this, and I got you off-track, but the observation that over half the drugs removed from the market in the last 15 years were safe when used as directed, which brings up the issue of using a drug off-label. Could you address that?

Dr. WOOSLEY. Yes. I wasn't really thinking so much of off-label, because again, this is one of the things I have learned over the years. The label is a very artificial piece of paper. It is something that is dependent upon what data were submitted to the FDA for review, and if someone doesn't submit data for a new use, it is not going to be in the label. And if we waited for all their uses to be submitted to the FDA, we would rarely use drugs very effectively.

Most of the pediatric use is off-label. Most cancer drug therapy is off-label, so we shouldn't look at that as good as bad. We should be looking at the use of the medications and the clinical outcome. The label is, as I said, a very artificial part of that analysis.

Mr. BURGESS. Well, just to finish up, the Ketek case study, is that a good example of the FDA disregarding safety?

Dr. WOOSLEY. I haven't followed that carefully enough. I think the hearings here and others are going to help really inform that. I would say, though, that everybody talks about Vioxx. I followed that one carefully, and I would say the only mistake made in Vioxx was when it was taken off the market by the company. Because the system really worked with Vioxx. It was a drug developed to prevent bleeding. It was a drug that we knew very early could cause heart disease, but we didn't know the risk-benefit. Only when it was put into a large enough trial to see if it prevented cancer did this come up. So again, I think it is another one of those drugs that if it could have been used when appropriate, it could have stayed on the market, and been a very important drug for many patients with arthritis at risk for GI bleeding, and keep it away from those people who could be harmed.

Mr. BURGESS. Yes.

Dr. PSATY. I just wanted to comment on Vioxx. I reviewed Vioxx in detail for the Finance Committee. The company was concerned about the possibility of adverse cardiovascular events back in 1996. They sought to design a large trial that would minimize the chance of finding any cardiovascular harm, and maximize the chance of finding benefit.

The FDA needs to make sure sponsors ask and answer the right questions. There were signals in the NDA for Vioxx, and they were not followed up with the appropriate well-designed studies.

Mr. BURGESS. So, did Merck Corporation deliberately set out to cause harm and cover it up?

Dr. PSATY. They didn't ask the question that a public health scientist would ask: "What is the risk and benefit of this drug? Who am I going to help, and who might I harm?"

Mr. BURGESS. But Dr. Woosley pointed out it wasn't until they began to use this in a widespread trial, looking for the prevention of colon polyps, that it actually, that the difficulties came to light.

Dr. PSATY. Well, the difficulties came to light in the bigger trial, and those results were available within about a year after the drug was on the market, and those signals were not, they were not pursued and not taken seriously.

Mr. BURGESS. Do you have a comment about that, Dr. Woosley?

Dr. FURBERG. Yes. I think the initial trials were not very informative. Focus was on low risk people, they did short-term studies, and follow them for a very short period of time, so it was fairly uninformative. So, that is how they got around detecting the problem. They should focus on the future users, but they are excluded from the pre-approval trials.

If you are on another drug, or if you have a concomitant condition——

Mr. BURGESS. Wait a minute. They have got to focus on the future users. There is no way of telling when you bring a drug to market what some clinician or some patient is going to do.

Dr. FURBERG. No, future users are those that are most likely to use the drug after it is marketed, and you know that if you have a painkiller, it is older people who have multiple conditions, taking multiple drugs, and they excluded those from the studies.

Dr. PSATY. Six week trials, many of the trials were 6 weeks long, and arthritis doesn't go away in 6 weeks. And Vioxx doesn't cure arthritis. So, people are going to use these drugs for a long time, until they had a joint replacement or something.

Dr. WOOSLEY. I would add, though, I think it is all human nature. It always comes back to that in making decisions, and if you are in a company, and you are looking at your options, would I invest money into seeing if a drug prevented colon cancer, or see if it is causing heart attacks, or go after the colon cancer, and hope that it doesn't cause heart attacks, expect the public to find out what is wrong with those things?

The NIH is doing trials, and has done trials to find out the unknowns out there, and yes, there is a responsibility of the company to find out all they need to know about the drugs, but to go after every signal, and ignore potential benefits like preventing cancer, I think you have got to recognize that those are decisions along the way in drug development that are not easy, and we, as a society, have to do something to provide the balance. This is a free enterprise Nation. We want companies to succeed. If every company does every study to find out what is wrong with their products, we are not going to last as a free enterprise society very long.

Mr. STUPAK. I am going to call time. You are way over.

Mr. BURGESS. Sure. Thank you, Mr. Chairman.

Mr. STUPAK. And we have another member who wants to go, and we are getting pressured to leave the room here for the markup. We don't want to have them do every study. We just want the 1,200 done.

Mrs. Blackburn for 10 minutes.

Mrs. BLACKBURN. Yes. Kind of huffing and puffing, running between meetings.

Dr. Crosse, I want to come to you. And this goes along the same line of questioning that I had with the Commissioner, as we started looking at efficiencies, and the way the FDA works, and the frustration that we hear from individuals who are going through the FDA process, and then, also from constituents when they know something is in the pipeline over there, they are hearing this.

But making the FDA workable for everyone, and one of the things that we like to focus on is being certain that we do this, and just not throw money at it. I think all too often, when we look at dealing with the bureaucracy, reforming the bureaucracy and making it workable, what Congress has a tendency to do is just go throw some money at something.

So, do you have, for lack of a better word, a checklist of things that you feel like we could do legislatively or statutorily, or through rulemaking authority, or that would improve the system over there, and not be just throwing money at it?

Dr. CROSSE. Well, we did recommend in our report that FDA be given additional authority to require post-market drug studies, and we believe that is something that would not be a burden, in terms of the finances of the Agency. It would, however, cost drug companies to pay for studies that FDA has evidence are needed, if there are strong indications of some sort of problem once a drug is on the market.

There are clear problems with the resources that have been available for post-market drug safety, the kinds of data that the Agency has been able to acquire, and the resources needed to develop a better system of accessing some of the data.

Now, some of that effort is underway, and some of it is being proposed by the department in its PDUFA IV proposals, that would call for additional funding, that would allow for development of some databases. We certainly would be supportive of that, but we have not developed any sort of comprehensive checklist of all of the needs of the organization.

Mrs. BLACKBURN. OK. Sometimes, I think that if we were to have from you all those specific recommendations, that that would be helpful. And you just started touching on something, and I want to go back.

In your testimony, you had mentioned that most of the time, that the Office of New Drugs and the Office of Surveillance and Epidemiology agree on what actions to take with respect to drug safety, and I wanted to see if you could give us an estimate on the percentage of the number of times, or is it 20 percent, 50 percent, 80 percent?

Dr. CROSSE. Oh, I think it is more in the range of 80 percent or 90 percent of the time when there is agreement between those offices. It is only in a limited number of cases that have come to light where there has been extremely strong disagreement. I think that in the day to day course of reviewing information, there are likely more minor kinds of disagreements that may be worked out, as additional information comes in, but certainly, the vast majority of cases, there is agreement among those staff.

Mrs. BLACKBURN. OK. All right. Thank you.

Dr. Woosley, I want to come to you with one thing. Staying on the same topic, looking at the FDA, their structure, how we achieve efficiencies and make the system workable. In your testimony, you had talked a little bit about the cultural and the organizational problems that are currently facing the FDA, and you made a statement I think is worthy of note. Stable leadership and adequate resources, and that that positive change would follow if the FDA had that.

So, what do you think, how do you view this? Stable leadership, define that for me, as far as people goes, as far as a mission goes, as far as a direction, and do you think that the Commissioner fills that role, and then, what about adequate resources, and the availability for that, as far as that stable leadership? Go ahead.

Dr. WOOSLEY. I think that I fully support the IOM recommendation of a 6-year appointment for the Commissioner. I think that is the kind of endorsement that a leader of this kind of an organization really must have. I think the acting leadership positions below the Commissioner have to be given more stability.

They need to be given the resources. These are mostly scientists, or at least people trained in science and medicine and pharmacy, that come into this Agency, and they want, they are some of the most dedicated people that I have ever met. They want to do the right thing, they want to serve the public health, and they are crying for more data, more interaction with science. They are put in, it used to be the Parklawn Building, and isolated, and not able, they don't have a travel budget to go to scientific meetings.

If anybody wants to meet with the Agency, they have to have the meeting in Washington and bring everybody here. So, they are really isolated. They are given the science in a bolus, a big dump of data, and asked to act on it. They are not given any warning. They may see a new kind of test in the NDA that they have never heard of, because they have been reviewing NDAs for the last 5 years, not keeping up with the science.

And I don't mean that as criticism. I also don't mean that they should be doing research to be good scientists. I think you need a good science background, you need an opportunity to keep up to date by interacting with good people who do science.

Mrs. BLACKBURN. So, basically, you are saying continuing education or professional development.

Dr. WOOSLEY. That, but also interaction. I don't think you can learn these things in courses, and this group that we now have working, 160 scientists from industry and 20 regulators that get together, are talking science. They are not talking products, and they are learning about new methods of drug testing. That is the kind of interaction I think is the most effective.

Mrs. BLACKBURN. Thank you. Mr. Chairman, I will yield back.

Mr. STUPAK. I thank the gentle lady for yielding back. That concludes the questions for this panel. I want to thank this panel.

Mr. Whitfield and I were saying we enjoyed the interaction. I wish we didn't have these time constraints, because I think we could get a lot more done, but it is very important to have the record, and you helped build this record, so as we do PDUFA and pediatric exclusivity reauthorizations, when we look back at the record and your good suggestions, and the documents you provided us, so I want to thank this panel for their work in furthering the cause of drug safety in this country.

Thank you for your testimony, you can be dismissed now. I ask for unanimous consent that the hearing record remain open for 30 days. I also ask for unanimous consent to have items in our evidence binder, the binders before us here, be made part of the record. Without objection, so ordered.

I thank the panel again. The hearing is now adjourned.

[Whereupon, at 2:10 p.m., the subcommittee was adjourned.]

[Material submitted for inclusion in the record follows:]

STATEMENT OF ANDREW C. VON ESCHENBACH, M.D.

Mr. Chairman and members of the Committee, I am Andrew von Eschenbach, M.D., Commissioner at the United States Food and Drug Administration (FDA or the Agency). I am pleased to be here today to share my vision for the future of FDA's drug safety program and to present a few of the initiatives and opportunities that we have embraced. I also will discuss the Agency's approval of Ketek.

FDA'S DRUG SAFETY INITIATIVE

New drugs, devices, and diagnostics present a significant opportunity to improve health care. For many patients, the improvement in the quality of their life directly attributed to new therapies vastly outweighs the risks that such treatments pose. Ensuring the safety of drugs and other medical products regulated by FDA has always been a key focus of our commitment to protect and promote the public health. In the past few years, FDA has reassessed its drug safety programs because of rapid advances in science and technology that have resulted in increasingly complex medical products. We are aware of increased attention and take very seriously our response to safety-related issues raised by consumer advocates, health professionals, academic researchers, and Members of Congress.

FDA has a proud, 100-year record of being the world's gold standard and we have maintained this record by our willingness to look internally to see what transformations are necessary to sustain this standard. For this reason, the Agency asked the Institute of Medicine (IOM) to assess the U.S. drug safety system, with an emphasis on the post-marketing phase, and to assess what additional steps FDA could take to learn more about the side effects of drugs as they are actually used. We asked the IOM to examine FDA's role within the health care delivery system and to recommend measures to enhance the confidence of Americans in the safety and effectiveness of their drugs.

On September 22, 2006, the IOM released its report entitled, The Future of Drug Safety—Promoting and Protecting the Health of the Public. The report recognized the progress and reform already initiated by the Agency. We have implemented an aggressive effort, including developing new tools for communicating drug safety information to patients. Through our Critical Path initiative, we are working with our health care partners to improve the tools we use and to more effectively evaluate products and processes.

The IOM report makes substantive recommendations about additional steps FDA can take to improve our drug safety program. The recommendations are consistent with the Agency's commitment to drug safety, including: (1) strengthening the science that supports our medical product safety system, (2) improving communication and information flow among key stakeholders, and (3) improving operations and management. Our Prescription Drug User Fee Act (PDUFA) proposal will, in part, support some of these initiatives.

Strengthening the Science. First, I am committed to strengthening the science that supports our medical product safety system at every stage of the product life cycle, from pre-market testing and development through post-market surveillance and risk management. We will focus our resources on three areas of scientific activity: (1) those relating to improving benefit and risk analysis and risk management, (2) surveillance methods and tools, and (3) incorporating new scientific approaches into FDA's understanding of adverse events.

Specifically, new scientific discoveries are generating an emerging science of safety that will help prevent adverse events by improving the methods used in the clinic to target a specific drug for use in patients for whom benefits relative to risks are maximized. This new science combines an understanding of disease and its origins at the molecular level (including adverse events resulting from treatment) with new methods of signal detection, data mining, and analysis. This approach enables researchers to generate hypotheses about and to confirm the existence and cause of safety problems, as well as explore the unique genetic and biologic features of individuals that will determine how he or she responds to treatment. This science of safety encompasses the entire life cycle of a product, from pre-market animal and human safety testing to widespread clinical use beyond original indications and should be used for all medical products so that safety signals generated at any point in the process will robustly inform regulatory decision-making.

Improving Communications. Second, I am committed to improving communication and information flow among all stakeholders to further strengthen the drug safety system. This will require a comprehensive review and evaluation of our risk communication tools with the benefit of Advisory Committee expertise, improving communication and coordination of safety issues within FDA.

One example of our efforts to improve communication is establishing a new advisory committee to obtain input on how to improve the Agency's communication policies and practices and to advise FDA on implementing communication strategies consistent with the best available and evolving evidence. We will include patients and consumers on the committee as well as experts in risk and crisis communication and social and cognitive sciences. Although IOM's report recommends legislation to establish this Advisory Committee, we intend to implement this recommendation more expeditiously through administrative procedures.

Improving Operations and Management. Finally, I am committed to improving operations and management to ensure implementation of the review, analysis, consultation, and communication processes needed to strengthen the U.S. drug safety system. We are and will continue to be committed to drug safety. Consistent with the IOM recommendations, we will be implementing several reforms that, together, will improve the culture of safety at FDA, and in the Center for Drug Evaluation and Research (CDER). Under my direction, CDER has initiated a series of changes designed to effect a true culture change that will strengthen the drug safety system. CDER has moved to reinvigorate its senior management team and charged its members with the responsibility to lead the Center in an integrated manner that crosses organizational lines.

CDER has employed process improvement teams comprising staff in various organizations including the Office of Surveillance and Epidemiology (OSE) and Office of New Drugs (OND) to recommend improvements in the drug safety program. Their recommendations to (1) establish an Associate Director for Safety and a Safety Regulatory Project Manager in each OND review division within CDER and (2) conduct regular safety meetings between OSE and all of the OND review divisions are now being implemented. We are committed to providing the necessary management attention and support to effect sustained culture change in our drug safety program.

We have recently engaged external management consultants to help CDER develop a comprehensive strategy for improving CDER/FDA's organizational culture. In addition to the ongoing FDA activities to improve how our organization supports the individuals who work on safety issues in FDA, we are enlisting the help of external experts in organizational improvement to help us identify additional opportunities for change and assist us with carrying out those needed changes.

Ketek

This is the second part of a two part hearing on the adequacy of the safety of the U.S. drug supply. FDA's approval of the drug Ketek was discussed at your first hearing. I am glad to have the opportunity to elaborate today on the Ketek approval process. FDA maintains the highest worldwide standards for drug approval and a review of the approval package for Ketek substantiates this. See: *http://www.fda.gov/cder/foi/nda/2004/21-144—Ketek.htm*. In these materials, we acknowledged the problems with a large safety study, Study 3014, and confronted challenges which arose as a result, in a way which, at the time, seemed appropriate. Notwithstanding the fact that Study 3014 had to be disregarded, as explained below, the Agency proceeded to approve Ketek because the product was otherwise shown to be safe and effective.

Due to the emergence of antimicrobial resistance, it is essential that we have access to a number of antibiotics to treat microbial infections. If we were to rely on just a few drugs, the development of resistance to those drugs could have serious public health consequences. Antibiotic resistance has been called one of the world's most pressing public health problems.

Ketek is the first member of a new class of antibiotics known as the ketolides, antibiotics which are closely related to the macrolide class (e.g. azithromycin, clarithromycin and erythromycin). Ketek has activity against bacteria that cause upper and lower respiratory tract infections, including multi-drug resistant Streptococcus pneumoniae. The company that markets Ketek submitted its application for marketing approval to FDA in the year 2000. FDA's counterpart in Europe, the European Medicines Evaluation Agency, approved Ketek in July 2001 for use in the fifteen member countries. The drug was first launched in October 2001 in Germany and in 2002 in other European markets. By June 2003, Ketek was marketed in 36 countries around the world, including Canada and Japan. In the United States, FDA approved Ketek on April 1, 2004, after rigorous scientific evaluation but did not approve the product for the full range of indications approved elsewhere.

Notwithstanding the great need for new antibiotics, and contrary to some of the misimpressions that have circulated publicly, FDA did not rush to approve Ketek. The Agency approved Ketek after three cycles of rigorous scientific review.

First Cycle. The sponsor submitted its Ketek new drug application (NDA) on February 28, 2000, seeking approval for four indications (community-acquired pneumonia, acute bacterial sinusitis, acute bacterial exacerbation of chronic bronchitis, and pharyngitis), including a claim for drug-resistant Streptococcus pneumoniae. The Agency discussed the Ketek NDA at an April 2001 Anti-infective Drugs Advisory Committee meeting, and, except for the pharyngitis claim where substantial evidence of efficacy was not demonstrated, the Committee recommended that the clinical trials demonstrated similar efficacy for Ketek and comparator antibiotics for the other three claims. The April 2001 Advisory Committee recommended approval for the indication of community acquired pneumonia. At that time, safety concerns led Advisory Committee members and the Agency to ask the sponsor for additional safety and efficacy data for the claims for acute bacterial sinusitis and acute bacterial exacerbation of chronic bronchitis. The safety concerns included liver, heart, and visual side effects. The Committee also recommended more studies to demonstrate efficacy in patients with resistant Streptococcus pneumoniae, as well as more safety data to characterize more fully the benefit/risk of Ketek in the broad population. Nevertheless, rather than issue an approval letter for this indication, the Agency issued an approvable letter in June 2001, requesting more information.

Second Cycle. In late July 2002, the sponsor submitted additional safety and efficacy studies. The submission included multiple Phase I studies to address safety and pharmacokinetics in various populations; three Phase III studies in patients with community-acquired pneumonia and acute exacerbation of chronic bronchitis; and the results from Study 3014, a large controlled usual care trial in approximately 24,000 patients with outpatient respiratory tract infections at approximately 1,800 sites. Study 3014 was designed to address the need for additional safety information by examining potential toxicities of Ketek with regard to liver, heart, and visual adverse events. FDA scheduled a meeting of the Anti-Infective Drugs Advisory Committee for January 8, 2003, to discuss these new data, including Study 3014.

Shortly before this planned meeting, CDER's Division of Anti-Infectives and Ophthalmology Products (the Division) started to see preliminary results of inspections of clinical investigation sites from Study 3014. This began with information about the site with the highest enrollment that raised substantial concerns about data coming from that site. Shortly thereafter, results from investigations at other sites also showed deficiencies, though not nearly as concerning as those that had arisen in the first inspection. As this information began to come to light, in accordance with normal practice, the Division met with the sponsor. The sponsor informed the Division that it was aware of some data irregularities and concerns about processes at the first site and assured FDA that there were no similar problems at any other sites.

Please note that at the time of the January 8, 2003, Advisory Committee, inspections had occurred at only three of approximately 1800 sites, and the findings at that time were quite preliminary. To avoid compromising any ongoing investigation, it is Agency policy not to publicly disclose even the existence of a pending investigation. Therefore, we could not discuss the data integrity issues of Study 3014 at the public Advisory Committee meeting. However, we also believed, based on the best information available to us, that the concerns applied to only one site out of more than 1800. It is not unusual for data from some sites to be eliminated from a study but to accept data from the other sites. At the time, there was less information about the other sites under investigation.

After considering the fact that the investigation results were preliminary and we had not received formal recommendations about how to take the results into account in review of the application, and the fact that only in very rare cases do inspection results from individual sites lead to the exclusion of an entire large clinical trial, FDA decided to hold the Advisory Committee meeting as planned. The Agency made this decision, knowing that any advice from the Committee would have to be later taken into account in the context of additional information about the integrity of data from Study 3014. It is not unusual for more information to come to FDA for review after an Advisory Committee meeting is held about an application. The Advisory Committee voted that the safety and efficacy of the requested indications had been demonstrated, based on the information it was provided, including Study 3014, and limited international post-marketing data provided at the meeting.

Although the Advisory Committee recommended approval, on January 23, 2003, (two weeks after the Advisory Committee meeting) FDA issued another approvable letter to the sponsor because of the remaining questions about the safety of Ketek. The letter specifically noted the unresolved data integrity issues associated with Study 3014 (issues confirmed in the final clinical inspection summary of the Agency's audits of the first three clinical trial sites) and the incomplete post-marketing safety data from foreign countries. FDA noted that the final decision regarding approval of each indication would be made after a review of the information and analyses requested in this letter.

On March 3, 2003, during a closed session of the Advisory Committee convened to discuss other matters, FDA briefly explained that an approvable letter was issued because the Agency wanted to see more information about data from Europe and Latin America. With regard to Study 3014, FDA explained that there were unresolved inspectional issues.

Third Cycle. The sponsor submitted a complete response to the approvable letter in October 2003. The October 2003 submission addressed issues of Study 3014 and included post-marketing reports for spontaneous adverse events for approximately four million prescriptions for patients in other countries where Ketek had already been approved. Upon completing the review of the sponsor's October submission, including the findings from the additional audits of clinical trial sites summarized in a March 2004 memorandum from the Division of Scientific Investigations, the Agency decided that it could not rely on Study 3014 to support approval of Ketek because of the systemic failure of the sponsor's monitoring of the clinical trial to detect clearly existing data integrity problems. Accordingly, Study 3014 was dropped for consideration in making the decision whether to approve Ketek. The Agency considered data from other clinical trials and the international post-marketing experience to conclude there was adequate evidence of safety.

FDA approved Ketek for three indications on April 1, 2004, following a very thorough analysis of pre-clinical and clinical safety data.

FDA's Medical Officer Safety Review dated March 31, 2004, specifically reviews the post-marketing data from countries where Ketek had already been approved, and data from a Phase III visual adverse event re-analysis submitted on October 17, 2003. In addition, the reviewer evaluated data from Study 5001 (an intensive monitoring study conducted in Germany) and a five-month safety update that provided post-marketing data from August 2003-December 2003. The reviewer also referred to the second cycle safety review which included data from eight additional Phase I studies, three new Phase III studies, and post-marketing data from approximately 1 million prescriptions for telithromycin (the generic name for Ketek) in countries where the drug had been approved.

The safety information evaluated in the March 31, 2004, review included post-marketing safety reports generated from an estimated 3.7 million uses in countries where the drug was already approved. This post-marketing data was collected in 36 countries. The majority of prescriptions were dispensed in France and Germany (2.2 out of 3.7 million). Other countries with more than 100,000 prescriptions dispensed included Italy, Spain and Mexico.

In addition to review of cumulative adverse events by organ system, the safety reviewer conducted focused reviews of deaths, serious adverse events, hepatic toxicity, cardiac toxicity, visual toxicity, and use in Myasthenia Gravis, including review of individual reports.

Even with its limitations, post-marketing adverse event reporting has proven valuable in detecting rare adverse events that are not seen in a clinical trial database. Limitations, such as under-reporting, were taken into account in assessing the data derived from these reports. Experience has shown that the full magnitude of some potential risks do not always emerge during the mandatory clinical trials conducted before approval to evaluate these products for safety and effectiveness. An example in this very case was the finding of exacerbations of Myasthenia Gravis in the post-marketing reports from countries outside the U.S. for Ketek. These reports led to the inclusion of a statement in the warnings section of the Ketek product label about exacerbations of Myasthenia Gravis at the time of approval in the U.S.

FDA's belief that valuable information can be gained from the marketing of a drug in countries outside the U.S. is expressed in our drug regulations, which require an NDA applicant to provide information of foreign marketing history at the time of an NDA submission. We can provide the Committee with numerous examples where post-marketing adverse event reporting data has been used to inform FDA's approval and labeling decisions (e.g. Tindamax (tinidazole), Zonegran (zonisamide)). In most cases, post-marketing reports from other countries have provided evidence of toxicities that have led to either the non-approval of the drug by FDA (e.g. Thalomid (thalidomide), Angex (lidoflazine) or to re-labeling to include serious adverse events (e.g. Tasmar (tolcapone), Tamiflu (oseltamivir).

Ongoing Postmarket Surveillance. As noted previously, the full magnitude of some potential risks does not always emerge during the mandatory clinical trials conducted before approval. That is why Congress has supported, and FDA has created, a strong post-market drug safety program designed to assess adverse events identified after approval for all of the medical products it regulates. This life-cycle approach is a complement to the pre-market safety reviews required for approval of prescription drugs. Monitoring the safety of marketed products requires close collaboration between our clinical reviewers and drug safety staff to evaluate and respond to adverse events identified in ongoing clinical trials or in voluntary reports submitted to us by health care providers and their patients, or in mandatory reports submitted to us by manufacturers.

The evaluation of the safety of Ketek, as well as all FDA-approved drugs, is an ongoing process. FDA continues to evaluate spontaneous reports and consult with outside experts. In March 2005, FDA began a comprehensive safety review of Ketek to coincide with the completion of its first year of marketing. Although one case of liver failure that resulted in death was found, it was not clear that this represented a signal beyond what had been seen in the data available at the time of approval. A second annual review was planned for March 2006. In January 2006, FDA was informed that a collection of three cases of serious liver toxicity, including one death, were to be reported in the Annals of Internal Medicine. Those cases had previously been reported to FDA, although in less detail, making conclusions about them difficult to reach until the published information was available. With that information now available, on January 20, 2006, FDA issued a Public Health Advisory to advise the public about the cases and that the Agency was conducting a comprehensive review of all cases of liver toxicity reported for the drug.

That review was complex and included a review of additional data requested from the sponsor about Ketek, liver toxicity of similar drugs, assessments of drug utilization and more in-depth review of the three cases reported in the Annals of Internal Medicine, all of which had occurred in one region, an unusual phenomenon. On June 29, 2006, FDA issued a press release regarding completion of the safety review and to inform the public that a new warning about liver toxicity was being added to Ketek's label.

Most recently, in a December 14 and 15, 2006, joint meeting of the Anti-Infective Drugs Advisory Committee and the Drug Safety and Risk Management Advisory Committee, the joint panel advised that the available data, including data acquired since the initial approval of Ketek, support a conclusion that the benefits of Ketek outweigh the risks in patients with community acquired pneumonia, but not for patients with acute bacterial sinusitis or acute bacterial exacerbation of chronic bronchitis. They also recommended a boxed warning for the drug.

On February 12, 2007, FDA acted on the recommendations of the joint panel and announced revisions to the labeling and indications for Ketek designed to improve the safe use of Ketek by patients. The changes include the removal of two of the three previously approved indications—acute bacterial sinusitis and acute bacterial exacerbations of chronic bronchitis—from the drug's label. Based on the new evidence, the Agency has determined that the balance of benefits and risks no longer support approval of the drug for these indications. At present, Ketek remains on the market for the treatment of community acquired pneumonia of mild to moderate severity (acquired outside of hospitals or long-term care facilities).

In addition, the Agency has worked with Ketek's sponsor, Sanofi Aventis, to update the product labeling with a "boxed warning," FDA's strongest form of warning. The warning states that Ketek is contraindicated (should not be used) in patients with Myasthenia Gravis, a disease that causes muscle weakness. FDA also worked with the manufacturer to develop a Patient Medication Guide that informs patients about the risk of the drug and how to use it safely. The Medication Guide (an FDA-approved patient information sheet) will be provided to patients with each prescription.

Other labeling changes included a strengthened warning section regarding specific drug-related adverse events including visual disturbances and loss of consciousness. As noted previously, warnings for hepatic toxicity (rare but severe symptoms of liver disease) were strengthened in June 2006.

This most recent action is the result of comprehensive scientific analysis and thoughtful public discussion of the data available for Ketek, and includes important changes in the labeling designed to improve the safe use of Ketek by patients and give health care providers the most up-to-date prescribing information.The Ketek approval and post-approval process conformed to the high standard the American public has come to expect from FDA. Furthermore, we believe that the data integrity issues in connection with Study 3014 uncovered by FDA staff are a testament to our staff's unrelenting dedication and commitment to the processes we have in place to help ensure the safety of our drug supply. We always welcome suggestions on how to improve these processes.

CONCLUSION

At FDA, providing the American public with safe and effective medical products is our core mission. We base decisions to approve a drug, or to keep it on the market if new safety findings surface, on a careful balancing of risk and benefit to patients. This is a multifaceted and complex decision process, involving scientific and public health issues. The recent initiatives we have announced will improve our current system to assess drug safety. Moreover, we will continue to evaluate new approaches to advance drug safety. As always, we value input from Congress, patients and the medical community as we develop and refine these drug safety initiatives.

Let me assure you, Mr. Chairman, that I am deeply committed to ensuring the safety of drugs and other medical products regulated by FDA. Once again, thank you for the opportunity to testify before the Committee today. I am happy to respond to questions.

United States Government Accountability Office

GAO

Testimony

Before the Subcommittee on Oversight and Investigations, Committee on Energy and Commerce, House of Representatives

For Release on Delivery
Expected at 9:30 a.m. EDT
March 22, 2007

DRUG SAFETY

FDA Needs to Further Address Shortcomings in Its Postmarket Decision-making Process

Statement of Marcia Crosse
Director, Health Care

GAO
Accountability * Integrity * Reliability

GAO-07-599T

March 22, 2007

GAO
Accountability Integrity Reliability

Highlights

Highlights of GAO-07-599T, a testimony before the Subcommittee on Oversight and Investigations, Committee on Energy and Commerce, House of Representatives

DRUG SAFETY

FDA Needs to Further Address Shortcomings in Its Postmarket Decision-making Process

Why GAO Did This Study

In 2004, several high-profile drug safety cases raised concerns about the Food and Drug Administration's (FDA) ability to manage postmarket drug safety issues. In some cases there were disagreements within FDA about how to address these issues.

GAO was asked to testify on the effectiveness of FDA's postmarket decision-making process.
This testimony is based on *Drug Safety: Improvement Needed in FDA's Postmarket Decision-making and Oversight Process*, GAO-06-402 (March 31, 2006). The report focused on the complex interaction between two offices within FDA that are involved in postmarket drug safety activities: the Office of New Drugs (OND), and the Office of Drug Safety (ODS). OND's primary responsibility is to review new drug applications, but it is also involved in monitoring the safety of marketed drugs. ODS is focused primarily on postmarket drug safety issues. ODS is now called the Office of Surveillance and Epidemiology.

For its report, GAO reviewed FDA policies, interviewed FDA staff, and conducted case studies of four drugs with safety issues: Arava, Baycol, Bextra, and Propulsid. To gather information on FDA's initiatives since March 2006 to improve its decision-making process for this testimony, GAO interviewed FDA officials and reviewed FDA documents in February and March 2007.

www.gao.gov/cgi-bin/getrpt?GAO-07-599T.

To view the full product, including the scope and methodology, click on the link above. For more information, contact Marcia Crosse, (202) 512-7119, crossem@gao.gov.

What GAO Found

In its March 2006 report, GAO found that FDA lacked clear and effective processes for making decisions about, and providing management oversight of, postmarket drug safety issues. There was a lack of clarity about how decisions were made and about organizational roles, insufficient oversight by management, and data constraints. GAO observed that there was a lack of criteria for determining what safety actions to take and when to take them. Certain parts of ODS's role in the process were unclear, including ODS's participation in the meetings of scientific advisory committees organized by OND to discuss safety issues for specific drugs. In the case of Arava, for example, ODS staff were not allowed to present their analysis of postmarket safety at an advisory committee meeting held to review Arava's safety risks and benefits. Insufficient communication between ODS and OND hindered the decision-making process. ODS management did not systematically track information about ongoing postmarket safety issues, including the recommendations that ODS staff made for safety actions. GAO also found that FDA faced data constraints that contributed to the difficulty in making postmarket safety decisions. GAO found that there were weaknesses in the different types of data available to FDA, and FDA's access to data was constrained by both its authority to require certain studies and its limited resources.

During the course of GAO's work for its March 2006 report, FDA began a variety of initiatives to improve its postmarket drug safety decision-making process, including the establishment of the Drug Safety Oversight Board. FDA also commissioned the Institute of Medicine to examine the drug safety system, including FDA's oversight of postmarket drug safety. GAO recommended in its March 2006 report that FDA take four steps to improve its decision-making process for postmarket safety. GAO recommended that FDA revise and implement its draft policy on the decision-making process for major postmarket safety actions, improve its process to resolve disagreements over safety decisions, clarify ODS's role in scientific advisory committees, and systematically track postmarket drug safety issues. FDA has initiatives underway and under consideration that, if implemented, could address three of GAO's four recommendations. Because none of these initiatives was fully implemented as of March 2007, it was too early to evaluate their effectiveness. In the 2006 report GAO also suggested that Congress consider expanding FDA's authority to require drug sponsors to conduct postmarket studies, as needed, to collect additional data on drug safety concerns.

Mr. Chairman and Members of the Subcommittee,

I am pleased to be here today as you examine the Food and Drug Administration's (FDA) process for decision making regarding postmarket drug safety issues. In 2004, several high-profile drug safety cases raised concerns about FDA's ability to manage postmarket drug safety issues. Those cases showed that there were disagreements and potential delays within FDA about how to address serious safety problems. My remarks today are based on GAO's March 2006 report on FDA's postmarket decision-making process (*Drug Safety: Improvement Needed in FDA's Postmarket Decision-making and Oversight Process*, GAO-06-402). I will also discuss a number of FDA initiatives to improve its decision-making process, including some that respond to the recommendations we made in that report.[1]

In carrying out the work for our report between December 2004 and March 2006, we focused on two offices within FDA's Center for Drug Evaluation and Research (CDER) that are involved in postmarket drug safety activities: the Office of New Drugs (OND) and the Office of Drug Safety (ODS).[2] While there is some overlap in the activities of OND and ODS, they have different organizational characteristics and perspectives on postmarket drug safety. OND is involved in postmarket drug safety activities as one aspect of its larger responsibility to review new drug applications, and it has the ultimate responsibility to take regulatory action concerning the postmarket safety of drugs. ODS is primarily focused on postmarket drug safety, which includes the review of reports of adverse reactions to drugs. ODS operates primarily in a consultant capacity to OND and does not have any independent decision-making responsibility.

For our report, we interviewed ODS, OND, and other CDER managers and staff, as well as drug safety experts from outside FDA. We also analyzed documents describing internal FDA policies and procedures. In order to obtain an in-depth understanding of FDA's policies and procedures, we conducted case studies of four drugs—Arava, Baycol, Bextra, and

[1]The report is available online at www.gao.gov/cgi-bin/getrpt?GAO-06-402.

[2]ODS was renamed the Office of Surveillance and Epidemiology in May 2006. For the purposes of this testimony, we are referring to this office by its former name.

Propulsid—that help to illustrate the decision-making process.[3] Each of these drugs presented significant postmarket safety issues that FDA acted upon in recent years, and they reflect differences in the type of adverse event or potential safety problem associated with each drug, the safety actions taken, and the OND and ODS staff involved. To follow up with FDA about its responses to our recommendations and its initiatives to improve its postmarket safety decision-making process, we interviewed four FDA managers, including CDER's Associate Director for Safety Policy and Communication, in February and March 2007. We did not evaluate the effectiveness of FDA's efforts to respond to our recommendations. All of our work was conducted in accordance with generally accepted government auditing standards.

In summary, we found that FDA lacked a clear and effective process for making decisions about, and providing management oversight of, postmarket drug safety issues. There was a lack of clarity about how decisions were made and about organizational roles, insufficient oversight by management, and data constraints. We observed that there was a lack of criteria for determining what safety actions to take and when to take them, which likely contributed to disagreements over decisions about postmarket safety. Certain parts of ODS's role in the process were unclear, including ODS's participation in scientific advisory committee meetings that were organized by OND to discuss specific drugs. Although ODS staff presented their analyses during some of these meetings, we found examples of the exclusion of ODS staff from making presentations at several meetings. For example, in 2003 ODS staff, who had recommended that Arava be removed from the market, were not allowed to discuss their analysis of Arava's postmarket safety data at a scientific advisory committee meeting. This meeting was held to review Arava's safety risks and benefits in the context of other similar drugs. Insufficient communication between ODS and OND's divisions was an ongoing concern and hindered the decision-making process. For example, ODS did not always know how OND had responded to ODS's safety analyses and recommendations. ODS management did not systematically track information about the recommendations its staff made and OND's response. This limited the ability of ODS management to provide effective oversight so that FDA could ensure that safety concerns were addressed

[3]FDA approved Arava to treat arthritis; Baycol to treat high cholesterol; Propulsid to treat nighttime heartburn; and Bextra to relieve pain. Baycol, Bextra, and Propulsid have since been withdrawn from the market (in August 2001, April 2005, and March 2000, respectively), and the warnings on Arava's label were strengthened.

and resolved in a timely manner. FDA faced data constraints that contributed to the difficulty in making postmarket safety decisions. In the absence of specific authority to require drug sponsors to conduct postmarket studies, FDA has often relied on drug sponsors voluntarily agreeing to conduct these studies. However, these studies have not consistently been completed. FDA was also limited in the resources it had available to obtain data from outside sources.

FDA has undertaken a variety of initiatives to improve its postmarket drug safety decision-making process. Prior to the completion of our report in March 2006, FDA commissioned the Institute of Medicine (IOM) to examine the drug safety system, including FDA's oversight of postmarket drug safety. FDA also established the Drug Safety Oversight Board in CDER and made other internal changes. Since March 2006, FDA has continued to address its oversight and decision-making shortcomings. In January 2007, FDA issued a detailed response to IOM's recommendations. In our 2006 report, we recommended that FDA revise and implement its draft policy on the decision-making process for major postmarket safety actions, improve its process to resolve disagreements over safety decisions, clarify ODS's role in scientific advisory committees, and systematically track postmarket drug safety issues. FDA has since begun to implement initiatives that we believe could address the goals of three of the four recommendations in our 2006 report. FDA has made revisions to, but not finalized, its draft policy on major postmarket drug safety decisions. FDA has not improved its process to resolve disagreements over safety decisions and the agency is developing but has not finalized guidance to clarify ODS's role in scientific advisory committees. FDA is in the process of implementing a tracking system. Although FDA's initiatives are positive steps, they are not yet fully implemented and it is too soon to evaluate their effectiveness.

Background

Because no drug is absolutely safe, FDA approves a drug for marketing when the agency judges that its known benefits outweigh its known risks. After a drug is on the market, FDA continues to assess its risks and benefits. FDA reviews reports of adverse drug reactions (adverse events)[4] related to the drug and information from clinical studies about the drug that are conducted by the drug's sponsor. FDA also reviews adverse events

[4]Adverse event is the term used by FDA to refer to any untoward medical event associated with the use of a drug in humans.

from studies that follow the use of drugs in ongoing medical care (observational studies)[5] that are carried out by the drug's sponsor, FDA, or other researchers. If FDA has information that a drug on the market may pose a significant health risk to consumers, it weighs the effect of the adverse events against the benefit of the drug to determine what actions, if any, are warranted.

The decision-making process for postmarket drug safety is complex, involving input from a variety of FDA staff and organizational units and information sources, but the central focus of the process is the iterative interaction between OND and ODS. After a drug is on the market, OND staff receive information about safety issues in several ways. First, OND staff receive notification of adverse event reports for drugs to which they are assigned and they review the periodic adverse event reports that are submitted by drug sponsors.[6] Second, OND staff review safety information that is submitted to FDA when a sponsor seeks approval for a new use or formulation of a drug, and monitor completion of postmarket studies. When consulting with OND on a safety issue, ODS staff search for all relevant case reports of adverse events and assess them to determine whether or not the drug caused the adverse event and whether there are any common trends or risk factors. ODS staff might also use information from observational studies and drug use analyses to analyze the safety issue. When completed, ODS staff summarize their analysis in a written consult. According to FDA officials, OND staff within the review divisions usually decide what regulatory action should occur, if any, by considering the results of the safety analysis in the context of other factors such as the availability of other similar drugs and the severity of the condition the drug is designed to treat. Then, if necessary, OND staff make a decision about what action should be taken.

Several CDER staff, including staff from OND and ODS, told us that most of the time there is agreement within FDA about what safety actions should be taken. At other times, however, OND and ODS staff disagree

[5]Observational studies can provide information about the association between certain drug exposures and adverse events. In observational studies, the investigator does not control the therapy, but observes and evaluates ongoing medical care. In contrast, in clinical trials the investigator controls the therapy to be received by participants and can test for causal relationships.

[6]Health care providers and patients can voluntarily submit adverse event reports to FDA. Adverse event reports become part of FDA's computerized database known as the Adverse Event Reporting System.

about whether the postmarket data are adequate to establish the existence of a safety problem or support a recommended regulatory action. In those cases, OND staff sometimes request additional analyses by ODS and sometimes there is involvement from other FDA organizations. In some cases, OND seeks the advice of FDA's scientific advisory committees, which are composed of experts and consumer representatives from outside FDA.[7] In 2002, FDA established the Drug Safety and Risk Management Advisory Committee, 1 of the 16 human-drug-related scientific advisory committees, to specifically advise FDA on drug safety and risk management issues. The recommendations of the advisory committees do not bind the agency to any decision.

FDA has the authority to withdraw the approval of a drug on the market for safety-related and other reasons, although it rarely does so.[8] In almost all cases of drug withdrawals for safety reasons, the drug's sponsor has voluntarily removed the drug from the market. For example, in 2001 Baycol's sponsor voluntarily withdrew the drug from the market after meeting with FDA to discuss reports of adverse events, including some reports of fatalities.[9] FDA does not have explicit authority to require that drug sponsors take other safety actions; however, when FDA identifies a potential problem, sponsors generally negotiate with FDA to develop a mutually agreeable remedy to avoid other regulatory action. Negotiations may result in revised drug labeling or restricted distribution. FDA has limited authority to require that sponsors conduct postmarket safety studies.

[7]These committees are either mandated by legislation or are established at the discretion of the Department of Health and Human Services.

[8]21 U.S.C. § 355(e). FDA may propose withdrawal when, for example, it determines through experience, tests, or other data that a drug is unsafe under the conditions of use approved in its application, there is a lack of substantial evidence that the drug will have the effect that it purports to have or that is suggested in its labeling, or required patent information is not timely filed. Prior to withdrawal, FDA would need to notify the affected parties and provide an opportunity for a hearing. Approval may be suspended immediately, prior to a hearing, if the Secretary of Health and Human Services finds that continued marketing of a particular drug constitutes an imminent hazard to the public health.

[9]At this meeting FDA communicated to the sponsor that it was considering proceeding with a withdrawal of the highest dose of Baycol because of its increased risk for a severe adverse event involving the breakdown of muscle fibers.

FDA Lacked a Clear and Effective Decision-making Process for Postmarket Drug Safety

In our March 2006 report, we found that FDA's postmarket drug safety decision-making process was limited by a lack of clarity, insufficient oversight by management, and data constraints. We observed that there was a lack of established criteria for determining what safety actions to take and when, and aspects of ODS's role in the process were unclear. A lack of communication between ODS and OND's review divisions and limited oversight of postmarket drug safety issues by ODS management hindered the decision-making process. FDA's decisions regarding postmarket drug safety were also made more difficult by the constraints it faced in obtaining data.

Decision-making Process on Drug Safety Lacked Clarity about Criteria for Action and the Role of ODS

While acknowledging the complexity of the postmarket drug safety decision-making process, we found through our interviews with OND and ODS staff and in our case studies that the process lacked clarity about how drug safety decisions were made and about the role of ODS. If FDA had established criteria for determining what safety actions to take and when, then some of the disagreements we observed in our case studies might have been resolved more quickly. In the absence of established criteria, several FDA officials told us that decisions about safety actions were often based on the case-by-case judgments of the individuals reviewing the data. For example, in the case of Bextra, ODS and OND staff disagreed about whether the degree of risk for serious skin reactions warranted a boxed warning, the most serious warning placed in the labeling of a prescription medication. Similarly, in the case of Propulsid, some staff, from both OND and ODS, supported proposing a withdrawal of approval because of the cardiovascular side effects of the drug while others believed label modifications were warranted.[10] Our observations were consistent with two previous internal FDA reports on the agency's internal deliberations regarding Propulsid and the diabetes drug Rezulin.[11] In those reviews FDA indicated that an absence of established criteria for determining what safety actions to take, and when to take them, posed a challenge for making postmarket drug safety decisions.

We also found that ODS's role in scientific advisory committee meetings was unclear. According to the OND Director, OND is responsible for setting the agenda for the advisory committee meetings, with the

[10] Propulsid's label was modified multiple times, including the addition of a boxed warning, to warn consumers and professionals about cardiovascular risks.

[11] Rezulin was removed from the market in 2000 because of its risk for liver toxicity.

exception of the Drug Safety and Risk Management Advisory Committee.[12] This includes who is to present and what issues will be discussed by the advisory committees. For the advisory committees (other than the Drug Safety and Risk Management Advisory Committee) it was unclear when ODS staff would participate. Although ODS staff presented their postmarket drug safety analyses during some advisory committee meetings, our case study of Arava provided an example of the exclusion of ODS staff. In March 2003, FDA's Arthritis Advisory Committee met to review the efficacy of Arava, and its safety in the context of all available drugs to treat rheumatoid arthritis.[13] The OND review division responsible for Arava presented its own analysis of postmarket drug safety data at the meeting, but did not allow the ODS staff—who had recommended that Arava be removed from the market—to present their analysis because it felt that ODS's review did not have scientific merit. Specifically, the OND review division felt that some of the cases in the ODS review did not meet the definition of acute liver failure, the safety issue on which the review was focused.[14]

A Lack of Communication and Limited Oversight Hindered the Decision-making Process

A lack of communication between ODS and OND's review divisions and limited oversight of postmarket drug safety issues by ODS management also hindered the decision-making process. ODS and OND staff often described their relationship with each other as generally collaborative, with effective communication, but both ODS and OND staff told us that there had been communication problems on some occasions, and that this had been an ongoing concern. For example, according to some ODS staff, OND did not always adequately communicate the key question or point of interest to ODS when it requested a consult, and as ODS worked on the consult there was sometimes little interaction between the two offices. After a consult was completed and sent to OND, ODS staff reported that OND sometimes did not respond in a timely manner or at all. Several ODS staff characterized this as consults falling into a "black hole" or "abyss."

[12]ODS is responsible for setting the agenda for meetings of the Drug Safety and Risk Management Advisory Committee.

[13]The committee was asked to consider whether the data presented by the drug's sponsor supported improvement in physical function and whether the drug's labeling needed to be updated to add any additional warning about liver toxicity. Ultimately, the label was strengthened in 2003 to state that rare cases of severe liver injury, including cases of fatal outcomes, had been reported in Arava users.

[14]Similarly, other senior-level CDER staff, including ODS and OND managers, did not agree with the ODS staff's conclusions and recommendation.

OND's Director told us that OND staff probably do not "close the loop" in responding to ODS's consults, which includes explaining why certain ODS recommendations were not followed. In some cases CDER managers and OND staff criticized the methods used in ODS consults and told us that the consults were too lengthy and academic.

ODS management had not effectively overseen postmarket drug safety issues, and as a result, it was unclear how FDA could know that important safety concerns had been addressed and resolved in a timely manner. A former ODS Director told us that the small size of ODS's management team presented a challenge for effective oversight of postmarket drug safety issues. Another problem was the lack of systematic information on drug safety issues. According to the ODS Director, ODS maintained a database of consults that provided some information about the consults that ODS staff conducted, but it did not include information about whether ODS staff made recommendations for safety actions and how the safety issues were handled and resolved, such as whether recommended safety actions were implemented by OND.

Data Constraints Contributed to Difficulty in Making Postmarket Safety Decisions

Data constraints—such as weaknesses in data sources and FDA's limited ability to require certain studies and obtain additional data—contributed to FDA's difficulty in making postmarket drug safety decisions. OND and ODS used three different sources of data to make postmarket drug safety decisions. They included adverse event reports, clinical trial studies, and observational studies. While data from each source had weaknesses that contributed to the difficulty in making postmarket drug safety decisions, evidence from more than one source could have helped inform the postmarket decision-making process. The availability of these data sources was constrained, however, because of FDA's limited authority to require drug sponsors to conduct postmarket studies and its resources.

While decisions about postmarket drug safety were often based on adverse event reports, FDA could not establish the true frequency of adverse events in the population with data from adverse event reports. The inability to calculate the true frequency made it hard to establish the magnitude of a safety problem, and comparisons of risks across similar drugs were difficult.[15] In addition, it would have been difficult to attribute adverse events to particular drugs when there was a relatively high incidence rate in the population for the medical condition. It was also difficult to attribute adverse events to the use of particular drugs because data from adverse event reports may have been confounded by other factors, such as other drug exposures.

FDA can also use available data from clinical trials and observational studies to support postmarket drug safety decisions. Although each source presents weaknesses that constrained the usefulness of the data provided, having data from more than one source can help improve FDA's decision-making ability. Clinical trials, in particular randomized clinical trials, are considered the "gold standard" for assessing evidence about efficacy and safety because they are considered the strongest method by which one can determine whether new drugs work.[16] However, clinical trials also have weaknesses. Clinical trials typically have too few enrolled patients to detect serious adverse events associated with a drug that occur relatively infrequently in the population being studied. They are usually carried out on homogenous populations of patients that often do not reflect the types of patients who will actually take the drugs. For example, they do not often include those who have other medical problems or take other medications. In addition, clinical trials are often too short in duration to identify adverse events that may occur only after long use of the drug. This is particularly important for drugs used to treat chronic conditions where patients are taking the medications for the long term. Observational studies, which use data obtained from population-based sources, can provide FDA with information about the population effect and risk associated with the use of a particular drug. For example, in the case of Propulsid, an observational study showed that a 1998 labeling change warning about contraindications did not significantly decrease the percentage of users in one population who should not have been prescribed this drug. Because they are not controlled experiments,

[15]This is due, in part, to the underreporting of adverse events and inconsistency in how those reporting define cases. These limitations have been reported elsewhere. See, for example, D.J. Graham, P.C. Waller, and X. Kurz, "A View from Regulatory Agencies," in *Pharmacoepidemiology*, ed. Brian L. Strom (Chichester: John Wiley & Sons, Ltd., 2000), pp. 109–124.

[16]In these trials, patients are randomly assigned to either receive the drug or a different treatment, and differences in results between the two groups can typically be attributed to the drug.

however, there is the possibility that the results can be biased or confounded by other factors.

We found that FDA's access to postmarket clinical trial and observational data was limited by its authority and available resources. FDA does not have broad authority to require that a drug sponsor conduct an observational study or clinical trial for the purpose of investigating a specific postmarket safety concern. One senior FDA official and several outside drug safety experts told us that FDA needs greater authority to require such studies. Long-term clinical trials may be needed to answer safety questions about risks associated with the long-term use of drugs. For example, during a February 2005 scientific advisory committee meeting, some FDA staff and committee members indicated that there was a need for better information on the long-term use of anti-inflammatory drugs and discussed how a long-term trial might be designed to study the cardiovascular risks associated with the use of these drugs.[17]

Lacking specific authority to require drug sponsors to conduct postmarket studies, FDA has often relied on drug sponsors voluntarily agreeing to conduct these studies. But the postmarket studies that drug sponsors agreed to conduct have not consistently been completed. One study estimated that the completion rate of postmarket studies, including those that sponsors had voluntarily agreed to conduct, rose from 17 percent in the mid-1980s to 24 percent between 1991 and 2003.[18] FDA has little leverage to ensure that these studies are carried out.

In terms of resource limitations, several FDA staff (including CDER managers) and outside drug safety experts told us that in the past ODS has not had enough resources for cooperative agreements to support its postmarket drug surveillance program. Under the cooperative agreement program, FDA collaborated with outside researchers in order to access a wide range of population-based data and conduct research on drug safety. Annual funding for this program was less than $1 million from fiscal year

[17]This was a joint meeting of the Arthritis Advisory Committee and the Drug Safety and Risk Management Advisory Committee.

[18]Postmarket studies for approved drugs and biologics are included in the percent calculations. See: Tufts Center for the Study of Drug Development (Kenneth I. Kaitin, ed.), "FDA Requested Postmarketing Studies in 73% of Recent New Drug Approvals," *Impact Report: Analysis and Insight into Critical Drug Development Issues*, vol. 6, no. 4 (2004).

2002 through fiscal year 2005. In 2006, FDA awarded four contracts for a total cost of $1.6 million per year to replace the cooperative agreements.

FDA's Initiatives to Improve Postmarket Drug Safety Decision Making

Prior to the completion of our March 2006 report, FDA began several initiatives to improve its postmarket drug safety decision-making process. Most prominently, FDA commissioned the Institute of Medicine (IOM) to convene a committee of experts to assess the current system for evaluating postmarket drug safety, including FDA's oversight of postmarket safety and its processes. IOM issued its report in September 2006.[19] FDA also had underway several organizational changes that we discussed in our 2006 report. For example, FDA established the Drug Safety Oversight Board to help provide oversight and advice to the CDER Director on the management of important safety issues. The board is involved with ensuring that broader safety issues, such as ongoing delays in changing a label, are effectively resolved. FDA also drafted a policy that was designed to ensure that all major postmarket safety recommendations—including those that involve disagreements—would be discussed by involved OND and ODS managers, beginning at the division level.[20] The draft policy states that decisions about major postmarket safety recommendations would be documented. FDA implemented a pilot program for dispute resolution that is designed for individual CDER staff to have their views heard when they disagree with a decision—including the failure to take a drug safety action—that could have a significant negative effect on public health. In that program, the CDER Director would decide whether the process should be initiated, appoint the chair for a panel to review the case, and make the final decision on how the dispute should be resolved. Because the CDER Director is involved in determining whether the process will begin and makes the final decision, the pilot program did not offer employees an independent forum for resolving disputes. FDA also began to explore ways to access additional data sources that it can obtain under its current authority, such as data on

[19] Institute of Medicine of the National Academies, Committee on the Assessment of the U.S. Drug Safety System, Editors A. Baciu, K. Stratton, and S.P. Burke, *The Future of Drug Safety: Promoting and Protecting the Health of the Public* (Washington, DC: Sept. 22, 2006).

[20] The draft policy is entitled "Process for Decision-Making Regarding Major Postmarketing Safety-Related Actions."

Medicare beneficiaries' experience with prescription drugs covered under the prescription drug benefit.[21]

Since our report, FDA has made efforts to improve its postmarket safety decision-making and oversight process. In its written response to the IOM recommendations, FDA agreed with the goals of many of the recommendations made by GAO and IOM.[22] In that response, FDA stated that it would take steps to improve the "culture of safety" in CDER, reduce tension between pre-approval and post-approval staff, clarify the roles and responsibilities of pre- and postmarket staff, and improve methods for resolving scientific disagreements.

FDA has also begun several initiatives since our March 2006 report that we believe could address three of our four recommendations. Because none of these initiatives was fully implemented as of March 2007, it was too early to evaluate their effectiveness.

- To make the postmarket safety decision-making process clearer and more effective, we recommended that FDA revise and implement its draft policy on major postmarket drug safety decisions. CDER has made revisions to the draft policy, but has not yet finalized and implemented it. CDER's Associate Director for Safety Policy and Communication told us that the draft policy provides guidance for making major postmarket safety decisions, including identifying the decision-making officials for safety actions and ensuring that the views of involved FDA staff are documented. According to the Associate Director, the revised draft does not now discuss decisions for more limited safety actions, such as adding a boxed warning to a drug's label.[23] As a result, fewer postmarket safety recommendations would be required to be discussed by involved OND and ODS managers than envisioned in the draft policy we reviewed for our 2006 report. Separately, FDA has instituted some procedures that are consistent with the goals of the draft policy. For example, ODS staff now participate in regular, bimonthly safety meetings with each of the review divisions in OND.

[21]In October 2006, the Centers for Medicare & Medicaid Services published a proposed rule that would, when finalized, facilitate access by FDA and others to information about prescription drugs covered by Medicare. See 71 *Fed. Reg.* 61445 (Oct. 18, 2006).

[22]HHS, FDA, *The Future of Drug Safety—Promoting and Protecting the Health of the Public: FDA's Response to the Institute of Medicine's 2006 Report* (Rockville, Md.: January 2007).

[23]The original draft policy included the market withdrawal of a drug, restrictions on a drug's distribution, and boxed warnings as major postmarket drug safety decisions.

- To help resolve disagreements over safety decisions, we recommended that FDA improve CDER's dispute resolution process by revising the pilot program to increase its independence. FDA had not revised its pilot dispute resolution program as of March 2007, and FDA officials told us that the existing program had not been used by any CDER staff member.

- To make the postmarket safety decision-making process clearer, we recommended that FDA clarify ODS's role in FDA's scientific advisory committee meetings involving postmarket drug safety issues. According to an FDA official, the agency intends to, but had not yet, drafted a policy that will describe what safety information should be presented and how such information should be presented at scientific advisory committee meetings. The policy is also expected to clarify ODS's role in planning for, and participating in, meetings of FDA's scientific advisory committees.

- To help ensure that safety concerns were addressed and resolved in a timely manner, we recommended that FDA establish a mechanism for systematically tracking ODS's recommendations and subsequent safety actions. As of March 2007, FDA was in the process of implementing the Document Archiving, Reporting and Regulatory Tracking System (DARRTS) to track such information on postmarket drug safety issues. Among many other uses, DAARTS will track ODS's safety recommendations and the responses to them. CDER's Associate Director for Safety Policy and Communication told us that DAARTS would be fully operational by the end of April 2007.

We also suggested in our report that Congress consider expanding FDA's authority to require drug sponsors to conduct postmarket studies in order to ensure that the agency has the necessary information, such as clinical trial and observational data, to make postmarket decisions.

Mr. Chairman, this concludes my prepared remarks. I would be pleased to respond to any questions that you or other members of the Subcommittee may have.

For further information regarding this testimony, please contact Marcia Crosse at (202) 512-7119 or crossem@gao.gov. Contact points for our Offices of Congressional Relations and Public Affairs may be found on the last page of this testimony. Martin T. Gahart, Assistant Director; Pamela Dooley; and Cathleen Hamann made key contributions to this statement.

Testimony of Curt D. Furberg, M.D., Ph.D.
Before the House Committee on Energy and Commerce
Subcommittee on Oversight and Investigations
March 22, 2007

Mr. Chairman and Members of the Committee,

My name is Curt Furberg. I am a professor of Public Health Sciences at the Wake Forest University School of Medicine, with expertise in drug evaluation and safety. I also serve as a member of the FDA Drug Safety & Risk Management Advisory Committee. This testimony reflects my personal views.

I am a firm believer in law and order. Congress has a critical role in developing and passing laws to protect what is right and fair. Laws and regulations are effective because violations have consequences! Our citizens cherish the notion that no one is above the law; therefore it troubles me that drug makers can violate FDA regulations, commitments and public trust without apparent consequences.

Here are some examples:

One company testing its antidepressant in adolescents reported and made public only three of its 13 trials. The other ten did not support the company's claim for efficacy and safety. Despite this suppression, the FDA has taken no action against the sponsor.

Another company delayed for several years submitting unfavorable safety data from a trial of its COX-2 inhibitor for Alzheimer's disease. The FDA has taken no action.

A third company submitted falsified data for an FDA hearing of its antibiotic, as discussed at your previous hearing on drug safety. Again, the FDA has taken no action against the company.

Thus, it appears that regulatory violations have no consequences in the U.S.

A fourth company "stalled" negotiations for 14 months over label changes that would add an important Black Box Warning for its COX-2 inhibitor. Decisions about label warnings should take only one to two weeks. This irresponsible delay in warning prescribers and the public about serious drug risks had no consequences for the drug maker.

These cases illustrate industry's malfeasance. They are alarming and have serious implications for public health. Tragically, they represent only a small fraction of the total problem. These examples pale in comparison to the potential public harm caused by industry's unmet commitments to conduct post-market safety trials. The approval of many new drugs is based on these commitments. As of last Fall, there were 1,259 unmet commitments with more than two-thirds of the safety trials not even initiated. What has the FDA done? Nothing!

In my view, it is critical for Congress to:

1. Provide the FDA with enforcement tools.
2. Give the FDA the legal authority to change drug labels and to withdraw unsafe drugs without negotiation.
3. Ensure through Congressional oversight that the FDA utilizes this new authority appropriately and in a timely manner.

I was asked to comment on the FDA's responses to the IOM recommendations. Overall I find them disappointing. Although many of the responses have merit, there are several shortcomings.

- First, the agency's apparent unwillingness to ask Congress for more authority to enforce safety regulations is troubling.

- Second, the FDA plan lacks concrete and constructive steps to bring drug safety to parity with drug benefit in the evaluation process. After all, decisions about drug approval and later use of a drug are based on the balance between benefit and harm. The Office of Surveillance and Epidemiology needs more experts in drug safety, public health and surveillance. The Director of this Office should report directly to the Commissioner and the Office should have its own external Advisory Committee.

Third, another concern not addressed is the FDA's lack of transparency. Prescribers and the public are not given safety data known to FDA officials in a timely manner. The reasons for disapproving a new drug or the reasons for requesting post-marketing safety studies are kept secret.

- Fourth, also missing in FDA's response is an evaluation plan. Progress towards improvement of the drug safety problems needs to be closely monitored and reported, with corrective actions being taken if goals are not met.

- Finally, the measure of FDA's performance needs to be changed. It should not be based only on the number of drugs approved within certain time limits. Full credit should be given for disapproval of drugs for safety reasons.

There are additional problems highlighted in a recent article entitled "The FDA and Drug Safety -- A Proposal for Sweeping Changes," which I would like to attach to my testimony. This article was written by me and four other current and past members of the FDA Drug Safety & Risk Management Advisory Committee.

I. What ar your concerns about PDUFA IV?

1. PDUFA has created an unhealthy relationship between the FDA and the industry that the FDA is supposed to regulate.

2. The dependence on the user fees has made the FDA more "accommodating" towards drug makers' requests. We have a clear conflict-of-interest situation.

3. The size of the user fee magnifies the problem.

4. The problem is compounded by the restricted use of the fees to meet industry's self-serving interests. For every $13.50 slated for approval reviews and general expenses, only $1 is allocated to post-market safety activities.

5. No other user fees have such restrictions on their use, only PDUFA.

6. Recent analyses have shown that the rush to meet approval deadlines and to qualify for payments has subsequently brought to the market drugs with an excess of unrecognized safety problems.

7. The number of serious adverse events reported to the FDA since PDUFA II was enacted has increased more than 2.5-fold.

8. PDUFA benefits the drug makers but the price is paid by an increasing number of innocent patients suffering serious adverse drug reactions.

I am in favor of closing out PDUFA over the next few years and replacing the budget shortfall with a normal prescription drug fee of 5 cents.

II. How can the use of potentially harmful drugs be reduced?

1. In two ways: First, by restricting the number of prescriptions. The right to prescribe the drug can be limited to physicians within certain specialties, prescribers can be required to undergo special training related to the drug, prescriptions could be restricted to patients who are refractory to safer treatment alternatives, and the duration of drug treatment could be limited.

2. The second way to reduce use of potential harmful drugs is through patient education. Patients (or their parents) could be given a Medication Guide when they pick up the drug in the Pharmacy, which fully explains the beneficial and harmful effects of a drug. They could also be asked to sign a form every time they fill the prescription. This would state that they are fully aware of all the risks of their prescribed medication. These steps tend to discourage use.

Testimony of Bruce M. Psaty, M.D., Ph.D.
Before the House Committee on Energy and Commerce
Subcommittee on Oversight and Investigations
March 22, 2007

Mr Chairman and members of the Committee,

My name is Bruce Psaty. A professor of medicine and epidemiology at the University of Washington, I served on the Institute of Medicine (IOM) drug-safety committee (1,2). The IOM review was undertaken at the request of the FDA after the withdrawal of Vioxx had raised questions about the integrity of the US drug-safety system. This testimony reflects my views as a public-health scientist.

According to one former FDA commissioner, the only novel IOM recommendation was the proposed 6-year term for future commissioners [IOM recommendation 3.1 (1)]. All the other recommendations had been made in one form or another in a dozen previous reports. Yet, in the FDA response to the IOM report (3), all actions are listed as "recently initiated," "new," or "planned" in PUDFA IV. What happened to the scores of previous recommendations? Whether, this time, FDA responses will eventually improve drug safety remains to be seen.

The FDA, which has many outstanding scientists, has a difficult job. The interests of the pharmaceutical industry in risks and benefits are not symmetrical; there is little short-term economic interest in safety; and some sponsors lack imagination when it comes to safety: hence, the need for strong science-based regulation to protect the health of the public.

The current drug-safety system, in which approval largely signals the end of evaluation, could hardly be weaker. The FDA centerpiece, the Adverse Event Reporting System (AERS), creates a "case series," the weakest form of epidemiologic evidence. Other major drug-safety efforts are the post-market commitments made by sponsors. Their completion rate dropped from 62% in the 1970s down to 24% in recent years (4). As of September 2006, 899 (71%) of the 1259 post-market studies were still "pending" (5).

To improve the system, the IOM committee recommended a life-cycle approach to drug evaluation (1)--an on-going systematic effort to identify safety signals, translate them into high-quality studies, evaluate both health benefits and risks, integrate the information into risk-benefit analyses, and communicate the findings to patients and physicians.

FDA needs additional resources (IOM, 7.1). While some FDA responses to the IOM report were excellent or were limited by inadequate resources, others seem to embrace the culture, vision and values of the status quo at the Agency (3).

For all new molecular entities (NMEs), the IOM recommended a re-evaluation of post-approval data by FDA (IOM, 5.4), an idea will be pilot tested. Leaving the review of new safety data in the hands of industry may, on occasion, be a hazard to the health of the public.

The IOM recommended public release of the FDA's risk-benefit analysis after the completion of post-marketing studies (IOM, 4.13). FDA plans to do so only on a case-by-case basis. Transparency is, however, essential. Although the Agency usually needs to make one decision, physicians and patients deserve to hear, not one constrained voice, but the range and quality of evidence underlying regulatory decisions. Otherwise, FDA fails in its mission to serve as the trusted intermediary of complex information.

The IOM recommended joint authority for the Office of New Drugs (OND) and the Office of Surveillance and Epidemiology (OSE) in the post-approval setting (IOM, 3.4). The FDA planned a few pilot projects. This response, which fails to acknowledge even a future commitment to the spirit of joint authority for OSE, does not signal major cultural change at the FDA.

The IOM Committee recommended that a substantial majority of Advisory Committee members be free of significant financial conflicts (IOM, 4.10), yet FDA described no commitment to limit conflict of interest. The failure to recognize the importance of independent review provided by Advisory Committees is not in the spirit of broad cultural change.

These responses, taken together, do not represent "fundamental changes … [that will] entail a cultural shift within the FDA" (page 5). A fundamental change would involve actively embracing an on-going lifecycle evaluation that includes both transparency and independent review. Cultural changes need to come first, from the top, and include leadership that relies on science in its decision-making process, leadership that values and harnesses scientific disagreement to improve drug approval decisions, and leadership that is at once courageous under outside pressures and passionate about the health of the public.

References

1. Committee on the Assessment of the US Drug Safety System, eds Baciu A, Stratton K, Burke SP. The Future of Drug Safety: Promoting and Protecting the Health of the Public. The National Academies Press, Washington, DC.
2. Psaty BM, Burke SP. Protecting the health of the public--Institute of Medicine Recommendations on drug safety. N Engl J Med 2006;355:1753-55.
3. Food and Drug Administration. The future of drug safety--promoting and protecting the health of the public: FDA's response to the Institute of Medicine's 2006 Report. US Department of Health and Human Services, January 2007; http://www.fda.gov.
4. Tufts Center for the Study of Drug Development. FDA requested postmarketing studies in 73% of recent new drug approvals. Impact Report July/August 2004;6(4):1-4.
5. Food and Drug Administration. Report on the performance of drug and biologics firms in conducting postmarketing commitment studies; availability. Federal Register 2007 Feb 2;72(22):5069-70.

c:\work\hoi\PsatyTestimony032207.doc

Mr. Chairman, members. Thank you for the opportunity to provide testimony before the Subcommittee on this very important topic. I am Raymond L. Woosley, MD, PhD, President and CEO of The Critical Path Institute (C-Path) which is based in Tucson, Arizona and Rockville, MD. I am a physician and pharmacologist with over 40 years of experience in the study of medications. C-Path is a non-profit, publicly funded organization that operates under a Memorandum of Understanding with the FDA to create and facilitate collaborations that advance the FDA's Critical Path Initiative. The Critical Path Initiative began in 2004 because of a near doubling of the failure rates of drugs in clinical development and a development process that has evolved to the point that it now takes an investment of 15 years and $1.3 billion to bring a single innovative product to market. The critical path initiative is all about "process improvement," that is, improvements that will enable **innovative** medical products to be **safely**, quickly, efficiently and reliably brought to market for patients and the public.

Why is the consideration of innovation so important to this discussion drug safety? Quoting a colleague, Dr. Hugh Tilson, **"without innovation, all we will have are the products of yesterday."** Truly innovative new products have much greater potential for benefit compared to those products that are simply incremental improvements over those already on the market. However, innovative products also present special challenges for safety evaluation and surveillance because they may have new forms of unanticipated toxicity. All agree that we need to improve our ability to develop safe medical products. However, it is essential that we do so without threatening the opportunity for innovation or interfering with our ability to translate our nation's $90 billion annual investment in biomedical research and development into better health.

A Basic Principle: Essential to our understanding of drug safety is recognition that: Neither drug risk nor benefit can ever be fully defined before drugs reach the market. The enormous variability between people means that any reasonable premarket safety evaluation must be confirmed by an ongoing evaluation after products reach the marketplace where they will be used in many more people and in different ways than before. Drugs must be carefully evaluated throughout their life cycle. This is best shown in a recent example. As a result of a new clinical use for the old drug, methadone, we just recently detected a life-threatening adverse effect on heart rhythm that had been undetected for over 50 years. Thus, careful surveillance should be continuous and not confined to just the newest drugs. A corollary to this rule is that, when a drug has to be removed from the market due to toxicity, it is not necessarily the result of any mistakes made by anyone, including the developer or the FDA.

Premarket Evaluation of Safety: For decades we have needed better ways to evaluate drugs before they enter human testing. The methods that are recommended today are the same ones developed over fifty years ago. One of C-Path's first projects under the Critical Path Initiative, the Predictive Safety Testing Consortium (PSTC), was conceived by scientists at the FDA. PSTC is a collaboration that includes 160 scientists from the sixteen largest global biopharmaceutical companies in which they share and cross validate their safety testing methods. Regulatory scientists from the FDA and, their European counterpart, EMEA, are participating. Based upon the outcome of the work, the FDA will make recommendations for new standards for improved safety testing methods. I strongly encourage Congress to support the Critical Path Initiative and foster this kind of "precompetitive" collaboration. Congress has helped solve this type of issue before when it created Sematech in the 80's to preserve the competitiveness of the computer chip industry. Unfortunately, today the FDA has a limited numbers of scientists and few resources to participate in evaluation and setting of standards. In order to have greater safety, efficiency and predictability in new drug development, we must expand this type of work in public-private collaborations. Furthermore, the improved testing methods will result in safer drugs reaching the market and identification of biomarkers that can predict which patients are at risk for harm before they receive the drug.

Post-marketing Safety Assessment: Prior to the U.S. adoption of user fees and efforts to reach international harmonization on methods, the FDA's high approval standards and prolonged review times resulted in more new drugs being first marketed in Europe. In response, European countries developed post-marketing active surveillance systems to quickly detect adverse events. The UK's yellow card system and the General Practitioner Research Database are valuable and proven tools. The French developed a pharmacovigilance system that includes sixteen regional specialized centers that employ scientists trained to detect and accurately characterize adverse events that occur with newly marketed drugs. Unlike Europe, the U.S. does not have an effective active surveillance system capable of rapid and accurate detection of safety problems with new drugs. This is therefore a serious deterrent to the timely approval of important new therapies. Because the agency's budget requests for active surveillance have been denied in the past, the FDA is forced to rely solely on its voluntary Adverse Event Reporting System (AERS). It is not by choice that the FDA has placed so much reliance on the AERS system.

Even when the FDA is given adequate resources, we should not expect that the FDA will be able to singly address all aspects of post-market safety assessment of new drugs. Over half of the drugs removed from the market in the last 15 years were safe when used as directed. In 1997, Congress authorized the Agency for Healthcare Research and Quality to create Centers for Education and Research on Therapeutics (CERTs) with the mission of conducting programs to improve the health outcomes from drugs, biologicals and devices. There are now eleven CERTs that have established a network of health plans that serve approximately 100 million Americans.

With relatively modest additional funding, this network of health plans could serve as a sentinel network and conduct the active surveillance that is needed to assure the early and accurate detection of adverse effects of new drugs.

Calls for Change at the FDA: It is my firm belief that many of the current problems at the FDA can best be addressed by giving the agency the resources it needs to execute its mission and to gain access to the "science" that will better inform decision making. Most disagreements among agency scientists and subsequent criticisms of agency actions can be better addressed if the FDA has more staff and scientists with the time and resources necessary to make decisions that are based on better data and a fuller appreciation of the science. Today, the limited resources at the FDA means that there is no travel budget for attending scientific conferences or participating in meetings that would enable agency employees to keep current on the rapidly evolving technical advances for the products they regulate. I do not believe that FDA scientists must continue to be actively conducting research in order to stay abreast of scientific advances in their chosen field. However, they do need opportunities outside of their review work in which they gain a critical appreciation of the newest relevant scientific advances.

The Institute of Medicine, the Government Accountability Office and many others have called for a change in the "culture" and organizational structure at the FDA. In my interactions with the FDA, which span four decades and address issues important to drugs, devices, diagnostics and even dietary supplements, I have seen, first hand, the enormous scope of the scientific questions that the agency scientists must face in regulating the many products that consumers rely on. This broad mission will never be served well by a single or rigid organizational structure. Likewise, the culture will never be ideal, unless the FDA regulators, who began their careers as scientists, are given access to the scientific methods and the data they need to make their decisions. How can anyone expect an organization to have a healthy culture when it has interim leadership more than half of the time? How can anyone expect an organization to maintain a high level of productivity or take on more authority when it has only a small fraction of the people and resources required to accomplish its current mission? With stable leadership and adequate resources, positive changes in the culture will follow.

Some have called for post market safety assessment to be separate from the Office of New Drugs. I believe that post-market assessment of drugs must include an ongoing assessment of benefit and risk simultaneously. I would not recommend creating a system in which the "drug approvers" and the "drug removers" are pitted against one another. Drug approval decisions and subsequent evaluations are very difficult questions that require a consensus be reached by an interdisciplinary team based on the best possible scientific information. We should accept that there will often be dissent in this process. In an effective organizational structure, the dissenters should feel that they have been given a fair chance to express their opinions but at some point a single consensus and decision is required. Ties and minority opinions are not options.

In summary, the Food and Drug Administration is expected to protect the public health by regulating the industries that produce foods, drugs, biologicals, diagnostics, devices, veterinary products, etc but it has never been given adequate resources. If adequately funded, the FDA can also create a system to conduct active post-market surveillance of new medical products. I have no doubt that the FDA is protecting the public health as well as anyone could expect considering its often temporary leadership, complex and ever increasing mission and the severely constrained resources that it has been given. It is possible to have a world class safety surveillance system and, at the same time, pave the way for more innovative new therapies to reach patients.

Major Points

1. The future of the pharmaceutical industry is threatened by its inefficiency and an unacceptably high failure rate of drugs during development and after marketing.

2. Greater drug safety must be achieved without threatening the opportunities for innovation.

3. Biological differences between people will result in rare drug toxicities that could not have been predicted and must be detected early after marketing.

4. The FDA's Critical Path Initiative (CPI)includes important "precompetitive" work to develop better and more predictive safety testing during development. New biomarkers from this work will further enable therapies that are targeted for those who can benefit with lower risk of harm.

5. The FDA's Office of Drug Safety (ODS) needs an independent source of reliable, timely information from an active, electronic surveillance system like the one available in AHRQ's CERTs that includes a network of health plans serving 100 million Americans.

6. To be successful in its mission, the FDA requires:

    Stable leadership

    Increased funding for adequate numbers of scientists and staff for CPI and ODS

    Access to the science and technologies that enable optimal decision making

    Retain the single system to make benefit/risk assessment over each drug's life cycle

1 of 1 DOCUMENT

Newark Star-Ledger (New Jersey)

February 22, 2007 Thursday
FINAL EDITION

SECTION: BUSINESS; Pg. 55

LENGTH: 649 words

HEADLINE: Ex-FDA chief: Pharma goal at odds with safety

BYLINE: ROBERT COHEN, STAR-LEDGER WASHINGTON BUREAU

DATELINE: WASHINGTON

BODY:

The Food and Drug Administration's diminished credibility on drug safety is due in part to the pharmaceutical industry's tactic of mass marketing medicines, a former agency commissioner said yesterday.

"The notion that you can come up with a new drug and have millions and millions of people take it safely - the blockbuster - that is what got us in trouble," said David Kessler, who led the FDA from 1990 to 1997.

Kessler, one of four former FDA commissioners participating in a panel discussion at the George Washington University School of Public Health, said large-scale promotion of prescription drugs through direct-to-consumer advertising has been a mistake.

The former FDA leader said the agency looks at statistical evidence from relatively small numbers of patients in clinical trials to determine safety and effectiveness of drugs, and then seeks to balance risks and benefits. But he said the goal of the pharmaceutical companies has been to create "a mass market and sell as many drugs as they can."

Kessler said it was inevitable that there would be an increase in serious side effects from many heavily promoted drugs because the question of whether it is "the right drug, the right person, the right disease and the right dose" often hasn't been asked.

He said he doesn't believe this model is sustainable, and suggested "limits should be placed" on marketing medicines as "just another commodity." Kessler opposed direct-to-consumer advertising when he was commissioner.

Joining Kessler during the panel discussion were former commissioners Donald Kennedy (1977 to 1979), Frank Young (1984 to 1989) and Jane Henney (1999 to 2001).

All four expressed unhappiness that the agency's integrity and credibility has been under attack in the last few years. They attributed the problems to a lack of consistent and sustained leadership, a paucity of resources and insufficient power to deal with safety issues.

The FDA in the last three years has been assailed for being lax on drug and medical device safety, and being too cozy with those industries. It also has been accused of stifling scientific dissent and for letting political considerations guide decision-making.

A May 2006 public opinion poll showed the majority of Americans don't think the FDA is doing a good job.

Many of the FDA's problems came to public attention in the wake of its mishandling of Merck's blockbuster Vioxx pain medication, which was taken off the market after being linked to heart attacks and strokes. A number of FDA reform proposals are pending in Congress to strengthen drug-safety laws.

At a separate conference held yesterday by the Center for Medicine and the Public Interest, Andrew von Eschenbach, the current FDA commissioner, said he thinks trust in the agency can be regained through "honesty, openness, transparency and a recognition of vulnerabilities." He said "science" will be the foundation for all decisions.

Von Eschenbach also defended direct-to-consumer advertising as a First Amendment right as long as the ads remain truthful.

He said he is committed to insuring all different points of view within the agency are heard and part of the deliberative process. But he added he won't tolerate whistleblowers who go outside the agency just because they disagree with a final outcome.

"The people have to understand to go outside that process is not constructive. It is actually destructive," von Eschenbach said. (Emphasis Added)

At the GW panel discussion, Young said the "FDA needs to be a high priority for the administration and the Congress, and the administration must avoid political meddling."

He said the FDA has been consistently underfunded, and needs more money and added powers including greater ability to monitor drugs after they are on the market. Henney said the FDA needs the authority to order rather than negotiate labeling changes and recalls.

Robert Cohen may be reached at rcohen@starledger.com.

LOAD-DATE: February 22, 2007

March 14, 2007

An Open Letter to:

Chairman Edward Kennedy and Senator Mike Enzi,
Chairman John Dingell and Representative Joe Barton
Members of the Senate Health, Education, Labor and Pensions Committee
Members of House Energy and Commerce Committee

The Food and Drug Administration (FDA) is facing a serious crisis that has significant implications for the nation's health.

The panel of experts recently convened by the Institute of Medicine (IOM) identified serious problems in the nation's capacity to determine drug safety and made a series of recommendations, calling on the FDA to "embrace a culture of safety in which the risk and benefits of medications are examined during their entire market life." [1,2]

The Prescription Drug User-Fee Act (PDUFA), in which brand name drug manufacturers pay a fee for each new drug the agency reviews, is an important cause of the difficulties faced by the FDA. Last year, this amounted to over $300 million, or over one-third of the entire budget for FDA's Center for Drug Evaluation and Research. PDUFA has helped to foster the public's perception that industry has become the primary client of FDA rather than the American people; this perception has contributed to the erosion of trust in FDA.

Unlike other user fee programs in the federal government, PDUFA requires the FDA to negotiate with representatives of the users, in this case the Pharmaceutical Research and Manufacturers of America (PhRMA), about how the agency may allocate its resources. The negotiated arrangement finances the drug approval process but neglects the equally important task of risk management once these drugs are on the market. This negotiated arrangement, which has explicitly limited its ability to conduct post-marketing drug safety surveillance and other critical activities, clearly diminishes the capacity of FDA to do its work on behalf of the nation.

User fees may appear to save the taxpayers money, but at an unacceptable cost to public health. In one study, PDUFA-imposed deadlines on FDA staff to complete reviews quickly are associated with subsequent withdrawals, warnings and other post-approval regulatory actions.[3] In fact, premature approval of a drug with safety problems, or an inadequate means of detecting problems that emerge after marketing (as occurred with Vioxx) actually cost the taxpayers far more than the Treasury appears to save through user fees. The human costs of delayed detection of safety problems are considerable.

With the expiration of PDUFA this year, the FDA and PhRMA have negotiated terms for a five year reauthorization.[4] This negotiation, completed behind closed doors, had only limited input from the public. Unfortunately, the proposal crafted by the FDA and PhRMA does not come close to addressing the problems identified by the IOM.

In February, four former FDA Commissioners agreed that the nation would be better served if Congress directly appropriated the money the FDA needs to do its job right, without the constraints imposed by PDUFA.[5]

We oppose reauthorizing PDUFA and other user fee programs modeled after it in the form negotiated by the FDA and PhRMA; instead, we support increased direct appropriations for the FDA, as is done with most federal agencies. The supposed "savings" realized through user fees make no sense in light of the added medical and economic costs that are generated by an inadequate drug safety surveillance system. Direct appropriation is the most effective way to ensure FDA's independence and commitment to drug safety.

As called for by the IOM and a recent Government Accountability Office report[6] on this topic, Congress and the nation must carefully re-assess the system in which drugs are developed, tested, approved and followed post-approval. Ideally, the plans for new funding sources and for new activities to improve drug safety would be completed before Sept 30, 2007. But this re-assessment cannot be done in the very short timeframe scheduled for PDUFA reauthorization.

However, if PDUFA must be reauthorized this year, in order for the nation to be able to have the substantive debate required for such an important and complex issue, we call on you to re-authorize it for no more than one year, and immediately schedule a series of hearings and investigations to examine ways to ensure that our drugs are effective and safe, and that the FDA itself is sound.

This limited re-authorized PDUFA should be structured to enable the FDA to do the best job it can in advancing the health of Americans. Any reauthorized PDUFA must have the following characteristics:

- Allow FDA leadership to determine how the agency allocates the fees collected to fulfill ***all*** aspects of its mission.
- Deadlines or targets for speed of review must be eliminated or modified to allow flexibility and adequate time for evaluation and analysis by reviewers.
- New performance goals must be linked with safety or other public health outcomes, not just speedy approval decisions.
- Adequate resources must be made available for scientific research and training for FDA scientific and medical staff, including in drug safety epidemiology and risk management.

The FDA's mission is to protect and advance the public's health. As it currently exists, and would exist in its proposed form, PDUFA stands in the way of this objective.

Sincerely,

Marcia Angell, MD,
Senior Lecturer in Social Medicine
Harvard Medical School

Jerry Avorn, MD
Professor of Medicine, Harvard Medical School
Chief, Division of Pharmacoepidemiology and Pharmacoeconomics
Brigham and Women's Hospital

Eula Bingham, PhD
Professor
University of Cincinnati College of Medicine
Former Assistant Secretary of Labor for Occupational Safety and Health

Daniel Carpenter, PhD
Professor of Government
Harvard University

R. Alta Charo, JD†
Professor of Law and Bioethics
University of Wisconsin Law and Medical Schools

J. Richard Crout, MD*
Former Director
FDA, Bureau of Drugs

Curt Furberg, MD, PhD
Professor of Public Health Sciences
Wake Forest University School of Medicine

Melissa Goldstein, JD
Associate Research Professor
George Washington University School of Public Health and Health Services

Jerome P. Kassirer, MD
Distinguished Professor
Tufts University School of Medicine

Sheldon Krimsky, PhD
Professor
Tufts University

David Michaels, PhD, MPH
Research Professor and Director
Project on Scientific Knowledge and Public Policy
George Washington University School of Public Health and Health Services

Woodrow A. Myers Jr. MD†
Myers Ventures LLC

Carl Nielsen*
Former Director
FDA ORA Division of Import Operations and Policy

Steven E. Nissen, MD
Cleveland Clinic

Bruce M. Psaty, MD, PhD, MPH†
Professor of Medicine
University of Washington

Richard J. Riseberg, JD*

David Ross, MD, PhD*

Christopher H. Schroeder, MDiv, JD†
Professor of Law and Public Policy Studies
Duke University

Eric J. Topol, MD
Director
Scripps Translational Science Institute

Susan F. Wood, PhD*
Research Professor
Project on Scientific Knowledge and Public Policy
George Washington University School of Public Health and Health Services

Affiliations for identification purposes only
* Former FDA/ HHS staff; † Member IOM Committee on the Assessment of the US Drug Safety System

---

[1] Committee on the Assessment of the US Drug Safety System, Alina Baciu, Kathleen Stratton, Sheila P. Burke, *Editors.* The Future of Drug Safety: Promoting and Protecting the Health of the Public. Institute Of Medicine, National Academies Press, Washington DC 2006

[2] Psaty BM, Burke SP. Protecting the health of the public--Institute of Medicine recommendations on drug safety. *N Engl J Med.* 2006;355(17):1753-1755.

[3] Carpenter D. et al. Deadline Effects in Regulatory Drug Review: A Methodological and Empirical Analysis. Available at: http://defendingscience.org/newsroom/upload/Carpenter_FDA_Deadlines.pdf

[4] Federal Register January 16, 2007 (Volume 72, Number 9)pps1743-1753

[5] Transcript of SKAPP Policy Workshop on Strengthening the FDA, February 21, 2007. Available at http://www.kaisernetwork.org/health_cast/hcast_index.cfm?display=detail&hc=2043

[6] Government Accountability Office. Drug Safety: Improvements Needed in FDA's Postmarket Decision-making and Oversight Process. March 2006. Report no. GAO-06-402. Available at: http://www.gao.gov/new.items/d06402.pdf.

PEDIATRIC EXCLUSIVITY LABELING CHANGES AS OF SEPTEMBER 1, 2001

(Source: www.fda.gov/cder/pediatric/labelchange.htm)

Delay	Exclusivity Granted (Labeled)	Product	Indications	Label Changes
9 Months	12/6/99 (8/11/00)	Etodolac-Lodine (Wyeth Ayerst)	Relief of signs & symptoms of Juvenile Rheumatoid Arthritis	New indication in 6 years -16 years Higher dose (per kg basis) in younger children which is approximately 2 times the lower dose recommended for adults
2 Months	5/22/01 (7/19/01)	Buspirone - Buspar (Bristol-Myers Squibb)		• Safety and effectiveness **were not established** in patients 6 to 17 years of age for treatment of General Anxiety Disorder at doses recommended for use in adults • PK parameters (AUC and Cmax) of buspirone and its active metabolite were found to be equal to or higher in children and adolescents than that of adults
8 Months	1/3/00 (9/28/00)	Fluvoxamine-Luvox (Solvay)	Treatment of obsessions and compulsions in patients with OCD	Determined that a dose adjustment (increased dose) may be necessary in adolescents and girls 8 - 11 year of age may require lower doses
18 Months	8/11/99 (2/23/01)	Propofol - Diprivan (AstraZeneca)	Induction and/or maintenance of anesthesia	• Maintenance of anesthesia- age decreased down to 2 months from 3 years • Induction of anesthesia remains the same- 3 years of age and above • Concomitant administration with fentanyl may result in serious bradycardia • Abrupt discontinuation following prolonged infusion may result in flushing of hands and feet, agitation, tremulousness and hyperirritability • Propofol is not indicated for pediatric ICU sedation as safety has not been established. In a single multicenter trial of ICU sedation in critically ill pediatric patients (patients with upper respiratory tract infections excluded), the incidence of mortality (causality not established) was 9% in the propofol arm versus 4% in the standard sedative agents arm

GAO Responses to Questions from the Honorable Bart Stupak, Chairman, Subcommittee on Oversight and Investigations, House Committee on Energy and Commerce

1. What is the most important reform that Food and Drug Administration (FDA) should undertake to address drug safety?

Our work has identified three important reforms that are needed to improve FDA's postmarket decision-making and oversight process. First, FDA should increase its resources for access to data sources to help monitor postmarket drug safety and inform its decision-making process. Several FDA staff, including managers within the Center for Drug Evaluation and Research (CDER) and outside drug safety experts, told us in the past that FDA has not had enough resources to support its postmarket drug surveillance program. We found that annual funding for FDA's program to access a wide range of population-based data and conduct research on postmarket drug safety is currently $1.6 million per year. Second, FDA needs stronger oversight of postmarket safety issues, including a mechanism for tracking postmarket safety recommendations and subsequent actions. In 2006 we reported that FDA management had not effectively overseen postmarket drug safety issues, in part, because FDA lacked systematic information on drug safety concerns. As a result, it was unclear how FDA could know that important safety concerns had been addressed and resolved in a timely manner. Third, Congress should consider expanding FDA's authority to require drug sponsors to conduct postmarket studies, such as clinical trials or observational studies, as needed. FDA lacks specific authority to require drug sponsors to conduct postmarket studies. While FDA has often relied on drug sponsors voluntarily agreeing to conduct postmarket studies, the postmarket studies that drug sponsors agree to conduct have not been consistently completed.

2. How has FDA addressed the major problems with drug safety the Government Accountability Office (GAO) identified a year ago?

FDA has only partially addressed the problems we identified in our 2006 report. When we interviewed FDA officials in February and March 2007, they told us that FDA has initiatives underway and under consideration that, if implemented, could address three of the four recommendations we made in our report. Because none of these initiatives is fully implemented, it is too early to evaluate their effectiveness. First, to make the postmarket safety decision-making process clearer and more effective, we recommended that FDA revise and implement its draft policy on major postmarket drug safety decisions. CDER has made revisions to the draft policy, but has not yet finalized and implemented it. Second, to help resolve disagreements over safety decisions we recommended that FDA improve CDER's dispute resolution process by revising the pilot program to increase its independence. FDA has not revised its pilot dispute resolution program. Third, to make the postmarket safety decision-making process clearer, we recommended that FDA clarify the Office of Drug Safety's (ODS) role in FDA's scientific advisory committee meetings involving postmarket drug safety issues. (ODS is now called the Office of Surveillance and Epidemiology). The agency intends to, but has not yet, drafted a policy to describe ODS's role in scientific advisory committee meetings. Fourth, to help ensure that safety concerns were addressed and resolved in a timely manner, we recommended that FDA establish a mechanism for systematically tracking ODS's recommendations and subsequent safety actions. FDA is in the process of implementing a system to track information on postmarket drug safety issues.

3. Has the dispute resolution process instituted by FDA been used yet?

In November 2004 FDA implemented a program for dispute resolution that is designed for individual CDER staff to have their views heard when they disagree with a decision that could have a significant negative effect on public health, such as a proposed safety action or the failure to take a safety action. An FDA official told us in March 2007 that the program had not been used by any CDER staff member.

4. What are your concerns about the independence of the dispute resolution process?

According to the dispute resolution pilot program, the CDER director is involved in determining whether the dispute resolution process should be initiated. If it is decided that the process will proceed, the CDER director is responsible for appointing the chair for a panel to review the case. The panel would then make a recommendation to the CDER director, who would then decide how the dispute should be resolved. Because the CDER director is involved in deciding whether the process should be initiated, appoints the chair of the panel, and is the final adjudicator, the pilot program does not offer employees an independent forum for resolving disputes.

5. What additional authority should Congress grant FDA to improve its drug safety programs?

In order to ensure that FDA has the necessary information to make postmarket decisions, we recommended in our 2006 report that Congress should consider expanding FDA's authority to require drug sponsors to conduct postmarket studies, such as clinical trials and observational studies, as needed.

6. Did your GAO team learn of any cases where Office of Drug Safety (ODS) personnel were excluded from advisory committee meetings by Office of New Drugs (OND) personnel?

In our 2006 report we described two examples where ODS personnel were excluded from advisory committee meetings. In March 2003, FDA's Arthritis Advisory Committee met to review the efficacy and safety of the drug Arava in the context of all available drugs to treat rheumatoid arthritis. The OND review division responsible for Arava presented its own analysis of postmarket drug safety data at the meeting, but did not allow the ODS staff—who had recommended that Arava be removed from the market—to present their analysis because it felt that some of the cases in the ODS review did not meet the definition of acute liver failure, the safety issue under consideration. As another example, in February 2004 an ODS epidemiologist was not allowed to present his analysis of safety data at a joint meeting of the Psychopharmacologic Drugs Advisory Committee and the Pediatric Subcommittee of the Anti-Infective Drugs Advisory Committee that was held to discuss reports of suicidal thoughts and actions in children with major depressive disorder for various antidepressant drugs. OND believed that the ODS staff member's analysis, which showed a relationship between the use of antidepressants and suicidal thoughts and behaviors in children, was too preliminary to be presented in detail. The ODS epidemiologist had recommended an interim plan to discourage the use of all but one antidepressant in the treatment of pediatric major depressive disorders.

7. Did FDA ever define the role of ODS in advisory committee meetings involving postmarket safety issues?

We recommended in our report that FDA clarify ODS's role in its scientific advisory committee meetings involving postmarket drug safety issues. An FDA official told us in March 2007 that the agency intends to, but has not yet, drafted a policy to describe ODS's role in scientific advisory committee meetings.

8. In your case study reviews, was there any pattern of OND resistance to instituting labeling changes or other safety measures?

For our 2006 report we conducted case studies of four drugs—Arava, Baycol, Bextra, and Propulsid—to illustrate FDA's current decision-making process. Our case studies provide examples of disagreements over the evidence that was required to warrant certain safety actions, such as a labeling change. For example, in March 2004 ODS staff recommended that Bextra, an anti-inflammatory drug, carry a boxed warning on its label about its risk of serious skin reactions. The ODS staff based their recommendation on the finding that Bextra's risk for serious skin reactions was significantly higher than that for other similar drugs. The OND review division responsible for Bextra did not initially agree that a boxed warning was warranted, but agreed about five months later after ODS conducted another analysis. We believe that if FDA had established criteria for determining what safety actions to take and when, then some of the disagreements might have been resolved more quickly. Without established criteria, decisions about safety actions are often based on case-by-case judgments of the individuals reviewing the postmarket safety data.

The Honorable Bart Stupak

1. *What problems do you see in connection with the restricted use of fees contained in Prescription Drug User Fee Act (PDUFA) IV?*

   The overemphasis on meeting "deadlines" for approval has shifted FDA efforts away from drug safety. Pursuing safety signals during the pre-approval phase takes time and could, at times, delay approval. Since more safety problems are now detected post-approval, it suggests that the pre-approval safety evaluation is less thorough. The presence of an adequately staffed and funded Drug Safety Office could restore the balance.

2. *Do the deadlines in PDUFA contribute to an excess of unrecognized safety problems in connection with new drug applications?*

   As stated above more safety problems are now detected post-approval. Today, 20% of new drugs have a Black Box warning added after they are on the market and 4% are withdrawn. This should not be considered acceptable public health practice.

3. *Has PDUFA affected the "culture" of the Food and Drug Administration (FDA)?*

   It would be hard to prove. However, it would not be overreaching to conclude that the degree to which PDUFA dictates how FDA must interact with industry could create tensions within a public health agency.

   One reason for the isolation and alleged mistreatment of the small drug safety staff may be that they can delay approval by bringing up potential safety concerns. These concerns may require more sponsor and FDA analysis of trial data and possibly even new studies. Any such delays may be at odds with management's need to meet PDUFA deadlines in order to realize user fee revenue.

4. *What changes in FDA's drug safety structure would be most likely to obviate another "Vioxx" tragedy?*

   Drug safety has to be brought to parity with drug benefit. This can not be accomplished without the creation of an *independent* Office of Drug Safety with a Director who reports directly to the Commissioner. This Office needs adequate funding to secure sufficient numbers of appropriately skilled staff and its own Advisory Committee.

5. *Should the Office of Surveillance and Epidemiology share authority with the Office of New Drugs in postmarket setting?*

   Since monitoring of drug safety is the main FDA mission post-approval, there ought to be an independent Office of Drug Safety responsible for post-marketing. The currently weak and understaffed Office of Surveillance and Epidemiology lacks authority. Sharing authority is fine in principle and should be done both pre-and post-approval. But, the final decisions pre-approval ought to rest with the Office of New Drugs and decisions post-approval with a new Office of Drug Safety, or alternatively, an expanded Office of Surveillance and Epidemiology.

6. *What is your opinion of direct-to-consumer marketing of new drugs?*

DTCA has led to over-utilization of very costly and typically non-essential drugs. There are often much better understood and less expensive alternatives are available. If DTCA is a first amendment commercial free speech right and cannot be restricted, then new rules requiring thorough FDA reviews of the advertisements for scientific accuracy prior to them being aired or printed should be introduced.

7. *How can the use of new drugs, with relatively unknown safety records, be reduced?*

Absolutely.

(a) Strict risk management programs should be linked to their approval.

(b) When there is inconclusive or incomplete data to support safety, drugs should only receive time-limited conditional approval.

(c) The rationale for the conditional approval due to safety concerns should be made public.

(d) Restrictions ought to be placed on DTCA. A prominent Black Box warning detailing any potential safety concern ought to be included in the advertisement.

8. *What are the problems associated with post marketing safety studies?*

(a) There are no legal consequences (fines, drug withdrawal) for drug companies who choose to ignore or stall the completion of a post-market safety study commitment.

(b) Every study commitment should have a clear deadline for completion and submission to FDA.

(c) Cleaning up the current backlog ought to be of highest priority.

9. *Does the FDA have sufficient authority to sanction pharmaceutical companies that suppress or delay submission of unfavorable trial information?*

FDA appears to believe it does, however it fails to behave accordingly and take meaningful action against regulatory violations by industry. Whether it actually has sufficient legal authority may be a question for regulatory experts to determine. However, FDA does need an expanded toolbox of available sanctions so it can deal appropriately with different kinds and degrees of violations.

May 1, 2007

The Honorable Bart Stupak

Question 1. Were there recommendations to which the FDA was especially responsive?

The answers to relevant to this question and to several other of the other questions listed below appear in a commentary published by the *Journal of the American Medical Association* (1). Brief answers to all questions are also provided here. The FDA clearly engaged the IOM report (2-4), but offered no opinion on the recommendations that would require Congressional action. Some of the excellent responses include the plans for: (1) the review of AERS (IOM, 4.1); (2) the access to study data from large automate health-care databases (IOM, 4.2); (3) the evaluation of the Risk Minimization Plans (IOM, 4.4); (4) the plans to develop and systematically improve risk-benefit analyses (IOM, 4.5); (5) the new Advisory Committee on communication with patients and consumers (IOM, 6.1); and (6) the development of the risk communication plan (IOM, 6.2);

Question 2. You listed a number of "incomplete" responses to IOM recommendations. Are there others?

The IOM recommended additional regulatory powers in the post-approval setting (IOM, 5.1 and 5.2), yet the FDA did not comment publicly on this recommendation.

Under the assumption that PUDFA might continue, the IOM suggested safety-related performance goals (IOM, 4.3). The FDA, however, described no specific safety-related performance goals.

The recommendation to involve Advisory Committees in the review of all NMEs was essentially ignored (IOM, 4.8).

The IOM recommendation to post all new-drug-application review packages on the Agency's website (IOM, 4.12) was not accepted.

The IOM recommended the review of all new molecular entities by Advisory Committees that included expertise in pharmacoepidemiology and public health (IOM, 4.9). The FDA plan for an occasional increase in the involvement of experts missed the point that the effort to assess risk and benefit almost always involves safety issues that might benefit from a public-health perspective.

The IOM recommended that the Secretary of HHS appoint an external Management Advisory Board to help transform the Center's culture (IOM, 3.2 and 3.3), but the management consultants mentioned in the FDA response, though perhaps a good start, were not the comprehensive approach recommended by the Committee.

The IOM Committee recommended building internal epidemiologic and informatics capacity to improve post-market studies (IOM, 4.6), but it appears that the FDA lacked the resources to respond to this recommendation.

The IOM recommended a public-private partnership to prioritize, plan and organize funding for confirmatory drug safety and efficacy studies of public health importance (IOM, 4.3). The effort still lacks a champion (5).

Question 3. Why is the public-private partnership recommended by the IOM necessary?

In the US, the tradition of leaving to the pharmaceutical industry the task of evaluating the efficacy and safety of its products has permitted manufacturers to make study design choices that largely pre-determine the answers provided by the trials. In active-treatment comparison trials, for instance, sponsors have often chosen inadequate doses or inferior comparison treatments that will make their products look good (5,6). More marketing than science, these studies do not answer important public health questions. The IOM Committee envisioned a public-private partnership that would help define the key public health questions that merit investment in large, long-term trials. This partnership would not only identify studies of greatest interest but also recommend the best design features through an independent unbiased process.

Question 4. You mentioned that 899 post-market commitments are still pending. Why are so many pending?

The number of pending post-marketing commitments has remained fairly constant, about 800 or more, over the past three years (7-9). Some are old and do not have an agreed-upon start date, so they can never be classified as "delayed," and many of them will remain "pending" in perpetuity. These post-market commitments, which are intended to address important questions, often come up so late in the approval process that they are not well designed. Some pending studies should be dropped, others redesigned, and all of those that remain need a start date. Additionally, many FDA reviewers are uncertain about the types of post-market commitments to request (10). The last minute rush to finalize the product label and design post-market commitments has contributed to the weakness of the US drug-safety system.

Question 5. You referred to the value of scientific disagreement. How is it that disagreement helps the FDA in its mission?

FDA has to make binary decisions, often with incomplete information. Uncertainty is the usual source of scientific disagreement, often best resolved by the conduct of additional studies. Scientific disagreements within the Agency during the pre-approval evaluation, as occurred with Ketek, are likely to be excellent predictors of drugs that eventually have post-market safety problems. The disagreement itself is useful information that should not be concealed. Some FDA views--for instance about the need to present a single public voice--seem to be unnecessary and even inappropriate in a science-based organization. IOM reports make a single set of consensus recommendations, yet when necessary, they allow for dissenting opinions. Law courts do so as well. What physicians and patients want is honest information, including legitimate scientific disagreements. Under the PDUFA timelines, 18% of FDA medical officers "felt pressure to approve … a drug despite reservations about its safety, efficacy or quality" (10,11). Suppression of healthy scientific disagreement has perhaps helped to erode the culture at the FDA.

Question 6. You have raised the question of transparency at the Agency. If you could look at internal FDA documents, which ones would you like to see?

I would like to see the approvable letter for muraglitazar and the internal correspondence leading up to the approvable letter. Muraglitazar is the diabetes drug that Dr Nissen talked about at the Oversight and Investigations Subcommittee hearing on February 13, 2007 (12). His work in this area was a great public health service (13). I would also point out that the safety and efficacy reviews by FDA medical officers were also outstanding (14,15). The FDA questions to the Advisory Committee, however, were not well designed to encourage a serious integration of risks and benefits or to elicit a formal risk-benefit analysis (16). The approvable letter for muraglitazar and the other correspondence, if they were written before Dr Nissen's publication, might provide some insight into the FDA division's understanding the public-health risk-benefit problem that Dr Nissen so eloquently described.

Question 7. One of the IOM's recommendations concerned risk-benefit. What did you think of the FDA response to this recommendation?

The FDA response was fairly comprehensive, but surprisingly late for an agency that has made determinations, for many years, about which drugs are "safe and effective for the intended use." Admittedly, risk-benefit analyses present a number of difficulties (17), but they are essential to the health of the public, and the FDA seems committed to adopting a new approach. In addition to their usefulness in counseling patients, risk-benefit analyses are also especially useful for identifying missing information and, thus, important for isolating the scientific questions that merit further study. At several stages, risk-benefit analyses are thus an integral part of the lifecycle approach to drug evaluation. An important corollary to risk-benefit analysis is, of course, transparency--making this information available to the physicians and the public.

Question 8. What is your view of direct-to-consumer (DTC) advertising?

The IOM Committee recommended the use of a symbol like the black triangle used in the United Kingdom to signal the uncertain safety associated with new drugs and a limitation on DTC advertising for up to two years (IOM, 5.3). As a public-health scientist, I would recommend abandoning DTC advertising altogether. It is an indiscriminate marketing technique that helps and harms (18-20)--like a fire department that hoses down all the homes in a neighborhood to put out a kitchen fire in one house. I have clinic on Monday mornings, and one day, all 5 men on my schedule came in asking for a prescription for the same drug. This epidemic of perceived erectile dysfunction was precipitated by Super Bowl ads the previous day. None of these men had ED. When a truly important and innovative therapy such as imatinib (Gleevec) arrives, word about it gets around fairly fast these days without any need for DTC advertising. I myself would not count, for instance, purple pills among the truly important and innovative therapies. The GAO report has also identified problems in the FDA review of DTC ads (21).

Question 9. Is there a conflict-of-interest problem on FDA Advisory Committees?

There is certainly the perception of a problem. Physicians and scientists are notoriously naïve about conflict of interest (22). In one survey of medical residents (23), 61% said that their colleagues were likely to be affected by gifts from industry, but only 16% admitted that they themselves might be affected. How can that be? Well, we tend view ourselves in such a favorable light that conflict of interest is harder to discern in ourselves than our colleagues. The IOM Committee recommended that a substantial majority of Advisory Committee members be free of significant financial conflicts (IOM, 4.10). In the FDA response, there was no commitment to limit conflict of interest. The recent guidance from the FDA on conflict of interest did not go far enough (24). The drug-review process will benefit from truly independent outside review. The more independent, the better. Regardless of whether conflicts may have affected FDA decisions, the issue of public confidence demands that even an appearance or suspicion of the adverse effects of conflicts must be addressed, otherwise the FDA's overall credibility decline.

Question 10. You referred to the industry's lack of interest in safety. Can you provide any examples?

The pharmaceutical industry has a structural conflict of interest. The need to recover their investments in research and development and their fiduciary duty to shareholders lead to pressure or bias in favor of promoting drugs and potentially discounting ambiguous risk signals for as long as possible. Sometimes, the effects on public health can be devastating. Baycol (cerivastatin), a lipid lowering "statin" drug, was voluntarily withdrawn from the market in August 2001 because of a high incidence of rhabdomyolysis, a breakdown of muscle that causes pain and sometimes kidney failure and death (25). The sponsor knew about the high risk of rhabdomyolysis but did not adequately inform the FDA, patients or physicians for about 20 months. When the company's scientists brought this problem to the attention of the head of the pharmaceuticals business group one year before the drug was finally withdrawn, he ignored their concerns and told his marketing staff to "promote the hell out this product" (26). America needs a strong well-funded FDA capable of regulating drugs from manufacturers that are ethical or behavioral outliers.

In a review of materials before my testimony at the Senate Finance Committee in November 2004, it was clear that the sponsor was aware of the possibility that Vioxx, compared with aspirin, might be associated an excess of cardiovascular events as early as 1996 (27). The sponsor sought to design a large study that would selectively maximize the chances of showing favorable results for the prevention of gastrointestinal bleeding and selectively limit the chances of finding any unfavorable results about increases in cardiovascular events. Under these circumstances, the FDA needs to make sure that sponsor's studies ask and answer the right questions in a manner that protects and advances the health of the public (28). Decisions about the study questions and designs are best made by scientists independent of the sponsor.

Question 11. Why did the IOM recommend clinical trial registration?

Some sponsors selectively publish favorable findings (29), sometimes with ghost authors (30); and some fail to publish unfavorable findings, sometimes by omitting data from published studies (31,32) and sometimes by failing to publish the study at all (25,28). They treat scientific data obtained from human subjects, who volunteered to help advance medical knowledge, as if they were mere marketing efforts. This selective approach to publication distorts the publicly available evidence base and undermines any efforts at genuine risk-benefit analyses. The IOM recommendations about registering clinical trials and eventually making the results public are important for public health (IOM, 4.11).

Question 12. Do you favor the continuing appropriations from user fees?

Under PUDFA, the US became increasingly the country of first launch, the public testing ground for new medicines without any efforts to improve the drug-safety system. Indeed, during the first 10 years, PUDFA prohibited the use of user fees for improvements in drug safety. According to Dr David Kessler, head of the FDA from 1990 to 1997, "PDUFA should have had funding on the safety side from the beginning, but the industry refused to accept that.... We wanted it. The industry said no" (33). When Congress created PUDFA, safety activities were largely entrusted to the pharmaceutical industry, and they were not adequately funded at the FDA. In its implementation, PUDFA has also created at least the appearance that the FDA has industry rather than the public as its primary client. Particularly troublesome is the fact that the FDA enters into negotiations with industry to develop the next round of PUDFA goals and funding (34). No other regulator in the federal government (to my knowledge) negotiates in this way with the regulated. The IOM Committee expressed its preference for funding from general appropriations because drug safety is a public good.

DEPARTMENT OF HEALTH & HUMAN SERVICES

Food and Drug Administration
Rockville MD 20857

The Honorable John D. Dingell
Chairman
Committee on Energy and Commerce
House of Representatives
Washington, D.C. 20515-6115

MAY 30 2007

Dear Mr. Chairman:

Thank you for your April 25, 2007, letter containing a follow-up question for the record from the March 22, 2007, hearing entitled, "The Adequacy of FDA to Assure the Safety of the Drug Supply – Part II," before the Subcommittee on Oversight and Investigations. Below we have reprinted the question from Representative Greg Walden in bold followed by our response.

Question

Notwithstanding the legitimate concerns that have been raised in connection with the use of non-inferiority studies to support certain product approvals, it remains that for certain conditions such as serious infections caused by resistant microbes, other study designs may be unethical and for these conditions well-designed non-inferiority trials may remain appropriate. Will changes in FDA policy concerning the agency's reliance on non-inferiority evidence take account of these considerations and will FDA continue to permit the use of such evidence in appropriate cases?

Response

Over the last few decades most antibacterial drugs have been approved based upon non-inferiority studies. Recently the use of non-inferiority studies has been called into question, for studies of less serious infectious diseases that typically resolve over time in the absence of antibacterial therapy, where the effectiveness of standard drugs compared to placebo is not well-established. In such cases, a non-inferiority study may not be informative. However, in more serious infectious diseases where antibacterial drugs are reliably known to have a large treatment effect and prevent the serious consequences of untreated infection, non-inferiority studies remain an appropriate type of study for evaluating the safety and efficacy of antibacterial drugs.

For these serious infectious diseases, e.g., acute bacterial meningitis or acute bacterial endocarditis, non-inferiority studies are both scientifically valid and an ethically acceptable study design because in these cases, it is known that the test drug is an active treatment and would be effective in the non-inferiority study.

When considering the use of a study designed to show non-inferiority to an active comparator, it is essential to know what the effect size of a comparator would be relative to placebo in order for the non-inferiority study to be informative.. It is important to carefully develop an estimate of the effect size for the active comparator treatment at the time when the study is being designed.

An active controlled study designed to show non-inferiority compares the treatment effect of a test drug with the treatment effect of an active comparator drug. The difference between the effect of the active comparator and the effect of placebo or no treatment is the effect size. When the effect size of the active comparator drug relative to placebo is reliably known, one can conclude a test drug would have been better than placebo if the test drug is non-inferior to the comparator (i.e., by demonstrating an effect for the test drug that is within a pre-determined margin relative to the effect of comparator). Essentially, the conclusion is that if A (the active comparator) is better than placebo and B is not inferior to A, then B (the test drug) is superior to placebo and therefore B is an active treatment. This approach depends upon the validity of the assumption that A would reliably beat placebo.

FDA is committed to providing advice to sponsors to establish acceptable approaches for determining non-inferiority margins in diseases where non-inferiority designs are appropriate. In some circumstances this may require a careful review and synthesis of data derived from older medical literature in order to understand the effect of treatment with an active antibacterial drug on survival or other outcomes in the disease of interest.

FDA is aware of the ethical concerns related to studying certain types of infectious diseases in placebo-controlled trials. FDA would not require a study design that we believe would compromise patient safety. However, there may still be circumstances in serious diseases where no drugs are known to be effective and for which a non-inferiority trial design would be non-informative, and therefore inappropriate. In these situations a superiority trial, e.g., either against placebo or a non-approved comparator, may be an appropriate study design.

Appropriate design of investigational studies is essential to conducting informative and ethical studies that provide for patient safety and evaluate the safety and efficacy of investigational drugs. FDA is committed to working through these important and often challenging issues.

Please let us know if there are further questions.

Sincerely,

Stephen R. Mason
Acting Assistant Commissioner
for Legislation

Questions from the Honorable Bart Stupak (from Dr. Ray Woosley):

1. In an article you co-authored in 1998 entitled "Making Medicines Safer," you cited figures indicating that adverse effects of drugs is one of the top six causes of death in this country. Is that still the case?

> I am not aware of more recent data and I suspect that it has changed significantly. The estimates that I cited in 1998 were based on the rates of adverse events in hospitalized patients. There is another component that occurs in outpatients and nursing facilities that has not been quantified and should add substantially to the number of deaths.

2. In the same 1998 article, you noted that, given the state of information technology in 1998, it was remarkable that the Food and Drug Administration (FDA) lacked a systematic program of post-marketing drug surveillance. Does it exist today?

> Not at this time. However, a potential program of post-marketing surveillance does exist but it is only partially utilized. The eleven AHRQ-funded Centers for Education and Research on Therapeutics (CERTs) have the potential to serve as such a system. They have the potential to establish access to the electronic medical records for over 100 million patients and they have the required medical and pharmacologic expertise. They are not now funded to conduct independent post-marketing safety surveillance but could do so if adequately supported. In addition to conducting post-marketing safety assessments, these Centers could also confirm drug effectiveness in the real world of medical practice, assess comparative effectiveness and confirm appropriate use. All of these functions are included in the authorizing language for the CERTs. AHRQ and FDA simply need the appropriations to jointly implement an active surveillance system utilizing the existing network of CERTs. Funding for FDA is an essential component of such a network so that the surveillance can be fully informed and any necessary regulatory action can be taken promptly.

3. How does FDA's voluntary reporting system (AERS – Adverse Event Reporting System) compare with France's post-approval drug safety surveillance system?

> France has an active surveillance system of 31 regional pharmacovigilance centers positioned throughout the nation at major universities and hospitals. They are staffed with scientists who are trained to detect, analyze and characterize the risk factors associated with adverse drug events. The centers receive spontaneous adverse event reports and gather the data to better understand the reliability and nature of any reports. Unlike AERS which relies only on voluntary reporting, the French system actively examines the medical records of patients who receive newly marketed drugs and obtains comprehensive information about those who have adverse experiences that might be drug reactions.

.4. How does FDA's voluntary reporting system compare with the United Kingdom?

According to experts at the FDA, the UK's General Practice Research Database (GPRD) is the largest pharmacoepidemiologic database in the world with the highest quality data. The database covers about 3 million lives with data going back 10 years. The data are collected from the computerized medical record systems of 5% of all general practitioners in the UK. This database resource is superior in many ways to any US-based database known to the FDA.

The UK also has a "yellow card" system in which they ask physicians to complete a survey reporting outcomes for a fixed number of patients who receive a newly marketed drug. This system allows the UK's regulatory body (MHRA) to, not only detect adverse events quickly, also provide an estimate of the frequency of the adverse event.

The AERS system can never accurately estimate incidence because of under-reporting. Mandatory reporting would not be a solution to the problem because of the likelihood of over-reporting of events that could obscure the detection of real adverse events.

5. The article you co-authored entitled “A New System for Moving Drugs to Market,” contains your recommendation that newly approved drugs should be given to a defined population under observed conditions only. Wouldn’t this require an initial ban on most direct-to-consumer marketing since a newly approved drug would be approved for a carefully defined population?

Yes, but not necessarily in every case. The original intent of those who approved direct to consumer (DTC) ads was to enable patients to learn that a new treatment for their illness had become available and that they should contact their physician to determine if it would be of value in their care. It was not their intention for the ads to be used to market the drugs. The attempts to balance the marketing components by requiring that the ads convey risk/benefit information in the limited time available is, not only futile, it raises false expectations that understanding will result.

DTC ads promote drugs to the general public although prescription drugs, by their very nature, require a trained intermediary to diagnose whether the drugs are likely to be safe and effective for the patient. Such broad promotion fosters overuse of the drugs and a lack of true appreciation of their potential risk. In the system of accelerated but limited access that we proposed, the ads could be prohibited unless the public needs to be informed that a new drug is now available. However, the ads should not be promotional in nature and should be more in accord with the original concept of a "public service announcement." The ad should also emphasize that the newly approved product is only recommended for a limited population, i.e. the types of patients for whom it has been studied and found to have an acceptable risk/benefit ratio.

6. How would the FDA enforce such a limitation on drug prescriptions given that states regulate medical practice not the FDA?

The FDA should not be expected to try to guide the use of prescription drugs, other than by providing information about the safety and efficacy of drugs. AHRQ is the element of government responsible for improving the outcomes in healthcare. The educational and research programs of the AHRQ-funded CERTs could be better utilized to help provide the data/information needed to adequately guide and manage the use of new medications.

Professional societies can also become even more involved in setting prescribing standards through the use of guidelines for the appropriate prescription and monitoring of new therapies. Professional societies establish standards of therapy but they need to be more specific. For example, they recommend a "beta blocker" for treating hypertension, but which of the many should be tried first. It is not always the least expensive to purchase. HMOs have effective systems to monitor and guide the use of therapies. The major problem is the absence of data to inform those who wish to guide therapy. The lack of data on comparative effectiveness and comparative safety is the limiting factor.

As Alastair Wood has suggested, in order for companies to receive market exclusivity for innovative new therapies, companies should be expected to conduct reasonable post-marketing studies (and, I would add, use their detail force to encourage the appropriate use of their drugs by rewarding the sales force when the drug is prescribed appropriately). In order to provide an incentive for companies to fully evaluate their drugs for safety early after entry into the market, the FDA should encourage companies to also monitor for evidence of effectiveness as a basis for expanded claims to treat broader populations.

Unfortunately, regulation of use is likely to be ultimately left to the plaintiffs bar. However, most Health Maintenance Organizations, the Veterans Affairs Medical Systems and others are increasingly able to track drug use and reward those who prescribe drugs appropriately.

7. Does providing warnings, product labels or package inserts adequately protect patients from adverse events?

No. We need better ways to manage risk by informing and protecting patients. Also we must recognize that some risk management tools that appear to be reasonable may not be effective and could cause unanticipated and unintended harm. Restrictions on the use of the drug, dofetilide, led to greater use of other drugs that had lower efficacy and even greater risk of harm. Also, the "Black triangle" warning for newly released prescription drugs has never been tested to be certain that it will produce a net positive impact. We should not assume it will work for every product and could result in non-compliance to therapy and patient

8. In your 1998 article, entitled "Making Medicines Safer," you called for establishment of a post-marketing drug-safety program independent of the FDA to assure objectivity and to avoid conflicts of interest. Do you still recommend the creation of an independent body responsible for oversight and investigation of post-market drug safety?

Yes, we recommended the creation of an independent Board to evaluate the overall safety process and programs available to the FDA and to inform the FDA of its findings from active surveillance. However, we did not recommend that this body assume any of the responsibility for regulating the industry and its products. Our suggestion was to have the Board gather data, submit it to the FDA and make recommendations on safety, not take away the regulatory responsibility. The regulatory decisions are best made by those government employees who have been trained in medicine and the regulatory sciences and who are experts in the science of simultaneously assessing benefit and risk for populations. Physicians are trained in assessing risk and benefit for a patient, not populations.

9. Given that the FDA permits the same reviewers in the Office of New Drugs who approve a drug to make the final decision on post-market status of the drug, is this not an inherent conflict of interest?

I think it is can be a "perceived" conflict of interest, not an "inherent" conflict of interest. The reviewers' responsibility must include the counterbalancing assessment of effectiveness in addition to safety. Post-market assessment must include an ongoing assessment of benefit and risk simultaneously. I don't believe it would be wise to change the current system and create one in which the "approvers" and the "removers" are pitted against one another. Recommendations for the market status of drugs require complex assessments, a synthesis of the scientific information and a consensus decision. It is very likely that there will be dissenters on the team that makes these assessments. The dissenters must be given a opportunity to express their opinions but at some point, only one recommendation can be made by the Agency. Public airing of "split decisions" only result in chaos and loss of credibility for the FDA. The best way to minimize disagreements and maximize the accuracy of the decision making process is to have an independent source of highly accurate information on the post-market experience with new drugs.